Randomized Clinical Trials

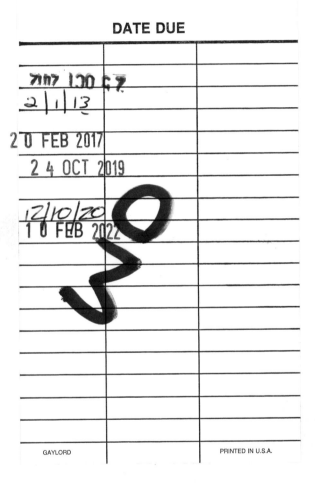

Randomized Clinical Trials
Design, Practice and Reporting

David Machin

Medical Statistics Group, School of Health and Related Sciences,
University of Sheffield, UK
Children's Cancer and Leukaemia Group,
University of Leicester, UK

Peter M Fayers

Department of Public Health, University of Aberdeen, UK
Faculty of Medicine, Norwegian University of Science and Technology,
Trondheim, Norway

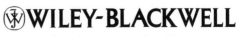

A John Wiley & Sons, Ltd., Publication

Library of Congress Cataloging-in-Publication Data

Machin, David, 1939–
 Randomized clinical trials : design, practice and reporting / David Machin, Peter M Fayers.
     p. ; cm.
 Includes bibliographical references and index.
 ISBN 978-0-471-49812-4 (pbk.)
 1. Clinical trials. 2. Clinical trials—Statistical methods. I.
 2. Fayers, Peter M. II. Title.
 [DNLM: 1. Biomedical Research—methods. 2. Randomized Controlled
Trials as Topic—methods. 3. Data Interpretation, Statistical. 4.
Research Design. W 20.5 M149r 2010]
 R853.C55M337 2010
 610.72′4—dc22
                          2009054234

A catalogue record for this book is available from the British Library.

ISBN: 978-0-471-49812-4

Set in 10.5/12.5pt Minion by Integra Software Services Pvt. Ltd., Pondicherry, India
Printed and bound in Singapore by Fabulous Printers Pte Ltd.

First impression—2010

Christine Machin
and
Tessa and Emma Fayers

Contents

Preface

Clinical trials play a key role in developing strategies for healthcare, whether in the development of a new drug or medical device, modifying existing approaches to better effect, improving care in the community or, as at the time we write this preface, vaccines for swine flu and many other situations. Many trials are conducted by pharmaceutical and allied healthcare organizations, many by academic and charity-supported research groups and many with support from multiple agencies. Trials vary in size from those including tens of subjects to many thousands, and consume a correspondingly wide range of resources – both financial and in terms of specialist personnel required to conduct the trial.

Trials concerned with the later development of a new drug for a particular condition will often be preceded by a long programme of laboratory, preclinical and early clinical research, whereas other trials may arise more directly from clinical experience whether in the hospital clinic, operating theatre or elsewhere.

It is not possible in a single text to cover the whole range of areas in which clinical trials are conducted. Nor can we cover the plethora of clinical trial designs which are in current use, the choice of which will crucially depend on the stage of the development. Consequently, we have focused on the late stage of the process when, at least in many situations, the relative efficacy of a new or test intervention is compared with a current standard in a randomized comparative trial.

The context in which we are writing is for those directly concerned with patient care, not because we wish to exclude from our readership those in the pharmaceutical and allied industries, but rather to enable us to focus on issues which might not be so clear for new investigators who wish to become involved with clinical trials research. In general, these investigators will not come with the type of support available from industry, either in monetary terms or with the ready and extensive clinical trials expertise that industry has at hand. We believe, however, that even for those who work on clinical trials in full collaboration with industry, a broad view of the whole process will lead to a better understanding.

In this book we have tried to give an overview of the key issues to consider in designing, conducting, analyzing and reporting clinical trials. We have used a parallel two-group randomized design as a basis for this in Chapters 2–10. The subsequent chapters extend this basic design to consider, for example, cross-over trials and trials comparing more than two groups. A suggested first reading of the book is the introductory Chapter 1, then Chapters 2–7, omitting Chapters 8 and 9 concerned with the more statistical issues of analysis and trial size, and finally Chapter 10.

Many thanks are due to Simon Day who generously allowed us to copy freely from his *Dictionary for Clinical Trials* in constructing the Glossary. Thanks are also due to Nicky Cullum, University of York and Jane Nixon, Clinical Trials Research Unit, University of Leeds who have allowed us to extensively quote from the PRESSURE protocol funded by the NHS Health Technology Assessment Programme.

David Machin
Peter M Fayers
Leicester and Sheffield and Aberdeen and Trondheim

CHAPTER 1

Introduction

A very large number of clinical trials have been conducted with human subjects in a wide variety of contexts. Many of these have been concerned, for example, with improving (in some way) the management of patients with disease and others the prevention of the disease or the condition in the first place. The essence of a clinical trial is the comparison of a standard strategy with an alternative (perhaps novel) intervention. The aim of this chapter is to illustrate some of the wide variety of clinical trials that have been conducted and to highlight some key features of their design, conduct and analysis.

1.1   Introduction

The aim of this book is to introduce those who are to become involved with randomized clinical trials to the wide range of challenges that are faced by those who conduct such trials. Our intended readership is therefore expected to range from health care professionals of all disciplines who are concerned with patient care to those more involved with the non-clinical aspects such as the statistical design, data processing and subsequent analysis of the results. We assume no prior knowledge of clinical trial processes and we have attempted to explain the more statistical sections in as non-technical a way as possible. In a first reading of this book, these sections could be omitted. Throughout the book we stress the collaborative nature of clinical trials activity and would hope that readers would consult their more experienced colleagues on aspects of our coverage.

   The business of clinical trials is an ongoing process and, as we write, trials are currently being designed, opened, conducted, closed, analyzed and reported. Results are being filtered into current practice and the next trials planned. It is difficult to know where to start in describing the key features of this process, as each stage interacts to some extent with the others. For example, in designing a trial the investigators need to be mindful of the eventual analysis to be undertaken as this governs (but it is only one aspect) of how large a trial should be launched. Some of the steps are intellectually challenging, for example, defining the key therapeutic question, while others may perhaps appear more mundane, such as defining the data forms or the data entry procedures. However, all steps (whether large or small, major or minor) underpin the eventual successful outcome – the influence on clinical practice once the trial results are

Randomized Clinical Trials: Design, Practice and Reporting   David Machin and Peter M Fayers
© 2010 John Wiley & Sons, Ltd

available. Entire books have been written for many of these aspects we can only provide an introduction to the process.

Numerous terms need to be introduced, including 'clinical trial' itself. As a consequence we have included a Glossary of Terms, which is mainly extracted from Day (2007) *Dictionary of Clinical Trials*. The Glossary defines clinical trial: any systematic study of the effects of a treatment in human subjects. These definitions may not be exhaustive, in the sense that 'treatment' used here may be substituted by, for example, 'intervention', depending on the specific context of the clinical trial under consideration.

Clinical trials require a multidisciplinary approach in which all partners play a key role at some stage of the trial process. Furthermore, this is the era of evidence-based medicine (EBM), in which it is important to consider critically *all* the available evidence about whether, for example, a treatment works before recommending it for clinical practice. In this respect it is therefore vital that we can clearly see that a proposed trial addresses a key question which will have a clinically meaningful outcome, is well designed, conducted and reported and the results are persuasive enough to change clinical practice if appropriate.

Despite perhaps having a professional interest in the science of clinical trials, everyone has an additional vested interest as potential patients. How many of us have never been to see a doctor, had a hospital admission or taken medication? All of us may be, have been or certainly will be recipients of clinical trial results whether at pre-birth or birth, childhood for vaccination and minor illness, as an adult for fertility, sports injuries, minor and major non-life threatening or life-threatening illnesses and in old age for care related to our mental or physical needs.

1.2   Some completed trials

As we have indicated, there are countless ongoing trials and many have been successfully conducted and reported. To give some indication of the range and diversity of application, we describe a selection of clinical trials that have been conducted. Their designs include some features that we will draw upon in later chapters.

The examples of successfully completed clinical trials illustrate a wide range of topics investigated. These include patients with disease (breast cancer, colon cancer, eczema, glaucoma, malaria and diabetes mellitus), those requiring coronary artery stents or hand surgery, elderly residents of nursing homes, children with dental caries, healthy individuals and those requiring vaccinations. Although not included here, trials are also conducted to evaluate different diagnostic procedures, different bed mattresses to reduce the incidence of bed sores, different dressings for wounds of all types and fertility regulation options for male and females of reproductive potential, for example.

These trials are often termed Phase III trials in contrast to Phase I and Phase II trials, which are concerned with early stages of the (often pharmaceutical) development process. Although the trials differ in aspects of their design, the majority have the general structure of a two (or more) group parallel design in which eligible patients are assigned to receive the alternative options (often treatments but more generally termed interventions) and then at some later time assessed in a way which will be indicative of (successful) outcome. The outcomes measured in these trials include: survival time,

Example 1.1   Recovery of gastrointestinal function after elective colonic resection

Lobo, Bostock, Neal, *et al.* (2002) describe a randomized trial in which 20 patients with colonic cancer either received postoperative intravenous fluids in accordance with current hospital standard practice (S) or according to a restricted intake regimen (R). A primary endpoint measure in each patient was the solid-phase gastric emptying time on the fourth postoperative day. The observed difference between the median emptying times was shorter with R by 56 minutes with 95% confidence interval (CI) from 12 to 132 minutes. The trial also included pre-operative and postoperative (days 1, 2, 4 and 6) measures of the concentrations of serum albumin, haemoglobin and blood urea in a repeated measures design.

Key features include:

- **Design:** randomized comparison of a standard and test, single centre participation, unblinded assessment;
- **Endpoint:** gastric emptying time;
- **Size:** 21 patients following colonic resection;
- **Analysis:** Mann–Whitney-U test* for comparing two medians;
- **Conclusion:** The restricted group had shorter delays in returning to gastrointestinal function.

*This can also be referred to as the Wilcoxon Rank-Sum Test.

Example 1.2   Azathioprine for the treatment of atopic eczema

Meggitt, Gray and Reynolds (2006) randomized 63 patients with moderate-to-severe eczema to receive either azathioprine or placebo in a double-blind formulation to ascertain the relative reduction in disease activity determined by the six-area six-sign atopic dermatitis (SASSAD) score between the groups. They reported a 5.4 unit advantage with azathioprine. In this trial patients were randomized, using a minimization procedure, in the ratio of 2 to 1 in favour of azathioprine in order to '... encourage recruitment, to reduce the numbers receiving pharmacologically inactive systemic treatment, and to increase the likelihood of identifying infrequent adverse events'.

Key features include:

- **Design:** single centre, randomized double-blind, placebo-controlled, 2 : 1 allocation ratio using minimization;
- **Endpoint:** SASSAD;
- **Size:** 63 patients with moderate-to-severe atopic eczema;
- **Analysis:** comparison of mean group regression slopes over a 12-week period;
- **Conclusion:** azathioprine produces a clinically relevant improvement.

Example 1.3   Anacetrapib and blood pressure

Krishna, Anderson, Bergman, *et al.* (2007) describe a randomized placebo (*P*) controlled, 2-period cross-over trial of anacetrapib (*A*) in 22 healthy volunteers. Half of the individuals were randomized to receive the sequence *AP* (i.e. *A* in Period I of the trial followed by *P* in Period II) and half *PA*. The primary endpoint recorded was the blood pressure on day 10 of Period I and of Period II. The healthy individuals and investigators were blinded to the order in which the trial medication was administered. The authors state: 'A one-sided test was applied, since another molecule in this class was found to increase blood pressure . . .'. They reported a difference in mean systolic blood pressure between *A* and *P* as 0.6 mm Hg (90% CI -1.54 to 2.74, *p*-value $= 0.634$) and concluded that: '. . ., anacetrapib seems not to increase blood pressure, . . .'.
   Key features include:

- **Design:** single centre, randomized placebo controlled, 2-period cross-over trial;

- **Size:** 22 healthy volunteers;

- **Endpoint:** ambulatory blood pressure;

- **Analysis:** comparison of means using analysis of variance;

- **Conclusion:** anacetrapib seems not to increase blood pressure.

Example 1.4   Topical medication and argon laser trabeculoplasty for glaucoma

The Glaucoma Laser Trial Research Group (1995) recruited 271 subjects with newly diagnosed primary-angle glaucoma. One eye of each patient was randomly assigned to argon laser trabeculoplasty (LT) or to a stepped medication (TM) as initial treatment. They treated 261 eyes with LT first followed by TM and the same number with TM first then LT. They found that measures of visual field status for eyes treated by LT-MT were slightly better than those treated by MT-LT. The authors state: 'Statistical significance was attained for only some of the differences, and the clinical implications of such small differences are not known.'
   Key features include:

- **Design:** multicentre, paired design, compares alternative schedules for administering two procedures – the schedule was randomized to one eye with the other eye receiving the alternative;

- **Endpoint:** visual field status;

- **Size:** 271 patients with primary open-angle glaucoma;

- **Analysis:** comparison of means at particular time points following initiation of treatment using the paired *t*-test;

- **Conclusion:** eyes treated with laser trabeculoplasty first were judged to have slightly more improvement and slightly less deterioration.

Example 1.5   Use of glass-ionomer for atraumatic restorative treatment

Lo, Luo, Fan and Wei (2001) conducted a trial in 89 school children from two schools, who had bilateral matched pairs of carious posterior teeth requiring atraumatic restorative treatment (ART). A split-mouth design was used in which the two materials, ChemFlex and Fiji IX GP 49, were randomly placed on contralateral sides. From a total of 101 bilateral matched teeth-pairs included in the trial, the authors concluded that the clinical performance of both materials over a 2-year period was similar.

Key features include:

- **Design:** two schools, split mouth, random allocation;
- **Endpoint:** clinical examination at 24-month recall;
- **Size:** 89 children with 101 pairs of bilateral carious posterior teeth;
- **Analysis:** comparison of mean occlusive wear between materials using a paired *t*-test;
- **Conclusion:** the clinical performance of different materials was similar.

Example 1.6   Use of hip protectors in elderly people in nursing homes

Meyer, Warnke, Bender and Mülhauser (2003) conducted a trial involving 942 residents from 49 nursing homes. In this cluster design, the nursing homes contain 'clusters' of residents and the homes (not the individual residents) were randomized. Twenty-five homes comprising a total of 459 residents were assigned to the intervention group, and 24 homes with 483 residents were assigned to the control group. The intervention comprised a single education session for nursing staff, who then educated residents, and the provision of three hip protectors per resident. The control clusters gave usual care optimized by brief information to nursing staff about hip protectors and the provision of two hip protectors per cluster for demonstration purposes. The main outcome measure was the incidence of hip fractures. There were 21 hip fractures in 21 (4.6%) residents in the intervention group and 42 in 39 (8.1%) residents in the control group – a difference of 3.5% (95% CI 0.3 to 7.3%, *p*-value = 0.072). The authors concluded: 'The introduction of a structured education programme and the provision of free hip protectors in nursing homes may reduce the number of hip fractures'.

Key features include:

- **Design:** multicluster, randomized;
- **Size:** 49 nursing homes comprising 942 residents with high risk of falling;
- **Endpoint:** hip fractures;
- **Analysis:** chi-squared test adjusted for cluster randomization but not for the second fractures in some residents;
- **Conclusion:** increasing the use of hip protectors resulted in a relative reduction of hip fractures of about 40%.

Example 1.7   Treatment of uncomplicated falciparum malaria

Zongo, Dorsey, Rouamba, *et al.* (2007) conducted a randomized non-inferiority trial to test the hypothesis that the risk of recurrent parasitaemia was not significantly worse with artemether-lumefantrine (AL) than with amodiaquine plus sulfadoxine-pyrimethamine (AQ+SP). A total of 826 patients were screened, of which 548 were found to have uncomplicated malaria, and were randomized (273 to AQ+SP and 275 to AL). A primary endpoint was the risk of treatment failure within 28 days of randomization. The authors concluded that AQ+SP with a failure rate of 1.7% (4/233) was more effective than AL with a rate of 10.2% (25/245), representing a difference of 8.5% (95% CI 3 to 12%). These results suggest that the hypothesis of 'non-inferiority' should not be accepted.
   Key features include:

- **Design:** multicentre, two-group comparison, non-inferiority trial;
- **Endpoint:** time to recurrent parasitaemia;
- **Size:** large trial of 521 patients with uncomplicated falciparum malaria;
- **Analysis:** comparison of Kaplan–Meier failure-time curves;
- **Conclusion:** AL was less effective than AQ+SP.

Example 1.8   Trastuzumab for HER2-positive breast cancer

Smith, Procter, Gelber, *et al.* (2007) showed that 1 year of treatment with trastuzumab after adjuvant therapy in HER2-positive patients with breast cancer was superior to observation alone. They reported a hazard ratio, $HR = 0.67$ (95% CI 0.47 to 0.91, p-value $= 0.0115$) for overall survival in favour of adjuvant treatment. This comparison was from two arms of a 3-arm large multicentre international randomized trial comprising 1698 patients randomized to observation alone, 1703 to trastuzumab for 1 year and 1701 to trastuzumab for 2 years: a total of 5102 patients.
   Key features include:

- **Design:** randomized, multicentre, observation versus active treatment;
- **Size:** large trial of 5102 women with HER2-positive breast cancer;
- **Endpoint:** overall survival;
- **Analysis:** comparison in 3401 women from the control and 1-year trastuzumab groups using survival curves;
- **Conclusion:** treatment with 1-year trastuzumab after adjuvant chemotherapy has an overall survival benefit.

Example 1.9 Pain prevention following hand surgery

Stevinson, Devaraj, Fountain-Barber, *et al.* (2003) conducted a randomized double-blind, placebo-controlled trial to compare placebo with homeopathic arnica 6C and arnica 30C to determine the degree of pain prevention in patients with carpel tunnel syndrome undergoing elective surgery for their condition. Pain was assessed postoperatively with the short-form McGill Pain Questionnaire (SF-MPQ) at 4 days. A total of 64 patients were randomized to the three groups resulting in median scores of 16.0 (range 0–69), 10.5 (0–76) and 15.0 (0–82) respectively. From these results, the authors suggest that homeopathic arnica has no advantage over placebo in reducing levels of postoperative pain.

Key features include:

- **Design:** single centre, randomized double-blind, placebo-controlled, three-group dose response;

- **Endpoint:** pain using the MPQ;

- **Size:** 64 patients undergoing hand surgery for carpal tunnel syndrome;

- **Analysis:** Kruskal–Wallis test;

- **Conclusion:** irrespective of dose, homeopathic arnica has no advantage over placebo.

Example 1.10 Newly diagnosed patients treated for type 2 diabetes

The randomized trial of Weng, Li, Xu, *et al.* (2008) compared, in newly diagnosed patients treated for type 2 diabetes, three treatments: multiple daily insulin injections (MDI), continuous subcutaneous insulin infusion (CSII) and oral hypoglycaemic agent (OHA).

Key features include:

- **Design:** nine centres, randomized three-group comparison;

- **Endpoint:** time of glycaemic remission;

- **Size:** 410 newly diagnosed patients with type 2 diabetes;

- **Analysis:** Cox-proportional-hazards regression model;

- **Conclusion:** early intensive therapy has favourable outcomes on recovery and maintenance of β-cell function and protracted glycaemic remission compared to OHA.

Example 1.11   Recombinant hepatitis B vaccine

Levie, Gjorup, Skinhøj and Stoffel (2002) compared a 2-dose regimen of recombinant hepatitis B vaccine including the immune stimulant AS04 with the standard 3-dose regimen of Enderix-B in healthy adults. The rationale behind testing a 2-dose regimen was that fewer injections would improve compliance.
Key features include:

- **Design:** two centres, randomized two-group comparison;
- **Endpoint:** seroprotection rate;
- **Size:** 340 healthy subjects aged between 15 and 40 years;
- **Analysis:** Fisher's exact test;
- **Conclusion:** the 2-dose regimen compared favourably to the standard.

Example 1.12   Temporary scaffolding of coronary artery with bio-absorbable magnesium stents

Erbel, Di Mario, Bartunek, *et al.* (2007) describe a non-randomized multicentre trial involving eight centres in which 63 patients were enrolled with single de novo lesions in a native coronary artery. In these patients, a total of 71 biodegradable magnesium stents were successfully implanted. The (composite) primary endpoint was the rate of major adverse cardiac events (MACE) defined as any one of: cardiac death, Q-wave myocardial infarction or target lesion revascularization at 4 months post stent implant. This was to be compared with an anticipated rate of 30%. They reported a rate of MACE of 15/63 (23.8%); all of which were attributed to target lesion revascularization (there were no deaths or Q-wave myocardial infarctions) and concluded: '... stents can achieve an immediate angiographic result similar to ... other metal stents ...'. Nevertheless, the authors also commented in their discussion: 'The absence of randomization precludes direct comparison with other techniques of percutaneous revascularization'.
Key features include:

- **Design:** no comparison group hence non-randomized, multicentre;
- **Size:** 71 stents in 63 patients;
- **Endpoint:** composite endpoint – MACE;
- **Analysis:** proportion experiencing MACE with 95% confidence interval;
- **Conclusion:** bio-absorbable stents can achieve an immediate angiographic result similar to other metal stents and can be safely degraded.

gastric emptying time, reduction in disease activity, visual field status, recurrent parasitaemia, major adverse cardiac events, pain, the number of hip fractures, systolic blood pressure and standard criteria used to assess dental restorations. In the trial of homeopathic arnica for pain relief following hand surgery, assessment was made in a double-blind or double-masked manner in which neither the patient nor the assessor were aware of the treatment received.

The methods used for the allocation to the options included simple randomization of equal numbers per group, a 2 to 1 allocation, a minimization procedure taking into account patient characteristics, randomization to nursing homes (clusters) rather than to individual residents and, in one case, the non-random allocation to a single arm study using a new bio-absorbable stent for coronary scaffolding. In this example, the trial data were compared to that of historical data. For the split-mouth design used for the dental caries trial, a 'random number table was used to determine which tooth of a pair was to be restored with ChemFlex and which with Fiji IX GP'.

The trials ranged in size from 21 patients with colonic cancer to 5102 women with HER2-positive breast cancer. One trial involved 522 eyes from 271 subjects, another 202 teeth from 89 children. Although not fully detailed in the above summaries, methods of statistical analysis ranged from a simple comparison of two proportions to relatively complex methods using techniques for survival time outcomes.

In general, trials are designed to establish a difference between the (therapeutic) options under test, were one to exist. Consequently, they are sometimes termed *superiority* trials. However, in certain circumstances, as in the trial for the treatment of uncomplicated falciparum malaria, the research team were looking for *non-inferiority* implying that the two treatment strategies of AQ + SP and AL would give very similar risks of failure. In the event, the trial suggested that AL was (unacceptably) less effective, implying that non-inferiority was not established. Such designs usually imply that a satisfactory outcome is that the test treatment does not perform worse than the standard to an extent *predefined* by the investigating team. Use of a non-inferiority design often implies that, although some therapeutic loss may be conceded on the main outcome variable, other factors favouring the new therapy will have some features (*gain*) to offset this. For example, if the new compound was a little less effective (not equal to) but had a better toxicity profile, this might be sufficient to prefer it for clinical practice.

1.3 Choice of design

1.3.1 Biological variability

Measurements made on human subjects rarely give exactly the same results from one occasion to the next. Even in adults, our height varies a little during the course of the day. If we measure the blood sugar levels of an individual on one particular day and then again the following day, under exactly the same conditions, greater variation compared to that observed in height would be expected. Hence, were such an individual to be assessed and then receive an intervention (perhaps to lower blood sugar levels), any lowering recorded at the next assessment cannot necessarily be ascribed to the intervention itself. The levels of inherent variability may be very high. This implies that where a subject has an illness, the oscillations in symptoms may disguise the beneficial effect of the treatment given to improve the condition (at least in the early stages of treatment).

With such variability it follows that, in any comparison made in a biomedical context, differences between subjects or groups of subjects frequently occur. These differences may be due to real effects, random variations or both. It is the job of the experimenter to decide how this variation should be considered in the design of the ensuing trial. Once at the analysis stage, the variation can be suitably partitioned into that due to any real effect of the interventions on the difference between groups, and that from the random or chance component.

Example 1.13   Azathioprine for the treatment of atopic eczema

The considerable between-patient variability in the trial of Example 1.2 is illustrated in Figure 1.1. In the 41 patients receiving azathioprine, the reduction in disease activity (SASSAD) ranged from −10 to 32. There is considerable overlap of these values with those from the 20 patients receiving placebo, whose values range from −12 to 20. This figure clearly illustrates that, although there is considerable variation, the majority of patients in both groups improve. Further, the corresponding reduction in percentage body area affected with azathioprine was reported to range from approximately −15 to 85% and for placebo approximately −20 to 45%. Nevertheless, even with the majority of patients improving in both groups, the trial of Meggitt, Gray and Reynolds (2006) indicated a better outcome, on average, for those receiving azathioprine.

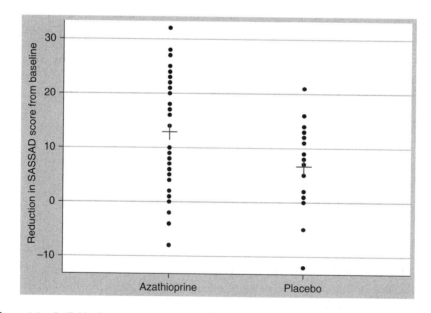

Figure 1.1   Individual patient reductions in disease activity (SASSAD) for the azathioprine and placebo treatment groups with the corresponding means indicated (data from Meggitt, Gray and Reynolds, 2006)

1.3.2   Randomization

In laying the foundations of good experimental design (although more in an agricultural and biological context), Ronald A Fisher (1890–1962) advocated the use of randomization in allocating experimental treatments. For example, in agricultural trials, various plots in a field are randomly assigned to the different experimental interventions. The argument for randomization is that it will prevent systematic differences between the allocated plots receiving the different interventions, whether or not these can be identified by the investigator concerned, before the experimental treatment is applied. Once the experimental treatments are applied and the outcome observed, any differences between treatments can be estimated objectively and without bias. In these and many other contexts, randomization has long been a keystone to good experimental design.

The need for random allocation extends to all experimental situations, including those concerned with patients as opposed to agricultural plots of land. The difficulty arises because clinical trials (less emotive than experiments) do indeed concern human beings who cannot be regarded as experimental units and so allocated the interventions without their consent. The consent process clearly complicates the allocation process and, at least in the past, has been used as a reason to resist the idea of randomization of patients to treatment. Unfortunately the other options, perhaps a comparison of patients receiving a 'new' treatment with those from the past receiving the 'old', are flawed in the sense that any observed differences (or lack thereof) may not reflect the true situation. In the context of controlled clinical trials, Pocock (1983) concluded, more than 25 years ago and some 30 years after the first randomized trials were conducted, that:

> The proper use of randomization guarantees that there is no bias in the selection of patients for the different treatments and so helps considerably to reduce the risk of differences in experimental environment. Randomized allocation is not difficult to implement and enables trial conclusions to be more believable than other forms of treatment allocation.

As a consequence, we focus on randomized controlled trials and do not give much attention to less scientifically rigorous options.

1.3.3   Design hierarchy

The final choice of design for a clinical trial will depend on many factors. The key factors are clearly the specific research question posed, the practicality of recruiting patients to such a design and the resources necessary to support the trial conduct. We shall discuss these and other issues pertinent to the design choice in later chapters. Nevertheless, we can catalogue the main types of design options available; these are listed in Figure 1.2. This gives a relative weight to the evidence obtained from these different types of clinical trial. All other things being equal, the design that maximizes the weight of the resulting evidence should be chosen. For expository purposes, we assume that a comparison of a new test treatment with the current standard for the specific condition in question is being made.

Evidence level	Type of trial
Strongest	Double-blind randomized controlled trial (RCT) Single-blind RCT Non-blinded (open) RCT Non-randomized prospective trial Non-randomized retrospective trial Before-and-after design (historical control)
Weakest	Case-series

Figure 1.2 The relative strength of evidence obtained from alternative designs for comparative clinical trials

The design that provides the strongest type of evidence is the *double-blind (or double-masked) randomized controlled trial* (RCT). In this, the patients are allocated to treatment at random. This ensures that, *in the long run*, patients will be comparable in the test and standard groups before treatment commences. Clearly, if the important prognostic factors that influence outcome were known, we could match the patients in the standard and test groups in some way. However, the advantage of randomization is that it balances the *unknown* as well as the *known* prognostic factors, and this could not be achieved by matching. The reason for the attraction of the randomized trial is therefore that it is the *only* design that can give an absolute certainty that there is no bias in favour of one group compared to another at the start of the trial. Indeed, in Example 1.12, Erbel, Di Mario, Bartunek, *et al.* (2007) admitted that failure to conduct a randomized comparison compromised their ability to draw definitive conclusions concerning the stent on test.

For the simple situation in which the attending clinician is also the assessor of the outcome, the trial should ideally be double-blind. This means that neither the patient nor the attending clinician will know the actual treatment allocated. Having no knowledge of which treatment has been taken, neither the patient nor the clinician can be influenced at the assessment stage by such knowledge. In this way, an unprejudiced evaluation of the patient response is obtained. Thus Meggitt, Gray and Reynolds (2006) used double-blind formulations of azathioprine or placebo so that neither the patients with moderate-to-severe eczema, nor their attending clinical team, were aware of who received which treatment. Although they did not give details, the blinding is best broken only at the analysis stage once all the data have been collated.

Despite the inherent advantage of this double-blind design, most clinical trials cannot be conducted in this way as, for example, a means has to be found for delivering the treatment options in an identical way. This may be a possibility if the standard and test are available in tablet form of identical colour, shape, texture, smell and taste. If such 'identity' cannot be achieved, then a single-blind design may ensue. In such a design the patient has knowledge of the treatment being given but the clinical assessor does not. In trials with patient survival time as the endpoint, double-blind usually means that both the patient and the treating physician and other staff are blinded; assessment is objective (death) and blinding of the assessor is irrelevant.

Finally, and this is possibly the majority situation, there will be circumstances in which neither the patient nor the assessor can be blind to the treatments actually received. Such designs are referred to as 'open' trials.

In certain circumstances, when a new treatment has been proposed for evaluation, all patients are recruited prospectively but allocation to treatment is not made at random. In such cases, the comparisons may well be biased and hence are unreliable. The bias arises because the clinical team choose which patients receive which intervention and in doing so may favour (even subconsciously) giving one treatment to certain patient types and not to others. In addition, the requirement that all patients should be suitable for all options may not be fulfilled; if it is known that a certain option is to be given to a particular subject then we may not rigorously check if the other options are equally appropriate. Similar problems arise if investigators have recruited patients into a single arm study and the results from these patients are then compared with information on similar patients, having (usually in the past) received a relevant standard therapy for the condition in question. However, such historical comparisons are also likely to be biased and to an unknown extent so again it will not be reasonable to ascribe the difference (if any) observed entirely to the treatments themselves. Of course, in either case, there will be situations when one of these designs is the only option available. In such cases, a detailed justification for not using the 'gold standard' of the randomized controlled trial is required.

Understandably, in this era of EBM, information from non-randomized comparative studies is categorized as providing weaker evidence than that from randomized trials.

The before-and-after design is one in which, for example, patients are treated with the Standard option for a specified period and then, at some fixed point in time, subsequent patients receive the Test treatment. This is the type of design used by Erbel, Di Mario, Bartunek, *et al.* (2007) to evaluate a bio-absorbable stent for coronary scaffolding. In such examples, the information for the Standard group is retrospective in nature, in that often the information is in the clinical records only and was not initially collected for trial purposes. If this is the case, the before-and-after design is likely to be further compromised. For example, in the 'before' period the patient selection criterion, clinical assessments and data recorded may not meet the standards required of the 'after' component. Such differences are likely to influence the before-and-after comparison in unforeseen and unknown ways.

Example 1.14   Non-randomized design – glioblastoma in the elderly

Brandes, Vastola, Basso, *et al.* (2003) describe a study comparing radiotherapy alone (Group A), radiotherapy and the combination of procarbizine, lomustine and vincristine (Group B) and radiotherapy with temozolomide (Group C) in 79 elderly patients with glioblastoma. The authors state:

> The first group (Group A) was enrolled in the period from March 1993 to August 1995 . . . .
> The second group (group B) was enrolled from September 1995 to September 1997 . . . . The
> third group (Group C) was enrolled from September 1997 to August 2000 and . . . .

The authors conclude:

> Overall survival was better in Group C compared with Group A (14.9 months v 11.2 months,
> P = 0.002), but there was no statistical differences found between Groups A and B or
> between Groups B and C.

However, since patients have not been randomized to groups, we cannot be sure that the differences (and lack of differences) truly reflect the relative efficacy of the three treatments concerned. This type of design should be avoided if at all possible.

A case-series consists of a study in which the experience of an investigator treating a series of patients with a particular approach reports on their outcome. This may be the only 'design' option available in rare or unusual circumstances, but is unlikely to provide clear evidence of efficacy. There are many criticisms of this design. Generally, we may not know how the patients have been selected. The clinical team may have an eye for selecting those patients to be given the treatment who are likely to recover in any event. Without further evidence of the natural history of the disease, we do not know whether the patients may have recovered spontaneously without intervention. Finally, we do not know whether their approach to treatment is better than any alternatives.

1.4 Practical constraints

Control of the 'experiment' is clearly a desirable feature – perhaps easy to attain in the physics laboratory where experimental conditions are tightly controlled but not so easy with living material, particularly if human. A good trial should answer the questions posed as efficiently as possible. In broad terms, this implies recruiting as few subjects as is reasonably possible for a reliable answer to be obtained.

Although good science may lead to an optimal choice of design, the exigencies of real life may cause these ideals to be modified. We can still keep in mind the hierarchy in the choice of designs of Figure 1.2, but where to enter this hierarchy will depend on circumstance. The investigators therefore do not aim for the best design, but only the best realizable design in their context.

Technical (statistical) aspects of experimental design can be used in a whole variety of settings; nevertheless, there are specific problems associated with implementing these designs in practice in the field of clinical trials. It is clear that trials cannot be conducted without human subjects (often patients); nevertheless, the constraints this imposes are not inconsiderable. Figure 1.3 lists some aspects that need to be considered when conducting such trials.

As we have indicated, the requirements for human studies are usually more stringent than in other research areas. For example safety, in terms of the welfare of the experimental units involved, is of overriding concern in clinical trials but possibly of little relevance in animal studies and of no relevance to laboratory studies. In some sense the laboratory provides, at least in theory, the greatest rigour in terms of the experimental design, and studies in human subjects should be designed (whenever possible) to be as close to these standards as possible. However, no consent procedures from the experimental units or from animals, if they are involved, are required, whereas this is a very important consideration in all human experimentation even in a clinical trial with therapeutic intent.

Constraints may also apply to the choice of interventions to compare. For example, in certain therapeutic trials there may be little chance that a placebo option will bring

Design feature	
Method of assessments	If invasive – may not be acceptable.
Treatment or Intervention	Implicit that treatment should do some good – thus an innocuous or placebo treatment may not be acceptable.
Subject safety issues	Overriding principle is the safety of the subjects
Protocol Review	Scientific and ethical
Consent	Fully informed consent mandatory
Recruitment	Usually, subjects recruited one-by-one over calendar time
Time scale	May be relatively long – rarely weeks, seldom months, quite often years
Trial size	Not too large or too small
Patient losses	Subjects may refuse to continue in the trial at any stage
Observations	Usually, subjects assessed one-by-one over calendar time
Design changes	Almost certainly requires new ethical approval
Data protection	Confidentiality and often National Guidelines for storage and transfer.
Reporting	CONSORT for Phase III trials (Moher, Shultz and Altman, 2001)

Figure 1.3 Special considerations for clinical trials in human subjects

any benefit (although this is certainly not the case in all circumstances). Comparisons may therefore have to be made between two allegedly 'active' approaches, despite little direct evidence that either of them will bring benefit. However, if a difference between treatments is demonstrated at the end of such a trial, activity for the better option is established so that comparison with a placebo is not necessary. In contrast, should the two treatments appear not to differ in their effectiveness, no conclusions can be drawn since we do not know whether they are equally beneficial or equally ineffective. An investigating team conducting this type of trial therefore needs to be fully aware of the potential difficulties.

Ethical considerations, as judged perhaps by a local, national or international committee, may also prevent the 'optimal' design being implemented. There are also issues related to patient data confidentiality which may, in the circumstances of a multicentre trial, make synthesis of all the trial data problematical. We address other components of Figure 1.3 in later sections of the book.

1.5 Influencing clinical practice

As we have indicated, an important consideration at the design stage of a trial is to consider whether, if the new treatment proves effective, the trial will be reliable enough in itself to convince clinical teams not associated with the trial of the findings. Importantly, if a benefit is established, will this be quickly adopted into national clinical practice? Experience has suggested that all too frequently trials have less impact than they deserve, although it is recognized that results that are adopted in practice are likely to be from trials of an appropriate size, conducted by a respected group with a multi-centre involvement. There are therefore considerations, in some sense outside the strict confines of the design, which investigators should heed if their findings are to have the desired impact.

Some basic or administrative features can help reassure the eventual readers of the reliability of the trial results. These include (some of these may be mandatory) registering the trial itself, involving and informing other clinical colleagues outside the trial team of progress, careful documentation of any serious adverse events, ensuring the trial documentation is complete, establishing procedures for responding to external queries, clarity of the final reporting document in the research literature and seeking avenues for wider dissemination of the trial results.

1.6   History

Probably the single most important contribution to the science of comparative clinical trials was the recognition by Austin Bradford Hill (1897–1991) in the 1940s that patients should be allocated the options under consideration at random, so that comparisons should be free from bias. Consequently, the first randomized trial was planned to test the value of a pertussis vaccine to prevent whooping cough. The results were subsequently published by the Medical Research Council Whooping-Cough Immunization Committee (1951). He later stated: 'The aim of the controlled clinical trial is very simple: it is to ensure that the comparisons we make are as precise, as informative and as convincing as possible.' This development by itself may not have led directly to more theoretically based statistical innovation, but was the foundation for the science of clinical trials.

Nevertheless, the history of clinical trials research precedes this important development by many years. Clinical trials were mentioned by Avicenna (980–1037) in *The Canon of Medicine* (1025), in which he laid down rules for the experimental use and testing of drugs and wrote a precise guide for practical experimentation in the process of discovering and proving the effectiveness of medical drugs and substances. His rules and principles for testing the effectiveness of new drugs and medications are summarized in Figure 1.4, and still form the basis of modern clinical trials.

---

(1) The drug must be free from any extraneous accidental quality.

(2) It must be used on a simple, not a composite, disease.

(3) The drug must be tested with two contrary types of diseases, because sometimes a drug cures one disease by its essential qualities and another by its accidental ones.

(4) The quality of the drug must correspond to the strength of the disease. For example, there are some drugs whose heat is less than the coldness of certain diseases, so that they would have no effect on them.

(5) The time of action must be observed, so that essence and accident are not confused.

(6) The effect of the drug must be seen to occur constantly or in many cases, for if this did not happen, it was an accidental effect.

(7) The experimentation must be done with the human body, for testing a drug on a lion or a horse might not prove anything about its effect on man.

Figure 1.4   Avicenna's rules for the experimental use and testing of drugs

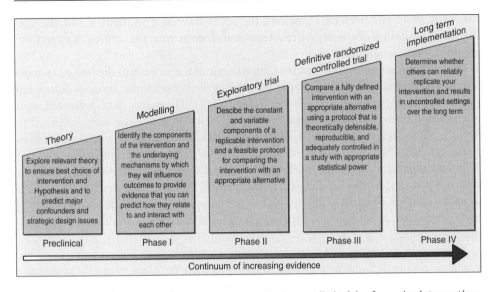

Figure 1.5 Sequential phases of developing randomized controlled trials of complex interventions (from Campbell, Fitzpatrick, Haines, *et al.*, 2000)

One of the most famous clinical trials was that conducted by James Lind (1716–1794) in 1747. He compared the effects of various different acidic substances, ranging from vinegar to cider, on groups of sailors afflicted with scurvy, and found that the group who were given oranges and lemons had largely recovered from their scurvy after 6 days. Somewhat later, Frederick Akbar Mahomed (1849–1884) founded the Collective Investigation Record for the British Medical Association. This organization collated data from physicians practicing outside the hospital setting and was an important precursor of modern collaborative clinical trials.

The very nature of clinical trials research is multidisciplinary in nature so that a team effort is always needed from the concept stage though design, conduct, monitoring and reporting. This collaborative effort has not only led to medical developments in many areas but also to developments of a more statistical nature. For those working in cancer and for whom survival was a key endpoint in the clinical trials, the two seminal papers published by Peto, Pike, Armitage, *et al.* (1976, 1977) in the *British Journal of Cancer* marked a new era. These papers provided the template for key items essential to the design, conduct, analysis and reporting of randomized trials, with emphasis on those requiring prolonged observation of each patient. In particular, these papers described the Kaplan and Meier (1958) estimate of the survival curve, logrank test and the stratified logrank test in such detail that any careful investigator could follow the necessary steps. A computer program (termed the Oxford program) had also been distributed (some time before the date of the publications themselves) and this allowed the methods suggested by the papers to be implemented. Certainly, for those working in data centres with responsibility for many (often reasonably large) trials, this program facilitated the analysis and helped to ensure that the ideas expressed in these articles were widely disseminated. These papers formed the basic text for those involved in clinical trials for many years and, as well as making the ideas accessible to medical statisticians, their role in easing the acceptance of statistical ideas into the clinical community cannot be underestimated.

It should not go unnoticed that DR Cox was one of the authors of the seminal papers referred to above, although his paper describing the proportional hazards regression model appeared some 4 years earlier (Cox, 1972). His paper was presented at a discussion meeting of the UK Royal Statistical Society and subsequently published in Series B of the Society's journals. This journal deals with the more theoretical aspects of statistical research; it does not make easy reading for many statisticians and would not be one to which clinical teams might readily refer. Despite this, this particular paper is probably one of the most cited papers in the medical literature. The methodology leads to easier analysis of trials, with survival time endpoints that include stratification in their design and/or baseline patient characteristics at the time of randomization which may affect prognosis.

As we have indicated, EBM requires that it is important to critically assess *all* the available evidence about whether an intervention works. More recently, systematic overviews have become a vital component of clinical trial research. They are routinely applied *before* launching new trials, as a means of confirming the need to carry out a clinical trial, and *after* completing trials, as a means of synthesizing and summarizing the current knowledge on the topic of interest. These reviews are the focal interest of the Cochrane Collaboration; the associated handbook by Higgins and Green (2005) provides the key to their implementation.

Some developments have not depended on technical advancement, such as the now standard practice of reporting confidence intervals rather than relying solely on p-values at the interpretation stage. Over this same time period the expansion in data processing capabilities and the range of analytical possibilities, made possible by the amazing development in computer power, have been of major importance. Despite many advances, the majority of randomized controlled trials remain simple in design – most often a two-group comparison.

1.7   How trials arise

Although the focus of this book is on comparative or Phase III trials to establish the relative efficacy of the interventions under test, it should be recognized that these may be preceded by an often extensive research programme. This programme may start with the laboratory bench, moving to animal studies and then to early and later stage studies in man. Also, once the Phase III stage itself is complete, there may be further studies initiated. Figure 1.5, taken from Campbell, Fitzpatrick, Haines, *et al.* (2000), succinctly summarizes the pathway of the whole trial process.

The steps range from studies to determine the pharmacokinetic profile of a drug in healthy volunteers (Preclinical) to establishing the appropriate dosage for use in man (Phase I), then the establishment of indications of activity (Phase II). However, some of these steps may be taken in parallel and even simultaneously in the same subjects.

These early studies are not usually randomized. However, the studies conducted by Krishna, Anderson, Bergman, *et al.* (2007) are described as 'randomized' and 'phase I'. Randomized they undoubtedly are, but their use of the Phase I nomenclature is not compatible with Figure 1.5. This highlights a difficulty when attempting to categorize trials using such a simple system. We may imagine that there will be clear stages in the development of a bio-absorbable coronary stent. These too will not exactly parallel those of drug development, although they may well involve laboratory and animal studies. Thus the single arm trial of Erbel, Di Mario, Bartunek, *et al.* (2007) may be considered as close to the Phase II type.

There are also parallels (although modifications will be necessary) for new approaches to, for example, surgical, radiotherapy or physiotherapy techniques and combinations of different procedures. They also extend beyond merely therapeutic trials to planning, for example, trials comparing alternative forms of contraception in women, and those evaluating alternative health promotion interventions. However in some instances, such as in trials comparing educational packages, they may start at the full Phase III stage without involving the earlier phases.

Alternatively, comparative trials may evolve from questions arising in clinical practice and not from a specific development process. We may therefore wish to compare different surgical timings, at 6 months or at 1 year of age, for reconstructive surgery in infants with cleft palette as is proposed in the trial being conducted by Yeow, Lee, Cheng, *et al.* (2007).

Whatever the pathway, the eventual randomized comparative trial to be conducted is clearly a major event. Only when this has been conducted will there be reliable (although not necessarily convincing) evidence of the efficacy of the intervention concerned. In certain situations, often for regulatory purposes, a Phase III trial may be followed by a confirmatory trial asking essentially the same question. In addition, following the regulatory approval of a product, so-called Phase IV or post-marketing trials may be initiated with the aim of gaining broader experience in using the new product.

1.8   Ethical considerations

For a trial to be ethical, at the time it is designed the ethical review committees will want to be convinced that there is collective uncertainty among clinicians as to which treatment is superior or more appropriate for the patients. They will also need to be persuaded that the sample size and other aspects of the study design are such that the trial is likely to provide information sufficient to reduce this uncertainty and therefore influence subsequent medical practice if one treatment or the other appears superior.

A clinical trial cannot go forward until the protocol has been through the appropriate ethical review processes, the exact nature of which varies from country to country. These should always include a very thorough review of the scientific aims as well as the more subject-oriented concerns to protect those who will be recruited to the trial. Briefly, this implies if a trial is not scientifically sound then it should not be judged as ethically acceptable.

1.9   Regulatory requirements

In addition to the more overtly scientific parts of the clinical trials process on which to focus, there are many regulatory requirements which a trial team are obliged to adhere to. For example, the regulations insist that informed consent is obtained from patients entering trials and on the preservation of personal data confidentiality. These regulations are generally referred to as requirements for Good Clinical Practice (GCP) as is described in ICH (1996). We will refer to specific aspects of GCP as they arise in the text, but readers are cautioned that the specifics are continually being changed. Principles to guide statisticians working on clinical trials have been laid down by ICH E9 (1998) and ICH E9 Expert Working Group (1999).

If the trial is seeking regulatory approval of (say) a new drug, then all the associated requirements for approval should be reviewed by the trial team *before, during* and *after* the development of the trial protocol to avoid the rejection of the application on what might be a technical detail. For example, there may be a regulatory requirement for some additional animal studies to be conducted before approval can be granted. These requirements are summarized in documents such as those of US Food and Drug Administration (FDA, 1988) and European Medicines Agency (EMEA, 2009).

In some circumstances, it is a requirement for regulatory approval that a confirmatory trial is conducted. Such a trial is essentially a repeat of an initial trial, perhaps in a different or wider patient group or with wider clinical teams involvement, but it must follow the essential features of the predecessor design. Clearly these details should be cross checked with the relevant authorities before the protocol is finalized and patients are recruited.

1.10   Focus

As we have illustrated, the size of clinical trials can range from the relatively few to as many as several thousands of subjects being recruited. Consequently, and leaving specific details aside, these will require a range of resources from the relatively modest to the very considerable. It must be emphasized that the size of a clinical trial is determined by the question(s) that are posed, and the resources allocated should reflect the importance of that question. Clearly a very experienced team is required to launch a large trial, but even the design team of an ultimately small-sized trial will need access to appropriate personnel including, at a minimum, those with clinical, statistical, data management and organizational skills as well as other specialist skills such as pharmacy or pathology. It is important that the design team do not underestimate the scale of the task.

The focus of this book is on the design of (randomized) comparative (usually termed Phase III) trials which are likely to be of a relatively modest size. We aim to provide clear guidance as to how these may be designed, conducted, (to some extent) analyzed and reported. However, it is also important that investigators contributing patients to clinical trials who are perhaps not part of the design team also understand the issues concerned; the very success of the trials depends crucially on their collaboration and understanding of the processes involved.

1.11 Further reading

Although Day (2007) provides a comprehensive list of books about clinical trials the following are particularly useful:

Day, S. (2007) *Dictionary for Clinical Trials*, 2nd edn, John Wiley & Sons, Ltd, Chichester.

Fitzpatrick, S. (2008a) Clinical Trial Design, ICR Publishing, Marlow, www.icr-global.org

Fitzpatrick, S. (2008b) The Clinical Trial Protocol, ICR Publishing, Marlow, www.icr-global.org

Girling, D.J., Parmar, M.K.B., Stenning, S.P., . Stephens, R.J., and Stewart, L.A.,(2003) Clinical Trials in Cancer, Oxford University Press, Oxford.

Institute of Clinical Research (2008) The Fundamental Guidelines for Clinical Research V2.0, ICR Publishing, Marlow.

Jadad, A. (1998) Randomised Controlled Trials, British Medical Journal, London.

Machin, D., Campbell, M.J., Tan, S.B. and Tan, S.H. (2009) Sample Size Tables for Clinical Studies, 3rd edn, Wiley-Blackwell, Chichester.

Redwood, C. and Colton, T. (eds) (2001) Biostatistics in Clinical Trials, John Wiley & Sons, Ltd, Chichester.

Senn, S. (2007) Statistical Issues in Drug Development, 2nd edn, John Wiley & Sons, Ltd, Chichester.

Wang, D. and Bakhai, A. (eds) (2006) Clinical Trials, A Practical Guide to Design, Analysis and Reporting, Remedica, London.

Hints on how to display medical data in tabular and graphical form are given by:

Freeman, J.V., Walters, S.J. and Campbell, M.J. (2008) How to Display Data, BMJ Books, Oxford.

For those specifically interested in health related quality of life issues:

Fayers, P.M. and Machin, D. (2007) *Quality of life: the assessment, analysis and interpretation of patient-reported outcomes*, John Wiley & Sons, Ltd, Chichester.

For those requiring a wide view of how randomised trials have impacted on clinical practice over a wide range of diseases and conditions:

Machin, D., Day, S. and Green, S. (eds) (2006) Textbook of Clinical Trials, 2nd edn, John Wiley & Sons, Ltd, Chichester.

CHAPTER 2

Design Features

This chapter gives an overview of the general structure of a randomized clinical trial. The key components are highlighted. These include the type of patients or subjects that are likely to be relevant to the objectives of the trial and, within this group, those who are specifically eligible for the trial in mind, the research question(s) and the choice of design. We emphasize the requirement of fully informed consent before a patient is entered into a trial, the determination of whether the interventions on offer are appropriate for the individual concerned, the method of allocation to the alternative interventions and the subsequent patient assessments required to determine the relevant trial endpoint(s). Aspects associated with analysis, reporting and interpretation of the results are also included. Finally, we introduce the basic ideas of a statistical model upon which the ultimate analysis of the clinical trial is based.

2.1 Introduction

Although we will focus on one particular design for clinical trials in this chapter, there are many features of the clinical trials process which are common to the majority of situations. We use the example of a parallel two-group randomized trial to overview some pertinent issues, ranging from defining carefully the research question posed (and thereby the type of subjects to recruit), the interventions used, the allocation of the trial participants to these interventions, endpoint assessment, analysis and reporting. In later chapters, however, we will expand on detail and also on other design options.

This basic design will often compare a test therapy or intervention with a standard (or control) therapy. Frequently, the patients will be assigned at random to the options on a 1 : 1 basis. In reality, the actual choice of design will be a key issue at the planning stage of the design and it should not be assumed that the common design used here for illustration best suits all purposes.

In the ensuing sections we will follow the sequence of Figure 2.1 even although this will not be entirely reflected in real-life situations of the planning stages where a more back-and-to process is more likely. In general, there will also be additional and trial-specific steps that we must also take.

Randomized Clinical Trials: Design, Practice and Reporting David Machin and Peter M Fayers
© 2010 John Wiley & Sons, Ltd

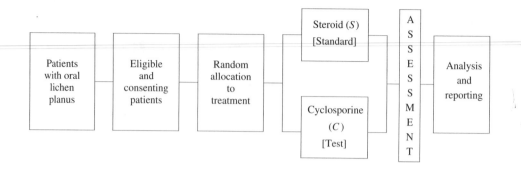

Figure 2.1   Randomized controlled trial of the effect of topical steroid (*S*) and topical cyclosporine (*C*) in patients with symptomatic oral lichen planus (after Poon, Tin, Kim, *et al.*, 2006).

Example 2.1   Two-group parallel design – topical steroid versus topical cyclosporine for symptomatic oral lichen planus

Poon, Tin, Kim, *et al.* (2006) describe a randomized trial of the comparative effect of topical steroid (*S*) and topical cyclosporine (*C*) in patients with systematic oral lichen planus. The basic structure of their trial is given in Figure 2.1.

This trial typifies the design and structure of the randomized parallel group comparative trial, which is used extensively. The key features include: defining the general types of subjects to be studied, identifying the particular subjects eligible for the trial and obtaining their consent, randomly allocating the standard and test interventions and, once the intervention is effected, making the appropriate assessments in order to determine outcome. The analysis of the data recorded for all patients will form the basis of the comparison between the intervention groups, (hopefully) provide a clear indication of their relative clinical importance and supply the framework for the subsequent clinical report describing the results.

2.2   The research question

Of fundamental importance before embarking on a clinical trial is to identify the research question(s) of interest. This question may range from a highly scientific-orientated objective to one focused on a very practical day-to-day clinical situation. For instance, the trial of Example 1.6 aims to reduce the number of hip fractures in elderly residents of nursing homes, whereas one objective of those reported in Example 1.3 is concerned with 24-hour ambulatory blood pressure in healthy subjects, and therefore is almost akin to a non-clinical laboratory-based investigation.

Two key issues are: is the question worth answering and is the answer already known? Clearly the answer to the first should unequivocally be 'Yes'. For the second, one might expect a 'No', although there are circumstances when an earlier result may need confirmation. For example Wee, Tan, Tai, *et al.* (2005) conducted a confirmatory trial of one previously conducted by Al-Sarraf, Pajak, Cooper, *et al.* (1990). The rationale for the repeat trial was based on the former trial involving mainly Caucasian patients; the repeat involved those of predominantly Chinese ethnicity and was conducted by different investigators in another part of the world. In the event, the advantage to chemo-radiation as compared to radiotherapy alone, in terms of overall survival of patients with advanced nasopharyngeal cancer, was confirmed thereby indicating wider generalization of the results from the two trials.

The question(s) posed must have important consequences in that the answer should inform research and/or influence clinical practice in a meaningful way. Further, before the trial is conducted there should be a reasonable expectation that the trial question will be answered. Otherwise, for example, patients may be subjected to unnecessary investigation and possibly discomfort without justification. An exception to this precondition may be when considering information from necessarily small randomized trials in truly rare diseases or conditions, where patient numbers will be insufficient for the usual rules for trial size determination to be applied. We return to this latter issue in Chapter 14.

Erbel, Di Mario, Bartunek, *et al.* (2007, p 1669) (see Example 1.12) state in the summary of their trial that:

> Coronary stents improve immediate and late results of balloon angioplasty by tacking dissections and preventing wall recoil. These goals are achieved within weeks after angioplasty, but with current technology stents permanently remain in the artery, with many limitations including the need for long-term antiplatelet treatment to avoid thrombosis.

This provides a clear rationale for testing a stent for coronary scaffolding made from a bio-absorbable material, which should provide an effective scaffold but would not be permanently retained in the artery.

Meyer, Warnke, Bender and Mülhauser (2003) (Example 1.6) point out that hip fractures in the elderly are a major cause of disability and functional impairment, so that reducing their incidence by encouraging the use of hip protectors within nursing homes may help to reduce this morbidity.

The use of homeopathic remedies is widespread, although there have been few randomized trials to establish their relative efficacy against conventional methods (including placebo). Consequently, the trial of Example 1.9 by Stevinson, Devaraj, Fountain-Barber, *et al.* (2003) compares daily homeopathic arnica against placebo in patients with carpal tunnel syndrome having elective surgery, as it has been claimed that:

> Homeopathic arnica is widely believed to control bruising, reduce swelling and promote recovery after local trauma . . . .

At least to the investigators, and also the corresponding journal editors and peer reviewers, these trials address important questions. The results of the trials suggest that the bio-absorbable magnesium stent is a useful development and encouraging the use of hip protectors reduces hip fracture rates, whereas homeopathic arnica appears no better than placebo.

2.3   Patient selection

Common to all clinical trials is the necessity to define precisely which types of subjects are eligible for recruitment purposes. This implies that even if healthy volunteers are to be the participants, then a definition of 'healthy' is required. This definition may be relatively brief or very complex, depending on the situation.

At the early stages of the design process, we may only have a general idea of the types of subjects required. Identifying the research question may already have made this reasonably clear. Elderly patients may therefore be the first target group for whom preventative action to reduce hip fractures may be considered. Then, when considering the trial question in detail, it might be decided to confine the elderly patient group to those resident in a nursing home. Further refinement may then define the elderly for trial purposes as those over 80 years of age, for example, and exclude those nursing homes who deal with psychiatric residents only. Considerations here might have been an anticipated very low fracture rate in those under 80 years of age and the difficulties associated with obtaining fully informed consent from patients with psychiatric illnesses. These selection criteria are easy to understand, easy to determine and therefore easy to apply in practice.

Eligible patients for the trial conducted (Example 1.2) by Meggitt, Grey and Reynolds (2006) in patients with atopic eczema had to satisfy an extensive list of criteria before they could be considered eligible for the trial. The general requirements specified patients 16–65 years of age with atopic eczema. However, only those with moderate-to-severe disease were to be included and this had to be determined according to the UK modification of the Hanifin and Rajka diagnostic criteria, suggested by Williams, Burney, Hay, et al. (1994), which involves a detailed examination of the patient. Further, they then excluded those: admitted to hospital for eczema; who had used phototherapy or sun beds; had been treated with cyclosporin, systemic steroids, Chinese herbal medicine, topical tacrolimus or evening primrose oil during the preceding 3 months; unstable or infected eczema in the previous 2 weeks requiring either highly potent topical steroids or oral antibiotics; thiopurine methyltransferase (TMPT) activity < 2.55 nmol/h/ml red blood cells (RBC); malignant disease; serious or uncontrolled systemic disease; HIV; pregnancy; lactation; mild eczema and concomitant drugs known to interact with azathioprine. The process of checking the eligibility criteria excluded one-quarter (24) from the 101 patients initially screened for entry to the trial, although it is not clear how many of these were excluded on the grounds of having mild eczema as opposed to being excluded for one or more of the other reasons. If the mild cases are not to be included, clearly the disease status should be determined early in the patient selection process to avoid unnecessary details from a patient who will not be eligible for the trial on that basis alone. We might also conjecture as to why those over 65 years are not included.

In general terms, it is not advisable to restrict the patient pool for entry into a clinical trial. If too many restrictions are in place, the patient pool reduces accordingly so that the required number of patients for the trial takes longer to identify and so trial duration may become prolonged. Also, if those that are eligible comprise only a small subgroup of the total patient pool (e.g. selecting only the moderate-to-severe cases from all those with atopic eczema), then the trial results will not have application to those with less severe disease. As a result, clinical teams are left wondering whether the trial findings are applicable to these patients. Of course, in this example extending the eligibility to less severe cases might not be sensible if useful treatments are already available for these patients.

In determining eligibility, investigators should give as much thought as possible to ensuring generalizability of the subsequent trial results. Simple and minimal eligibility and exclusion criteria should be defined which allow the widest range of patients into the trial who may benefit from the therapy. In many cases, these will include all the patient types for which the comparator in the trial is the current standard. If the eligibility criteria are too narrow then however good the test treatment, the clinical implications will only be relevant to those small groups.

In the context of trials in oncology, but equally applicable in all areas, Wright, Bouma, Dayes, *et al.* (2006) warn:

> In a highly selected trial population, the question of generalizability becomes: how useful are the results of such a study in a more typical population of patients? Unfortunately such information is rarely reported, and oncologists and patients are left estimating how selected the trial population is and what implications it may have for applying the results of the trial in practice.

A long list of eligibility criteria is also very time-consuming to produce and to verify. Nevertheless, and despite the requirement for as few restrictions as possible on the entry requirements to a trial, patient safety is of paramount importance and every care must be taken to ensure vulnerable patients are not entered into a trial. Those that are vulnerable are, for example, those who may be at high risk of a serious adverse event were they to take the trial medication or undergo the trial procedures. This is also often a major concern of the committees giving ethical approval for trials to be conducted.

There must be specific reasons given for why a patient should *not* be included. For example, in some circumstances pregnant women and those lactating (otherwise eligible) may be excluded for fear of impacting adversely on the foetus or the newborn child.

One aspect of selecting patients for inclusion to a trial is seldom explicitly reported in the literature. This is the need to verify that each individual considered for recruitment is suitable for *all* the treatments or interventions on offer within the clinical trial. Thus if there are three treatment options A, B and C, then not only must the attending physician be happy to prescribe every one of the options but also the patient must be willing to receive any of these options. If only two of these three are acceptable (by either the physician, patient or both) then the patient should not be regarded as eligible for the trial and so cannot be regarded as a potential recruit. Further, if the physician thinks that for a particular patient one of the options is preferable then, despite eligibility in all other respects, the patient should receive that option and so cannot be considered for the trial. In such circumstances, the clinician should not enter the patient in the hope that following the treatment assignment process the patient will be allocated the 'preferred' option. Neither should the physician expect, if the unacceptable alternative option is allocated by the randomization process, that he or she can simply withdraw the patient from the trial. Such action, certainly if repeated sufficiently often, will seriously undermine the trial and thereby a misleading outcome could arise. The difficulty is that we do not know to what extent the information or lack of information from such patients distorts or biases the estimate of the treatment effect that is obtained at the end of the trial.

Example 2.2   Trial eligibility – partial thickness burns

In a randomized trial by Ang, Lee, Gan, *et al.* (2001), patients with severe burns were emergency admissions into the specialist burns centre in Singapore, requiring immediate treatment. Once admitted to the burns centre, only those patients with partial thickness burns were eligible for the trial. Their consent was then sought and, once given, randomization was effected by telephone to the statistical centre. Nevertheless, in certain cases, the attending medical team felt that the option of conventional therapy was more appropriate than the test therapy. For those patients, details of the clinical trial were not explained and conventional therapy commenced immediately.

2.4   The consent process

Once a potential participant is deemed eligible for the trial, fully informed consent is required before the individual can be formally registered for the trial and the intervention allocation process implemented. Of course, before consent can be sought, those responsible for obtaining consent should regard the trial they are advocating as ethical from their own perspective. A simple ethical test that works for most researchers is: if your mother/father/child had this condition, would you be willing to enter them into the proposed trial? If not, are you sure the trial is ethical? Only if the consent seeker is in the state of equipoise (i.e. has an indifferent opinion about the relative merits of the alternative treatments), is the randomization considered ethical.

An integral part of the consent process is providing the individual concerned with full information pertaining to the trial including the potential benefits (if any) and risks. This information may be provided in a number of ways which will depend on the context, but will usually comprise written information as well as a verbal explanation of what is involved. The language of both the written and verbal components has to be chosen carefully and should be phrased in non-technical terms whenever possible. Clearly the consent process must provide full details of the intervention options and should explain what the objectives of the trial are and that the interventions will be allocated using a chance mechanism. If participating in the trial involves extra medical examinations or requires more (possibly invasive) samples to be taken from the patient than would be routine for the condition concerned in standard practice, then this needs to be made clear.

It is also a prerequisite of the process that the individual should not be pressurized into giving consent so that, for example, adequate time should be allowed by the investigating team for individuals to decide and, often in the case of patients, to discuss the situation with relatives or friends. It should also be explained that even if consent is given, the subject is free to withdraw that consent at any time without compromising in any way the quality of their care.

Regulatory requirements usually insist that the informed consent process is fully documented, and the consenting individual signs a consent form which is then appropriately witnessed. This part of the process will also need to be adapted to the particular circumstances. For example, in a trial concerning paediatric patients, the consent process will be directed at the parent or legal guardian of the child who then consents on the child's behalf. Other situations where the consent process may have to be carefully considered may be in accident and emergency situations, patients who are mentally compromised, have psychiatric conditions or who are frail and elderly.

It is important for the investigating team to be, and remain, fully conversant with local, national and even international regulations pertaining to the consent process. For international studies it may be sufficient to write in the protocol that patients must give fully informed written and signed consent, and participating clinicians must also conform to local requirements.

2.5   Choice of interventions

The particular interventions to be compared in a clinical trial will be determined by the choice of the specific research question concerned. We shall see in Chapter 9 that the size of a clinical trial, that is the number of subjects that need to be recruited, depends critically on the effect size. In loose terms, the effect size is the anticipated difference between (say two) interventions. If the effect size is small then trials have to be large, whereas if effect size is large then trials may be small. Setting all other aspects aside, small trials are preferable to large. They require fewer patients and therefore can be completed in a timely manner. From this fact, it follows that large effects are preferable to small. Of course, before the trial is conducted we do not know the *actual* size of the effect (indeed that is what we are trying to determine from the trial itself once completed). However, we can choose to make comparisons between interventions which, at the onset, are as different in their anticipated effect as reasonably possible. The way in which the comparator (often termed control and test) interventions are chosen is therefore critical.

2.5.1   Standard or control treatment

In the development of a new or alternative approach to therapy, it is important to compare this with the current standard for the disease or condition in question if at all possible. When no effective standard or alternative therapy exists, the new therapy may be compared against 'no-treatment' or a placebo control.

Example 2.3   Placebo controlled trial – advanced hepatocellular carcinoma

In a randomized controlled trial conducted by Chow, Tai, Tan, *et al.* (2002) in advanced liver cancer, patients were randomized to receive either placebo or tamoxifen. Tamoxifen, although not anticipated to influence survival outcome, is often used to palliate symptoms in such patients. No randomized trial has been conducted to measure its effectiveness, however, and this provided the rationale for the use of a placebo.

However, placebo controls and no-treatment controls are not possible in many circumstances. In this case, the control group may comprise those receiving current best practice. For example, in patients receiving surgery for the primary treatment of head and neck cancer followed by best supportive care, a randomized controlled trial may be assessing the value of adding post-operative chemotherapy to this standard (best supportive care only) approach. In this case, the control group are those who receive the current standard of no adjuvant treatment, while the test group receive chemotherapy in addition. In some situations, the no-intervention control may be a watch-and-wait policy while the comparator group receives an immediate intervention.

Example 2.4   Antipsychotic drugs in schizophrenia and schizophreniform disorder

In the trial described by Kahn, Fleischhacker, Boter, *et al.* (2008), four second-generation antipsychotic drugs were tested against haloperidol, a first-generation standard in first-episode schizophrenia. Although second-generation drugs had been in use for a decade, their clinical effectiveness compared with those of the first-generation was still debated.

2.5.2   Test treatment

If there are only minor differences in the actual type of interventions to be compared in a randomized trial, then outcome differences are likely to be small and only a very large-scale trial would detect any differences in efficacy, even if truly present. What is more, even if such small differences are demonstrated by a clinical trial, they may have little clinical or research consequence. It is therefore best (within the realms of practicability and safety considerations) if the treatment options are as different as possible so that clinically important differences may therefore be potentially established. For example, if a randomized trial is planned to test a drug (at dose d) against placebo (dose $d = 0$), then d should be set as high as possible. If in such a trial no effect is demonstrated, then we may be reasonably confident that the drug is not efficacious. On the other hand, if a lower dose $d/2$ (say) had been chosen to compare with placebo, then a 'no difference' outcome may be a result of the selected dose being too low rather than the drug being truly inactive. Another key question for the design team in this context is therefore to decide how high the dose should be while balancing potential efficacy against toxicity and safety issues. One may imagine the different scenarios when choosing the dose to include for a new analgesic if the patients are young (usually healthy) individuals compared to establishing the value of a drug suitable for those who are terminally ill.

An extreme example of a major difference in the interventions studied, which one may imagine would have been difficult to justify, is that of the hip-fracture prevention trial of Example 1.6 where the authors state the following:

> In homes allocated to usual care (control group) the nominated study coordinator received brief information (10 minutes) about and demonstration of the hip protector, and two hip protectors were provided for demonstration purposes.
>
> The intervention (intervention group) consisted of structured education of staff, who then taught patients, and provision of free hip protectors. We provided three hip protectors per resident . . ..

Clearly if an extreme intervention has little or no demonstrable effect then a less extreme intervention is also likely to be ineffective. Nevertheless, one has to be cautious in pushing the extent of the intervention too far as it may be that *less* intervention also has the desired effect. Thus one might be concerned, for example, that one of the components (structured education of staff or provision of three hip protectors per resident) of the intervention for elderly residents may not be essential to achieve the reduction in the hip fracture rates. As an extreme example, if cure can be achieved with dose $d/2$ then it would be foolish to give patients dose d. These issues have to be debated thoroughly by the trial design team.

2.6 Choice of design

The final choice of the design for the trial will depend crucially on the questions posed; these will be a key determinant of the interventions that are to be compared. Clearly, if there are only two interventions involved, then one option for the design is the two-group parallel trial illustrated in Figure 2.1. We discuss other options including cross-over and split-mouth designs in Chapter 12 and repeated measures, cluster and non-inferiority designs in Chapter 11.

However, even within the structure of the simplest of all comparative trial designs, there are options that have to be considered. Although randomization is mandatory for such a design, the choice of the allocation ratio of standard to test has to be agreed. Statistical considerations of efficiency usually favour a 1 : 1 allocation but other issues may predominate such as, for example, the availability of the test compound in a drug trial. The final choice of allocation ratio will influence the number of participants required to some extent, and may complicate the informed consent process if (say) an option other than equal allocation is chosen which may be more difficult to explain or justify in lay terms.

Further, as is suggested by the hierarchy of Figure 1.2, the options for presenting the interventions in a blinded or masked manner need to be discussed. In many circumstances, no blinding is possible and so an 'open' trial is conducted. In such cases, it is very important that the endpoint assessments are determined in as objective and reproducible manner as is possible.

If more than two interventions are to be compared, then the number of design options increases. Which to choose may crucially depend on the presence or absence of structure of the options under test. For example, if we are comparing three (or more) entirely different drugs, none of which can be considered as standard, the chosen design may obviously be a parallel three-group design with randomization of equal patient numbers assigned to each (although how to determine the appropriate trial size is less clear). Alternatively, if one of the drugs can be considered a standard then strategies for sample size calculation tend to be more clear-cut, as would be the case if the three drugs were in fact three different doses of the same drug. These issues are discussed in Chapter 13.

In certain situations it may be possible to ask two (therapeutic) questions within the same trial design rather than to conduct two separate two-group trials. For example, in the trial described by Yeow, Lee, Cheng, et al. (2007) which we expand on in greater detail in Chapter 13, infants are randomized to one of two types of surgery and also to whether the operation should be conducted at 6 months or 1 year of age. Thus, the two questions posed concern (i) the choice of surgery and (ii) when the surgery should be performed. The infants recruited to this so-called 2×2 factorial design are then randomized to one of the four options in equal proportions.

When the endpoint of concern is also a measure that can be assessed at baseline, immediately prior to randomization, then whatever the design structure such information may be used to improve the statistical efficiency of the design. Thus in the trial of Meggitt, Gray and Reynolds (2006) (Example 1.2), one endpoint was the disease activity of a patients' eczema as determined using the SASSAD score. This was assessed at -2 weeks and at baseline immediately prior to randomization, and then post-randomization at 4, 8 and 12 weeks during the course of treatment. This increase in efficacy accords with what clinicians would expect because we are then effectively evaluating within-patient change from baseline (albeit using a statistical analysis that does not explicitly use change scores). Such repeated measures designs are discussed in Chapter 11, where it is shown that increasing the number of pre- and post-randomization measurements has the effect of reducing the final numbers of subjects that need to be recruited. A reduction may be achieved even in the simplest situation of a single (baseline) measure together with one post-randomization assessment on every recruited individual.

However, obtaining the necessary regulatory approval of the trial may inhibit the choice of design that we may wish to conduct. For example, the committee may find the double-placebo arm in a proposed 2×2 factorial design unacceptable on ethical grounds, or may suggest that this makes obtaining consent difficult and could therefore compromise the ability to recruit the required numbers of patients. Thus, in some cases, the best experimental design may not be a practical option for the investigation and a balance has to be struck between what is statistically optimal and what is feasible.

We discuss details of how the size of a trial is determined in Chapter 9.

2.7 Assigning the interventions

A crucial role of randomization is to ensure that there are no systematic differences between the patient groups assigned to the different interventions. To preserve this situation we need to, at all cost, avoid losing patients subsequent to randomization, and we want to maximize the probability that the allocated treatment is indeed applied. It is therefore extremely important to minimize the delays between consent, randomization and the commencement of therapy.

In an ideal setting, once a patient has consented to take part in a clinical trial, randomization should take place immediately. Once the treatment allocation is known, therapy should begin immediately following that. This minimizes delay and avoids the patient having the opportunity to change his or her mind before therapy begins. This helps to prevent the dilution that can occur if a patient refuses the allocated treatment or switches to the comparator option in the period between randomization and starting treatment. As we will discuss later, for purposes of analysis such patients are retained in the treatment group to which they were allocated. Consequently, for example, a patient who switches from intervention A to B will still be retained in A for analysis, and this will make the effect of B appear more similar to that of A than might truly be the case. The prospect of dilution should therefore be anticipated at the design stage, and all steps taken to reduce this possibility to a minimum.

However, there will be many circumstances in which therapy cannot be initiated immediately. For example, in a trial comparing surgical options, there may be a delay until the surgery can take place because of the necessary preoperative workup procedures, although trials have been conducted in which randomization takes place while the patient is on the operating table. In life-threatening conditions, deaths may even occur before surgery can take place. For others there is at least the possibility that their disease progresses in the intervening interval and so the patient is no longer operable. As with those who refuse or switch the treatments allocated, such patients remain in the trial analysis within their randomized group and so these also dilute the estimate of the real difference (if any) between the interventions to be compared.

**Example 2.5   Delay between randomization and start of treatment –
radiotherapy for inoperable non-small cell lung cancer**

Although full details are not provided, there were unavoidable delays between randomization and the commencement of radiotherapy (RT) in a trial conducted by the Medical Research Council Lung Cancer Working Party (1996). This resulted in 3/255 (1.2%) patients allocated 2-fractions and 6/254 (2.4%) allocated 13-fractions not receiving any radiotherapy at all. However, these are relatively small proportions and so the consequences of the dilution caused by these 9 (1.8%) patients not receiving any radiotherapy is unlikely to have had any major impact on the trial conclusions.

2.8 Making the assessments

In the simplest situation, once the patient has been checked for eligibility, basic demographic and clinical variables recorded, consent obtained and randomization activated, treatment commences and is completed within a short time. If the trial endpoint is also defined to be observed within a relatively short time frame, the whole trial can be of very short duration and the data collection process should be relatively straightforward. Such a short-term situation could arise in a trial to study the immediate postoperative pain relief provided by a certain types of rapidly acting analgesics. However, most trials are more complex than this. For example, in many situations the period of treatment may be extensive and perhaps differ for each intervention and vary from patient to patient. In trials concerned with approaches to wound healing, the time to satisfactory closing of the wounds will vary and very detailed monitoring of the wound may be needed to determine when the outcome is indeed satisfactory. Further, some considerable time may be required before the endpoint can be determined. For example, trials testing potentially curative therapy for early prostate cancer might have to follow patients for more than a decade before any difference is detectable in an outcome such as survival. The trial design must therefore stipulate carefully exactly when assessments are to be made and the criteria used for determining the endpoint meticulously documented within the trial protocol.

2.9 Analysis and reporting

The main purpose of the statistical analysis at the end of the trial will be to compare the two intervention groups with respect to the endpoints specified in the protocol at the design stage. This comparison will involve estimating the difference between groups, the associated confidence interval and *p-value*. The statistical methods to be used will depend on the type of endpoint variable concerned. However, this basic analysis may need to take into account specific features of the design, such as whether a stratified or cluster randomization was used. It may also be appropriate to allow for patient or disease characteristics which may influence outcome in an important way. Further, there may be secondary outcomes to summarize, although these may or may not involve formal statistical comparisons. There may be unanticipated features such as serious adverse events (SAE) or unusual toxicities that were not anticipated at the protocol design stage. We describe some details of how the analysis of a trial is carried out in Chapter 8.

In addition, it is important to document patient progress through the different trial stages by, for example, tracking the number consenting to participate, the number randomized, those completing therapy and the number in which the endpoint assessment has been made in each intervention group. The CONSORT statement described by Moher, Schultz and Altman (2001) provides a framework for this. We referred to this in Figure 1.3 and we will expand upon the details in Chapter 10.

It is also usual to provide some basic demographic details, often a minimum of age and gender together with some pertinent clinical information (perhaps stage of the disease and a summary of clinical and/or diagnostic tests results) in tabular form and by allocated intervention group.

2.9.1   Which patients to analyze

We discussed in an earlier section the importance of initiating the intervention as soon after randomization as possible. Alternatively, it is best to delay the actual randomization until the time that treatment can be initiated. For those receiving homeopathic arnica in the trial of Example 1.9, for example, the treatment could commence immediately post-randomization. Indeed, the taking of the first medication could be supervised by the responsible investigator so that there was no delay and patients were less likely to withdraw immediately or refuse trial medication. In such a situation, it would not be in the best interest of the trial to randomize the patient and then not to have immediate access to the medication.

Example 2.6   Children with fever

In a randomized controlled trial reported by Hay, Costelloe, Redmond, *et al.* (2008), the median time between randomization and giving the first dose of study drug to children with fever was 8 min for paracetemol plus ibuprofen, 9 min for paracetemol and 9 min for the ibuprofen group. However, we suspect that this ideal state of affairs could not be replicated in too many situations.

2.9.1.1   *Intention to treat (ITT)*

Despite every effort to commence treatment as soon after randomization as possible, there will be circumstances when the patient nevertheless then refuses the treatment allocated or may even request the alternative option. In double-blind trials, requesting the other option at an early stage post-randomization would be very unlikely. In an open trial where the patient is fully aware (and can recognize the option) this will be more of a problem. However, even if a patient commences the intervention in question, they may subsequently refuse to continue with it and even wish to withdraw from the trial entirely.

The intention-to-treat (ITT) principle is that once randomized the patient is retained in the allocated group for analysis whatever occurs, even in situations where a patient is randomized to (say) A but then refuses and even insists on being treated by option B. As we have previously indicated, the effect of such a patient is to dilute the estimate of the true difference between A and B. However, if such a patient were analyzed as if allocated to treatment B, then the trial is no longer truly and totally randomized since patient choice rather than chance has determined the allocation in such cases. The resulting comparison may then be seriously biased to an unknown extent and direction. In contrast, analysis based on the ITT principle ensures that for a trial established to demonstrate superiority of one intervention over another, any estimate of their difference is if anything biased towards the null. In this case, although some bias may be present, we know what the consequences will be. For example in a trial in which there are patients who may have diluted the difference, yet an ITT analysis still demonstrates a clear difference between the treatment options, investigators can reasonably infer that there is indeed a difference.

In contrast, the difficulty with analyzing a trial by the treatment patients actually received is that we do not know the direction of the bias. If there are relatively few patients who do not receive their allocated intervention then clearly this is not likely to be a major issue. Conversely, if the numbers are large then this would be a major concern and may render the trial results untrustworthy.

One procedure that was once in widespread use was for the investigating team to review the trial data in detail after the protocol treatment and follow-up were complete and all the trial specific information collected, in order to decide which patients should be in the final comparison. This review would, for example, retrospectively check that all the patient eligibility criteria were satisfied and that there had been no important protocol deviations while on treatment. Only if eligibility and compliance to protocol (however defined) were confirmed, would the subject be deemed eligible for the analysis. Usually this review would not be blind to the treatment received. Even if the trial were double-blind, there may still be clues in the data which reveal the nature of the treatment received.

One problem is that this process tends to selectively exclude patients with the more severe disease. Evidence for selective exclusion of patients following such reviews is provided by Machin, Stenning, Parmar, *et al.* (1997) who examined the published and pioneering portfolio of the early randomized trials conducted by the UK Medical Research Council in patients with cancer. They showed that the earlier publications systematically excluded from analysis (and hence reported on) fewer patients in the more aggressive treatment arm, despite a 1 : 1 randomization. Thus, for example, any patient who had difficulties with this treatment (perhaps the more sick patients) was not included in the assessment of the efficacy of the treatment. This systematic exclusion would tend to bias the results in its favour.

2.9.1.2   *Per-protocol*

In certain circumstances, however, a per-protocol summary of the trial results may be more relevant. In such an analysis, the comparison is made only in those patients who comply (which has to be carefully defined in advance) with the treatment allocated. One example of a per-protocol analysis is if the toxicity and/or side-effects profile of a new agent are to be compared. In this case, an ITT analysis including those patients who were randomized to the drug but then did not receive it (for whatever reason) could seriously underestimate the true scale of the relative safety profiles. If a per-protocol analysis is appropriate for such endpoints, then the trial protocol should state that such an analysis is intended from the onset. One situation where a per-protocol analysis is important is when reporting the results of non-inferiority trials that we discuss in Chapter 11.

2.9.2   Trial publication

Once it is clear which patients are to be included in the final analysis, any exclusion after randomization should be accounted for, described and justified in accordance with the CONSORT statement. Only then can work on the analysis and the trial publication begin. However, it is usually expedient to plan and prepare preliminary analyses prior to the final endpoint analysis, so that the results of the trial can be disseminated with the minimum of delay. Since the structure of research publications often takes a familiar format (indeed investigators should have a target clinical journal in mind even at the design stage), key items can be prepared in advance and some of these will be based on sections of the trial protocol itself, as listed in Table 3.1. If nothing else, the protocol will provide much of the text outlining the background and purpose of the trial, details of eligible patients, interventions studied, randomization process, a sample size justification, key elements of the analytical methods and a list of some important references. Further, if the trial progress is monitored regularly with feedback reports to the investigating team, then these reports can form the basis for some tabular and graphical presentations that will be included in the final publication. Clearly the responsible writing committee will have to amend and update some of these details as appropriate, and the eventual presentation of results and ultimate discussion will depend on the trial findings.

2.10 Technical details

2.10.1 Statistical models

Whatever the type of trial, it is usually convenient to think of the underlying structure of the design in terms of a statistical model. This model encapsulates the question we are intending to answer. Once the model is specified, the object of the corresponding clinical trial (and hence the eventual analysis) is to estimate the parameters of this model as precisely as is reasonable.

Suppose that in a particular trial we wish to compare two treatment groups, C and T. We can use an indicator τ to identify the treatment received by a patient by setting $\tau = 0$ and $\tau = 1$ for the two treatments, respectively. If the outcome of interest is a continuous variable y then this is related to the treatment or intervention by the linear regression equation

$$y = \beta_0 + \beta_1 \tau + \varepsilon. \tag{2.1}$$

In this equation, β_0 and β_1 are constants and are termed the parameters of the model. (In later chapters, we will often refer to β_1 as β_{Treat}, the regression coefficient which is the major focus for clinical trials.) In contrast, ε represents the noise (or error) and is assumed to be random and have a mean value of 0 across all subjects recruited to the trial and standard deviation (SD) denoted σ. The object of a trial would be to estimate β_0 and β_1 and we write such estimates as b_0 and b_1 to distinguish them from the corresponding parameters.

On the basis of this model, the two fundamental issues in trial design to consider are:

(1) What levels of the design variable τ should be chosen?

(2) How many subjects should we recruit?

In this model, with $\tau = 0$ for the control treatment C, $y_0 = \beta_0$ and this represents the 'true' or population mean of this group, labelled μ_C. Alternatively, with $\tau = 1$, $y_1 = \beta_0 + \beta_1$ and this represents μ_T, the population mean of group T. The difference δ between those receiving C and T is therefore $y_1 - y_0 = \beta_0 + \beta_1 - \beta_0 = \beta_1$. From this, $\beta_1 = \mu_T - \mu_C$ and $\beta_0 = \mu_C$. Population means are estimated by sample means, in this case $\bar{x}_C$ and $\bar{x}_T$, so that the estimates of the parameters are $b_0 = \bar{x}_C$ and $b_1 = \bar{x}_T - \bar{x}_C$. The latter is the estimate of the true difference between treatments: $\delta = \mu_T - \mu_C$.

In this example, Equation 2.1 describes the two-group clinical trial of this chapter. Although this basic equation encapsulates the essential structure of all our analyses, we can extend this model to describe more complex clinical trial designs.

2.10.2   Randomization

In essence, one purpose of any experiment is to estimate the parameters of a statistical model analogous to that of Equation 2.1. We therefore conduct a trial in order to collect data with this purpose in mind. We would like to believe that the estimates we obtain reflect the true or population parameter values. In principle, if we repeated the study many times, then we would anticipate that these estimates would form a distribution that is centred on the true parameter value. If this is the case, our method of estimation is *unbiased*. For example, in a clinical trial comparing two treatments, the parameter β_1 corresponds to the true difference (if any) in efficacy between them, and the object of the trial is to obtain an unbiased estimate of this. The method of selecting which of the eligible patients is to be included in the trial does not affect this, but the way in which those patients who are recruited to the trial are then allocated to a particular treatment does. As we discussed in Chapter 1, of fundamental importance to the design of any clinical trial is the random allocation of subjects to the alternative treatments. Randomization also provides a sound basis for the ensuing hypothesis testing by the use of statistical tests of significance.

2.11   Guidelines

When planning a clinical trial of any size or complexity it is very important to establish the ground rules. Although many of these are based on common sense, it is very useful to have access to clear guidelines for all stages of the process. Such guidelines have been published, covering a wide range of topics ranging from regulatory requirements to what a statistical referee should look for when reviewing a clinical trial manuscript for publication.

We will refer to some of these guidelines at the relevant stages later in the book, but a useful start is the booklet provided by the Institute of Clinical Research (2008) which we list with some others below. However, readers are warned that many of these are constantly being updated and it is always useful to check if those referred to here are the most current.

2.12 Further reading

Craig, P., Dieppe, P.P., Macintyre, S., Mitchie, S., Nazarath, I. and Petticrew, M. (2008) Developing and evaluating complex interventions: the new Medical Research Council guidance. *BMJ*, **337**, 979–983.

Fuller details are provided by www.mrc.ac.uk/complexinterventionguidance

EMEA, Canary Wharf, London, www.emea.eu.int.

ICH E9 Expert Working Group (1999) Statistical principles for clinical trials: ICH harmonised tripartite guideline. *Statistics in Medicine*, **18**, 1907–1942.

This contains, for example, a clear statement of what distinguishes an ITT from a per-protocol analysis.

ICH E10 (2000). Choice of Control Group in Clinical Trials. CPMP/ICH/2711/99.

Contains information concerning what are regarded as suitable control groups for many situations.

Institute of Clinical Research (2008) The Fundamental Guidelines for Clinical Research V2.0, ICR Publishing.

This includes ICH Good Clinical Practice (1996), Declaration of Helsinki (2008), EU Directive 2001/20/EC (Clinical Trials Directive) and EU Directive 2005/28/EC (GCP Directive). Details are provided by www.icr-global.org.

CHAPTER 3

The Trial Protocol

It is a fundamental requirement to develop a formal protocol for any clinical trial and we describe, in general terms, the subject matter of such a protocol. The chapter focuses on the content common to all trial protocols such as the background to the trial, the basic design, the type and number of potential subjects to recruit, informed consent, details of the intervention options and other practicalities including the forms required for recording the data. We illustrate each section by extracts from activated protocols used for a variety of trials in different areas.

We also emphasize the need to check local regulations concerned with the conduct of trials and reference is made to some published guidelines to help in the protocol development process.

3.1   Introduction

Day (2007) defines a protocol as: 'A written document describing all the important details of how a study will be conducted. It will generally include details of the products being used, a rationale for the study, what procedures will be carried out on subjects in the study, how many subjects will be studied, the design of the study and how the data will be analyzed.' In our context, 'study' is replaced by 'trial' and commonly 'products' will be replaced by 'treatments' or 'interventions'. In particular, a clinical trial protocol is a document that will include sections addressing those design features highlighted in Chapter 2, as they relate to the specific trial in question.

As we have pointed out, the questions posed in a clinical trial must be important and so it is vital that the research team identify all the scientific, clinical and practical elements, together with the resources and skills necessary in order to achieve clear answers. This is no small task, even when embarking on a clinical trial of moderate size and complexity. A fundamental part of this process, and one that must be undertaken to obtain regulatory approval, is the development of the associated trial protocol. This document must be clear yet concise and contain all the elements necessary for all the members of the investigating teams to carry out their respective tasks. Thus for any

Randomized Clinical Trials: Design, Practice and Reporting   David Machin and Peter M Fayers
© 2010 John Wiley & Sons, Ltd

1.	Abstract (or Summary)
2.	Background (or Introduction)
3.	Research Objectives
4.	Design
5.	Intervention details
6.	Eligibility
7.	Randomisation
8.	Assessments and Data Collection
9.	Statistical considerations
10.	Ethical issues
11.	Organisational structure
12.	Publication policy
13.	Trial forms
14.	Appendices

Figure 3.1   Major components of a clinical
trial protocol

clinical trial, although the main features of the trial from design to analysis will be discussed in detail at the planning stage, the trial itself cannot be conducted unless the finalized plan is thoroughly documented. In broad terms, the range of features to be addressed in the trial protocol is indicated in Figure 3.1. There may be additional requirements dependent on the specifics of the actual trial to be undertaken, and the headings under which particular details fall will also vary with circumstance. For example, patient safety issues may be of paramount concern in one trial, which may warrant a dedicated section in the protocol. In another, this may not be the case and such issues may only require a brief mention.

It is very difficult for any one person to think of every detail of all the elements that are needed for a particular protocol and so it is important to involve as broad a team as possible (certainly to include members from a range of disciplines) in the development process.

Further, although this may be mandatory within many situations, a review of the document by two or more experienced but independent peers together with an independent statistician (and other experts as may be relevant) is also advisable. Such a group should also review the data forms to ensure they are clear and that they encapsulate the key features, do not overburden the clinical teams or trial subjects with unnecessary detail yet enable the trial endpoint(s) to be unambiguously recorded for each subject.

Finally the protocol should be dated, suitably bound in book form, and any subsequent amendments carefully documented. In the following sections we address the individual sections of a protocol as detailed in Figure 3.1 and, wherever possible, provide illustrative examples of how some of the sections have been phrased in activated protocols.

We cannot emphasize too strongly that the protocol must be a high quality document, in both scientific and clinical terms, and needs to be written in clear language with careful highlighting of important issues. The protocol serves many purposes; for example, it gives an overview of the trial process from beginning to end and details the specific interventions and how these are to be allocated. Importantly, it guides the clinician through when and how assessments are to be made, and where necessary provides a step-by-step guide to administering the precise interventions stipulated.

3.2 Protocol – abstract

This section of the protocol is intended to give a concise overview of the aims of the clinical trial. The precise structure will depend on the features of the protocol that need to be highlighted. Of particular importance will be the type of subjects concerned, the interventions planned and the chosen design. This may take a structured format, as when eventually submitting the trial for publication, or may be a bulleted list that is perhaps accompanied with a schema such as that of Figure 2.1, summarizing the design.

Example 3.1   Protocol SQGL02 (1999): Brimonidine as a neuroprotective agent in acute angle closure glaucoma (AACG)

This is an open-labelled, randomized, active-controlled prospective pilot study comparing the efficacy of Brimonidine 0.2% with Timolol 0.5% as a neuroprotective agent in preventing/reducing visual field defects in patients with acute angle closure glaucoma (AACG). 80 patients presenting with AACG at 4 centers (SGH/SNEC, TTSH, NUH and CGH) will be recruited into the study and randomized to Timolol or Brimonidine, in addition to the standard medical treatment and laser peripheral iridotomy (PI) for AACG. Baseline Humphrey visual fields program 24–2 will be performed after PI. The study medication will be continued for 1 month and the visual fields compared at the end of 4 months to determine if either group has better preservation of fields. If Brimonidine is found to be efficacious in preserving visual fields and hence offering neuroprotection, a larger prospective randomized clinical trial may be planned subsequently to follow.

This statement was followed by a sentence describing the trial objectives, very brief eligibility requirements of 'unilateral attack of AACG and informed consent' only, and finally a schema illustrating key aspects of the design to be implemented. The extract very clearly summarizes the main features of the planned trial.

An abstract within a scientific journal would not normally contain a schema of the trial design due to space limitations. However, within a trial protocol this may well be very helpful as an overview of the trial. SQCP01 (2006) of Example 3.3 therefore has an initial summary page (as opposed to an abstract), containing a structured review of objectives, eligibility, method and design, including an outline schema of their factorial trial. A more detailed schema is given in a later section of their protocol.

Example 3.2   Protocol SQCP01 (2006): Comparing speech and growth outcomes between two different techniques and two different timings of surgery in the management of clefts of the secondary palate (Figure 3.1)

Design

A multi-centre randomised controlled trail using a 2 × 2 factorial design to compare the efficacy of VWK type Palatoplasty with 2-Flap Palatoplasty and IVV, and the timing of surgery at 6 months or 1 year of age in infants with clefts of the secondary palate without associated cleft lip deformity.

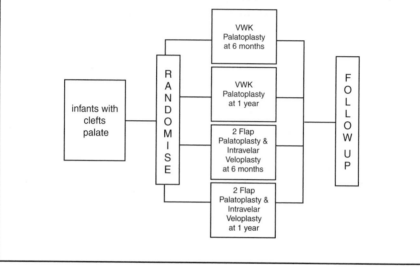

3.3   Protocol – background

Any individual or group concerned with answering an important clinical question by means of a clinical trial should be conversant with the medical speciality concerned and is likely to be expert within that discipline. Nevertheless, those planning a trial not only need to ensure they have the relevant team assembled but should still be prepared to seek outside assistance as appropriate. Even at the early stages of formulating the research question, discussions with peers from relevant disciplines will therefore always be valuable. Alongside this process, detailed reviews of the medical and related literature are required. These reviews can help formulate the research question itself and provide details on, for example, the safety of the interventions planned and information on many other aspects of the intended trial. Once the questions have been defined, a literature search may establish whether or not other trials have been conducted with the same or similar objectives and, if so, whether these either obviate the need for the trial in question or lead to some modification in its design.

The object of the background section within the trial protocol is to provide an in-depth summary of how the proposed trial arose, with references to relevant

published work as well as the consequences for clinical practice and/or research
once the trial results are known. Essentially, this section would contain the
information necessary for the introduction that will be needed for the future
research publication describing the trial results. Although it is difficult to be
precise about the content, the aim is to give an informed reader a clear rationale
for justifying the importance and relevance of the clinical trial to be conducted. It
must therefore be persuasive enough to convince those who will be part of the
formal approving process, for example, the local ethics committees of the participating clinical centres. It must also convince interested colleagues who may
wish to participate. It should therefore use language which is neither too specialized nor cluttered with unnecessary detail, yet it must provide a clear scientific/
clinical motivation for the randomized trial outlined.

3.4 Protocol – research objectives

In this section of the protocol, the research objectives of the trial are summarized in
broad outline and specifics with regard to the endpoints provided.

3.4.1 Objectives

The objectives need not be lengthy provided they encapsulate the major intentions,
essentially stating the hypotheses under test. The examples given below do not refer
explicitly to the design chosen, for example whether randomized or not, but do imply
they are comparative in nature.

**Example 3.3   Protocol SQNP01 (1997): Standard radiotherapy versus
concurrent chemo-radiotherapy followed by adjuvant
chemotherapy for locally advanced (non-metastatic)
nasopharyngeal cancer**

This trial aimed to compare the clinical response, distant metastases, disease-free
survival and overall survival of chemo-radiotherapy and adjuvant chemotherapy,
using combination chemotherapy comprising CisDDP and 5-Fluorouracil
(5-FU), with radiotherapy in patients with locally advanced nasopharyngeal
cancer (NPC).

The summary indicates the comparisons concerned, although omitting full
details of the (complex) chemotherapy regimen under test, and highlights that the
patients are those with a particular form of NPC. This statement also identifies the
several trial endpoints to be determined, which concern response (and the protocol includes details of how this is to be assessed), measures that require following the patients progress (and noting when distant metastases or recurrent disease
appears) and survival.

Example 3.4   Protocol PRESSURE (2000): Pressure relieving support surfaces: a randomized evaluation

RESEARCH OBJECTIVES

Primary objective

To determine whether there are differences between alternating pressure overlays and alternating pressure replacement mattresses with respect to:

(a) the development of new pressure sores;

(b) healing of existing pressure sores;

(c) patient acceptability of the surfaces;

(d) the cost-effectiveness of the different pressure relieving surfaces.

Secondary objective

To investigate the specific additional impact of pressure sores on patients' well-being.

The research objectives of the PRESSURE (2000) trial clearly distinguish between the primary, although multiple in nature, and secondary objectives. They also specify the two mattress types, overlay and replacement, that are to be compared.

3.4.2   Outcome measures

The eventual design chosen will have been influenced by the outcome measures, certainly by the primary one, and each endpoint measure must be explicitly defined. The trial structure in terms of, for example, the frequency and timing of the (possibly repeated) assessments should enable the endpoint for each individual subject on the trial to be determined. In the PRESSURE (2000) trial, in those patients admitted without pressure sores skin conditions were assessed daily by the ward nursing staff using the skin classification scale stipulated within the protocol.

Example 3.5   Protocol PRESSURE (2000): Pressure relieving support surfaces: a randomized evaluation

Primary endpoint

Development of new pressure sores

For each patient, the development of a Grade 2 or above pressure sore after randomization and before discharge or trial completion due to improved mobility/activity, transfer to non-participating centre, or 60 days from randomisation. This will include

---

Example 3.5 *(Continued)*

Grade 2 sores that develop from Grade 1a and 1b skin changes that were present at randomisation. For patients with existing Grade 2 sores, only sores developing at new sites will be considered as a new pressure sore. The surface area of new pressure sores will be recorded.

Secondary endpoints

Healing of existing pressure sores

Healing will be assessed in two ways:

(a) Changes of grade;

(b) Changes in surface area. The area encompassed by the acetate film tracings will be measured by computerised planimetry using a standardized technique to minimise error.

Patient acceptability

Two endpoints will be used to assess patient satisfaction:

(a) Amongst patients who remain eligible: patient request to be moved to a 'standard' mattress because they are dissatisfied with the alternating pressure device.

(b) The recording on discharge of whether or not ('yes' or 'no') patients experienced the following: excessive noise, interference with sleep, motion sickness, difficulty moving in bed, temperature and overall comfort.

The primary endpoint for Protocol AHCC01 (1997) in patients with inoperable hepatocellular carcinoma was their survival time, which is very short in such patients. Because of the multinational nature of this trial, assessing the secondary objectives was not stipulated as mandatory for all participating centres.

Example 3.6   Protocol AHCC01 (1997): Randomised trial of tamoxifen versus placebo for the treatment of inoperable hepatocellular carcinoma

The primary endpoint is survival from the date of randomisation. In addition, although these measures will be optional, Child-Pugh score and quality of life as assessed by the EORTC QLQ-C30 will be recorded immediately prior to randomisation and monthly thereafter. Changes in these scores over time will also be compared between the patients in the 3 treatment groups.

We emphasize that whenever possible all trials should explicitly declare one, or possibly two, so-called primary outcomes which are necessarily more specific than one or two objectives, as there may be multiple outcome measures per objective. Thus, for the four-component primary objective of PRESSURE (2000), it is not clear whether each of these complex objectives is associated with a single outcome measure or involves a combination of several different measures in order to define, for example, 'acceptability of the surfaces'. We note also in AHCC01 (1997) that use of EORTC QLQ-C30 implies 15 outcomes (scales), each outcome measured at multiple time points potentially resulting in a myriad of cross-sectional or longitudinal analyses. A more specific indication as to how this information will be summarized would be a necessary addition somewhere in the protocol.

3.5   Protocol – design

The choice of statistical design will reflect the (major) hypotheses being tested and the options for design will need to be discussed thoroughly by the design team and with other colleagues as appropriate. If not already included elsewhere, a schema of the trial is a useful addition to this section.

The important features here will include the number of interventions under test and the type of design; parallel group, fixed sample size or sequential or cross-over trial. If a parallel group design, then the allocation ratio should be specified. If this implies unequal numbers in the intervention groups, then a brief rationale for this should be included if not explained elsewhere. As appropriate, the standard (or control) intervention should be clearly identified. Further, if the design is to be stratified for one or more major prognostic factors this should be indicated. In addition, reference to the degree of blinding should be made with specific mention of 'open' trial if there are no masking mechanisms included. Importantly, it should be made very clear that the trial is randomized and when assessments are to be made.

Example 3.7   Protocol PRESSURE (2000): Pressure relieving support surfaces: a randomized evaluation

Design

This has been designed as a multi-centre, randomised, controlled, open, fixed sample, parallel group trial with equal randomisation. Patients will be allocated an alternating pressure mattress overlay or an alternating pressure mattress replacement.

The main trial design will be supplemented with a qualitative study involving a purposive sample of 20–30 patients who develop pressure sores, in order to assess the impact of the pressure sores on their well-being.

Here the design is clearly laid out as, for example, comparative and randomized specifically refer to a 'fixed sample' as opposed to a 'sequential' (see Chapter 14) design. They also indicate a supporting study to assess the impact of pressure sores that may develop. It might have been easier for the reader of the protocol if acronyms were given for 'alternating pressure mattress overlay' and 'alternating pressure mattress replacement' as each have a common three word stem. Perhaps simply 'overlay' and 'replacement' with the capitals R and O could have been used.

3.6 Protocol – intervention details

3.6.1 Interventions/comparisons

The alternative interventions or therapeutic options should be carefully described within the protocol, with details of what to do if these require modification or discontinuation for an individual participant. Interventions may be terminated for many reasons ranging from refusal of individuals to remain in the trial, or a clinical team's concern that the next stage in the intervention is no longer appropriate for the patient in question. Early stopping is of particular concern in trials where the interventions could result in serious untoward consequences. In some situations such events would not be anticipated, whereas in other circumstances they may be expected and are a known consequence of the treatments under test. There will always be occasions when the unanticipated occurs, and patient safety and well-being should be paramount in clinical trials just as in normal clinical practice.

Example 3.8 Protocol PRESSURE (2000): Pressure relieving support surfaces: a randomized evaluation

Table 1 Operational mattress definitions

	Alternating pressure mattress overlay	Alternating pressure mattress replacement
Alternating Cell Height minimum	3.5 inches/8.5 cm	8 inches/19.6 cm
Alternating Cell Height maximum	5 inches/12.25 cm	5 inches/29.4 cm
Cell Cycle Time	7.5–30 minutes	7.5–30 minutes
Cell Cycle	1 in 2 or 1 in 3 or 1 in 4	1 in 2 or 1 in 3 or 1 in 4

The overlay and replacement mattresses are easy to distinguish by their maximum height, if nothing else. This requires little explanation to busy ward teams, although their physical size would no doubt bring some difficulties. Nevertheless, elderly patients may be more likely to fall from the bed with the thicker mattress, which may cause some concern. In most situations, the interventions are likely to be more complex and hence need more detailed description.

An example of part of a more complex intervention is the concurrent therapy component of the concurrent chemo-radiotherapy and adjuvant chemotherapy of protocol SQNP01 (1997) for non-metastatic patients with NPC. For those familiar with the disease and its management in this single-centre trial, the tabular format highlights the main components of what is involved.

Example 3.9   Protocol SQNP01 (1997): Standard radiotherapy versus concurrent chemo-radiotherapy followed by adjuvant chemotherapy for locally advanced (non-metastatic) nasopharyngeal cancer

Therapy	Dose	Route	Days
CisDDP	i) 25 mg/m^2/day for 4 days	IV over 6–8 hours	1–4 (week 1) 22–25 (week 4) 43–46 (week 7)
	ii) Alternatively, 30/30/40 mg/m^2/day for 3 days, if patient starts RT on a Wednesday and only for the first cycle		1–3 (week 1) 22–25 (week 4) 43–46 (week 7)
RT	200 cGy/day	Mega-voltage with or without electrons	35 daily treatments

---

The design structure of the SQOLP01 (1999) trial in patients with oral lichen planus is illustrated in Figure 2.1 while the following panel from the protocol describes the treatments given together with dose modifications, should they be required. As was the case for the mattress types, the topical treatments concerned and how they should be applied are easily expressed. Clear guidance is given for dose reduction (and possibly cessation) should 'severe side effects' occur, although none were anticipated.

Example 3.10   Protocol SQOLP01 (1999): Comparison of steroid with cyclosporine for the topical treatment of oral lichen planus

Dose and duration

Steroid (S) – Triamcinolone acetonide 0.1% in oral base (Kenalog)

This is administered by topical application by the patients themselves. Patients are instructed to apply a small dab of the paste (about ½ cm) three times daily after meals. Treatment continues for 8 weeks.

Example 3.10   *(Continued)*

Cyclosporine (C) – Sandimmun neoral solution 100 mg cyclosporine/ml

The patients are instructed to apply the cyclosporine solution to the lesions with their fingers, three times daily after meals. Treatment continues for 8 weeks.

Application of topical medication

The topical medication is applied 3 times a day – after breakfast, after lunch and before going to bed. Patients will be advised to brush their teeth, gargle and dry the area/s of the lesion/s before each application. Emphasis will be made to use a mirror to see where the medication is to be applied. Patients will be asked to note each application in a patient diary, to monitor compliance. They are instructed not to eat, drink or smoke for 30 minutes after the application.

Dose modification

Topical application of the test drugs are not expected to produce severe side effects. However, if toxicity occurs following commencement of therapy, the number of applications of either *S* or *C* should first be reduced from 3 to 2 and then from 2 to 1 per day. Should the patient continue to experience the same, or greater levels of toxicity, *S* or *C* therapy should cease.

On the other hand, in protocol ENSG05 (1990) it was well understood by all the investigators and associated clinical teams that the chemotherapy schedule was indeed highly toxic and that many complex clinical situations could arise as a consequence. However, the teams concerned with treating these children and young adults were all in specialist paediatric oncology centres and there was an established network through which the clinical teams were constantly seeking each other's advice. Effectively, a 'virtual' case review would be established as and when necessary. However, this protocol was launched and completed some time ago and the statement contained within the protocol might be inadequate for current approval processes, which demand greater precision in the specification of details and mechanisms.

Example 3.11   Protocol ENSG5 (1990): Comparison of high dose rapid schedule with conventional schedule chemotherapy for stage 4 neuroblastoma over the age of 1 year

Modification of Therapy due to Toxicity

The aim of the protocol is to administer the maximally tolerated chemotherapy in both arms. There are no specifically determined toxicity modifications, but if significant toxicity occurs, please contact study co-ordinators.

3.7   Protocol – eligibility

Depending on the disease or condition in question, the precise mechanisms for determining which individuals are eligible for the protocol will vary considerably. The protocol should delineate with care the inclusion and exclusion criteria. For example, a general clinic may see many potential patients of a particular type, who will then need to be screened to determine whether they are truly eligible for the trial. In other situations, a clinic may be more specialized in nature so that everyone coming to the clinical has been pre-screened and is likely to satisfy the requirements of the protocol. The proportion of eligible subjects will vary from trial-to-trial. In Protocol UKW3 (1992), the number of operable children with renal (Wilms') tumours was likely to be less than half of those presenting with the disease.

**Example 3.12   Protocol UKW3 (1992) – preoperative chemotherapy
                 in Wilms' tumour**

Eligibility

All patients with renal tumours should be registered with the UKCCSG by the participating centres.

The following patients are eligible for this study:

Patients over 6 months and under 16 years at the time of diagnosis. Clinical and radiological evidence of unilateral Wilms' tumour considered to be operable – see Section 7.

No detectable distant metastases.

No previous treatment for Wilms' tumour.

Although criteria for eligibility to a trial can always be phrased as 'Inclusions', it may be appropriate sometimes to highlight some aspects of non-eligibility more forcibly as 'Exclusions'. In a trial of a new oral contraceptive, rather than phrase an eligibility condition as, for example: 'Women who are neither pregnant nor breast feeding'; one might state under a distinct heading of Exclusions: 'Women who are pregnant or breast feeding'. Then the clinical team can more readily identify those individuals who are, or are not, eligible. This section of the protocol is often better presented as a series of (short) bullet points rather than as prose. Further, it is also important to list these in as useful a sequence as possible, perhaps one that closely reflects the logistics of the clinical examination process. For example, if there is an age restriction on those patients who can enter the trial, this might be at the top of such a bulleted list as age is easily determined in most circumstances; for a patient outside the permitted range, there would be little point in checking further inclusion or exclusion criteria especially if these involve an invasive examination which is not part of routine clinical practice. Also high on the list might be ascertaining whether or not all the protocol treatment options are suitable for the potential trial recruit. This saves time and inconvenience for both the would-be trial patient and the protocol team. One example is the weight limit of 140 kg in the PRESSURE (2000) protocol, although it is listed as last amongst the specified Exclusion criteria. In this case, its priority may well be entirely justified, since this will be a relatively rare occurrence among the types of patients involved.

Example 3.13   Protocol PRESSURE (2000): Pressure relieving support surfaces: a randomized evaluation

Exclusion criteria

Patients will be excluded from the study if any of the following criteria apply. They:
– have pre-existing Grade 3, 4 or 5 (Table 1*) pressure sore on admission
– have participated in this trial during a previous admission
– are an elective surgical patient with a planned post-operative admission to ICU
– are an elective surgical patient admitted more than 4 days prior to surgery
– sleep at night in a chair
– weigh > 22 stones/140 Kg (upper weight limit for overlay mattress)

*This is similar to Figure 4.1 of the next chapter of this book

---

In addition to the Exclusion Criteria, in the PRESSURE (2000) protocol there were rather complex Inclusion Criteria as three general types of patients were to be included. These patients were those having an admission to one of the designated hospital wards and were also one of the following three types: (i) acute, (ii) elective with existing pressure sore or with reduced mobility and (iii) elective with neither a pressure sore or reduced mobility.

In the past, protocols tended to be restrictive about the patients admitted to trials and would focus on good-prognosis patients. Modern trials increasingly adopt the perspective that patients are eligible provided the clinician regards all treatments as potentially suitable for the patient under consideration, and provided the clinician acknowledges that it is objectively unclear as to which treatment is preferable. Thus, fewer eligibility criteria now specify an upper age limit new, but are more likely to emphasize that the patient should be fit enough to tolerate side effects and toxicity.

3.8   Protocol – randomization

There are two aspects of the randomization process that need to be described in the protocol. One is the structural features of the design while the other is the more procedural aspects of how patients will be randomized and hence allocated to a specific intervention. However, as we will discuss in Chapter 5, there is a difficulty in that if full details of a block-based or other restricted randomization scheme are made explicit in the protocol itself, then the objectivity of the randomization process may be compromised. We advise that such details are held in a confidential memo by the statistical team which is securely stored in the trial office files and, if need be, shared with the approving authorities but not with the clinical members of the protocol team until trial recruitment is complete.

3.8.1   Design

Although Protocol AHCC01 (1997) referred in the statistical methods to a 2 : 1 : 2 randomization between placebo (P), tamoxifen 60/mg/day (TMX60) and TMX120, no reference to 'randomization in blocks' was made. Nevertheless, the eventual trial publication of Chow, Tai, Tan, *et al.* (2002) stated:

> Randomization was performed in balanced blocks of 5, stratified by center, and corresponding to P, TMX60, and TMX120 in the respective ratios of 2:1:2.

In contrast to randomized blocks, the PRESSURE (2000) trial used a minimization method (see Chapter 5) with the four factors recruiting centre, skin condition, clinical specialty of the admitting hospital ward and whether an acute or elective admission.

Just as we have suggested that it is desirable not to reveal the block size, the precise amount of randomness in a minimization method should not revealed within the protocol itself, but should be documented in a separate memo by the statistical team.

Example 3.14   Protocol PRESSURE (2000): Pressure relieving support surfaces: a randomized evaluation

Mattress allocation method

Allocation to treatment will be by minimization and with respect to the factors listed in Table 4.

Table 4   Minimisation factors

Factor	Levels	
Centre	× 8	As Section 6[a]
Skin condition	× 2	No pressure sore
		Existing pressure sore
Ward speciality	× 3	Vascular
		Orthopaedic
		Elderly care
Admission type	× 2	Acute
		Elective

[a] Section 6 of the protocol named the eight participating centres.

3.8.2 Implementation

Whatever the design features of the randomization process, the protocol also has to address the method by which this is put into operation. This may range from a relatively unsophisticated telephone call or interchange of fax messages, to a voice-based response system. Thus the SQOLP01 (1999) protocol used a telephone-based randomization system (the details of which we give below), while a more recent trial opts for a web-based system with rather strict access provisions stipulated.

Example 3.15   Protocol SQOLP01 (1999): Comparison of steroid with cyclosporine for the topical treatment of oral lichen planus

Randomisation

After the potential OLP case has been confirmed according to the eligibility criteria and informed consent has been obtained, the patient should be randomized.

To randomise a patient telephone

NMRC CLINICAL TRIALS AND EPIDEMIOLOGY RESEARCH UNIT Tel: (65) 220-1292, Fax: (65) 220-1485 Monday–Friday: 0830–1730, Saturday: 0830–1230

Some brief details will be collected for identification purposes and the caller will be informed of the result of randomisation and at the same time the patient will be assigned a protocol Trial Number.

Example 3.16   Protocol ONGOING: Details remain confidential

Randomisation will be performed centrally using the Unit's automated 24-hour telephone randomisation system. Centre and authorisation codes, provided by the Unit, will be required to access the randomisation system. Access to the 24-hour randomisation system will only be provided on receipt of Ethics and Research Development (R&D) approvals, and signed Research Sponsorship Agreements.

Patients who fulfil the eligibility criteria will be randomised on a 1 : 1 basis to receive either X or Y and will be allocated a study number. A computer-generated minimisation programme that incorporates a random element to maintain allocation concealment will be used to ensure intervention groups are well-balanced for the following patient characteristics, details of which will be required at randomization:

[*A list then follows but is omitted here*]

The method of obtaining the randomization that is chosen will depend on circum-stances, but the trend is now towards more automated systems. However, this trend does not preclude simpler (yet reliable) approaches that are likely to be more viable for trials of a modest size. The SQCP01 (2006) protocol for management of clefts of the secondary palate in infants provides for both a telephone- and a web- based randomization option.

The use of sealed envelopes by the clinical teams, as opposed to contacting a trials office remotely, is not regarded as an optimal method of allocation and should be avoided if at all possible. Whenever employed, a clear justification for this is required. In the case of the investigators concerned with SQGL02 (1999), the nature of AACG, with its sudden onset and devastating consequences, provides the rationale.

Example 3.17   Protocol SQGL02 (1999): Brimonidine as a neuroprotective agent in acute angle closure glaucoma (AACG)

Procedure for randomisation

Due to the acute condition of AACG, sealed envelopes will be used for randomising the patients who will be more likely to be presented to the clinician after office hours.

3.9   Protocol – assessment and data collection

3.9.1   Assessments

At some place in the protocol an overview of the critical stages in patient management and key points of assessment needs to be provided. At each of these assessments, whether at the first presentation of the consenting individual prior to randomization, post-randomization at visits when active treatment will be given, or for visits merely for check-up purposes, the precise details of what examinations should be made and the details to recorded (on the trial data forms) must be indicated. In SQCP01 (2006) even those children randomized to delayed surgery will have the same assessment schedule as those randomized to immediate surgery as these time points represent important milestones in, for example, their speech development.

Example 3.18   Protocol SQCP01 (2006): Comparing speech and growth outcomes between 2 different techniques and 2 different timings of surgery in the management of clefts of the secondary palate

Method

Infants will be recruited at age less than 12 months and followed up until 17 years of age. They will be assessed at age 18 months, 3, 5, 7, 9, 15 and 17 years.

The PRESSURE (2000) trial lists the sequences of assessments under different headings, and for each provides details of precisely what is required. We have indicated these headings, but only for their section 8.2.3 specified the details. The number of assessments depends on whether or not the patient has or develops pressure sores and also on how long they remain in the hospital ward. As one would expect, this contrasts markedly with SQCP01 (2006) which stipulates seven assessment times scheduled at various growth and speech development stages of the children.

Example 3.19   Protocol PRESSURE (2000): Pressure relieving support surfaces: a randomised evaluation

ASSESSMENTS AND DATA COLLECTION

Registration and randomisation

Post randomisation assessments

Immediate

Daily

Twice weekly up to 30 days and then weekly up to 60 days

The research nurse or designated ward nurse will record the following details twice weekly up to 30 days and then weekly up to 60 days or trial completion/withdrawal:

- Skin assessment (sacrum, buttocks, heels and hips) using the skin classification scale.
- Mobility/activity/friction and shear/moisture/nutrition/sensory perception scores using Braden scale.
- Mattress checklist including: manufacturer, model, model number, type of mattress and confirmation that the mattress is alternating and working correctly. If the mattress has been changed by ward staff the reason for the change will be documented.
- Seating provision including model of chair or cushion.
- Confirm continued eligibility.

Weekly up to 60 days

Patients with pressure sores

At trial completion/and or discharge

3.9.2   Data collection

In contrast to the previous protocol section, here the precise details of the items required at each assessment should be specified. The items might not be listed exhaustively but are often indicated by reference to the trial forms with a set of specimen forms bound into the protocol. In PRESSURE (2000), skilled personnel were trained about detailed aspects of the protocol, including the examination and documentation procedures. Whenever possible, it is important to complete the documentation as the examination proceeds. Investigators should not rely on making routine clinical notes and completing the trial specific forms some time later, as the notes will not have been designed for trial specific purposes and important items may be omitted. The protocol should make clear which form or forms are applicable for each assessment; numbering the different trial forms in a logical manner is important for this. We return to data collection forms in Section 3.14 below and give some examples in Chapter 4.

3.10   Protocol – statistical considerations

Before formulating this section, the principle tasks of the statistical team is to debate issues relating to the final sample size chosen for the trial with the clinical teams, and to describe the main features of the subsequent analysis once the data are in hand. Straightforward statistical methods are preferable but not always feasible. The methods should be explained in lay terms and appropriate reference material, both understandable and accessible, indicated.

3.10.1   Number of subjects

The number of subjects required will depend on the hypotheses to test, the trial design, the type of endpoint variables and whether or not characteristics of the patients themselves need to be taken into account. An important consideration when deciding the eventual trial size is whether such a size can be achieved in a reasonable time frame. In many instances, developing teams are over-optimistic in this regard. Although some details of this process are somewhat routine, in that conventional wisdom dictates that the (two-sided) test size is set minimally at 5% and the power minimally at 90%, other details such as the anticipated effect sizes should be the subject of long discussion among the protocol development team. Neither should they accept the conventional wisdom indicated without debate. Test size is discussed in Chapters 8 and 9 and power in Chapter 9.

Example 3.20   Protocol SQGLO2: Brimonidine as a neuroprotective agent in acute angle closure glaucoma (AACG)

Statistical Considerations

Trial size

For sample size determination, it is anticipated that approximately 80% of patients receiving Timolol will experience visual field loss progression at 3 months post laser PI. With the hope that the proportion of patients treated with Brimonidine having visual field loss progression will be reduced to 40%, a two-sided test, with 5% level of significance and power of 90%, would require recruitment of 30 patients in each arm (Machin, Campbell, Fayers and Pinol, 1997*).

> **Example 3.20** *(Continued)*
>
> It is anticipated that after randomisation, 10% of the AACG patients may not respond to the initial medical treatment and will require surgery instead of laser PI, and thus will not continue in the trial. After PI, it is expected that a further 10% of patients may not complete the trial and may withdraw from the study (see Withdrawal from Treatment). Taking into consideration the patients expected to fall out at each stage, we therefore require approximately 80 AACG patients (40 patients per treatment group) for the trial
>
> *Now updated as Machin, Campbell, Tan and Tan (2009).

In this example, the protocol takes note of patient losses due to a relatively large proportion expected to need surgery (rather than laser peripheral iridotomy, PI) and compensates by adjusting upwards the number of patients to recruit. They do not stipulate however, how these patients will be dealt with in the final analysis and reporting. One option is to regard all these as failures when calculating the proportions in each group with visual field loss at 3 months post PI.

An alternative design possibility would have been to randomize patients after successful PI, in order to avoid recruiting patients who will provide little information on the relative merits of Timolol and Brimonidine. However, the design team may have discussed this (as well as other options) and rejected this for good reasons.

3.10.2 Analysis

As with determining the trial size, the format of the analysis will depend on the type of questions being posed, the trial design, the type of endpoint variables and whether or not characteristics of the patients themselves need to be taken into account. If there is only a single endpoint variable concerned, then the plan for the subsequent analysis may be described rather succinctly except in circumstances where the analysis may be unusual in format. Several endpoints will be included in most situations, so that a careful description of the analytic approach for each needs to be detailed. In these circumstances, multiple statistical tests may be concerned and cognisance of that may need to be taken into account.

> **Example 3.21 Protocol SQOLP01 (1999): Comparison of steroid with cyclosporine for the topical treatment of oral lichen planus**
>
> *Analysis plan*
>
> *Primary endpoints*
>
> Analysis of the primary endpoints of response and pain at 4 weeks will be made on an intention-to-treat basis.

Example 3.21   *(Continued)*

Clinical response at 4 weeks
Comparison of the observed clinical response rates in the two treatment groups will be made using the χ^2-test for the comparison of two proportions and a 95% confidence interval for the difference reported. In addition, logistic regression analysis will verify if this comparison requires adjustment for imbalance in the baseline clinical assessment values.

Pain score 4 weeks
Comparison of mean VAS in the two treatment groups will be made using the *t-test* with the appropriate degrees of freedom and a 95% confidence interval for the difference reported. (Should the VAS scores not follow an approximate Normal distribution shape, then this analysis may be replaced by the Wilcoxon test). In addition, regression analysis will verify if this comparison requires adjustment for imbalance in the baseline VAS values and clinical assessment values.

Secondary analyses
In those patients for which the marker lesion is measurable by the grid, the mean of the total area remaining affected at 4 weeks for each treatment group will be compared using the *t-test* and 95% confidence interval for the difference reported. In addition, regression analysis will verify if this comparison requires adjustment for imbalance in the baseline target lesion area values as well as its location and other clinical assessment values.

A more detailed longitudinal analysis will make use of all the individual measures (maximum 8 per patient) using the area under the curve (AUC) as the summary statistic for each patient. The mean AUC over all patients within the treatment group is calculated and between-treatment comparisons are made using the *t-test*. A full statistical modelling approach using generalized estimating equations (GEE) is also anticipated. However, details of this latter methodology may have to wait for the final data to become available. For example, this methodology would not be appropriate if all patients achieved complete response by week 4 and all subsequent target areas were then zero.

In a similar way, the complete VAS for burning sensation profile will be summarized.

Adverse events
It is not anticipated that a formal statistical analysis comparing the adverse event rates between groups will be conducted. However, full details will be presented and their presence (if any) used to contextualize any observed treatment differences.

Additional analysis
Clinical response at week 8 will also be associated with initial (week 4) response to give an indication of the duration of response and to report any recurrences.

This example details a number of analyses. Some of the repetition of essentially the same wording with respect to 'adjustment for baseline' values could have been avoided, as protocols should use succinct phrasing wherever possible. If the number of words can be reduced without loss of clarity, then this reduces the eventual size of the document, facilitates the proof reading and eases the job of the approving authorities.

3.10.3 Interim analysis

As part of the monitoring of the progress of trials, while recruitment is still ongoing many protocols include interim looks at the trial data. These may be reviewed by an independent Data Monitoring Committee (DMC). However, interim looks and DMCs may be irrelevant if innocuous interventions are being compared, if the trial is small-sized or if recruitment is rapidly completed. They should therefore be part of the protocol only when truly essential. One example of the remit given to a DMC is:

Example 3.22   Protocol ONGOING: Precise details remain confidential

An independent Data and Safety Monitoring Board (DSMB) has been established, through which the ongoing trial will be monitored and patient safety protected.
   The goals of the monitoring trial are to:

- help minimise the avoidable risks associated with a subject's participation;

- advise if the trial can be stopped early if there is evidence that a reliable conclusion can be drawn from the data accumulated to date;

- advise if the trial can be stopped early if there is accumulating evidence that it is unlikely to be able to answer the primary research question (trial 'futility');

- identify if the trial is underpowered and, if so, recommend an adjusted sample size.

In certain cases, special situations arise in which aspects of the trial need to be formally monitored. The investigators concerned with UKW3 (1992) wished to be reassured that the outcome had not been compromised by their decision to withhold radiation therapy from renal cancer patients who had been classified stage II, when it had previously been accepted practice to give it. As a consequence, they set out the details of appropriate interim analyses to facilitate the monitoring process.

Example 3.23   Protocol UKW3 (1992) – Preoperative chemotherapy in Wilms' tumour

Stopping rule for stage II patients

A specific stopping rule for stage II patients is included because the data from UKW2, in which these patients did not have radiotherapy, are not yet sufficiently mature to be assured of the safety of this reduction in therapy.

A total of about 70 stage II patients may be expected to be accrued. Their progress should be assessed for local relapse after every 14 patients, at one-year post diagnosis and subsequently at yearly intervals.

Local relapses should be fewer than 5 out of the first 14, 7 out of the first 28, 9 of the first 42, 11 of the first 56 and 13 out of the first 70. More relapses than these numbers will be an indication to resume the use of local radiation therapy.

The panel provides very specific guidance with respect to monitoring for local relapses, which the responsible trials office would have to incorporate into their routine systems. However, we stress that the clinical participants, especially those recruiting or treating patients, must not know the results of interim analyses as this may compromise their ability to continue with the trial.

3.11   Protocol – ethical issues

There are both general and specific issues that should be addressed in this section. These may range from ensuring that the protocol conforms to the internationally agreed Helsinki agreement and more recent Good Clinical Practice (GCP) regulations that have been adopted by many countries, through to obtaining local approval of the informed consent processes being applied.

3.11.1   General

There are internationally agreed standards under which clinical trials are conducted and these are encapsulated in GCP (ICH E6 (R1) 1996). There are also the more specific requirements, perhaps national as well as local, that must be adhered to. The precise details of these will vary with: the geographical location of the trial; whether single or multicentre in design; local, national or international; the type of interventions under study; and the intended target participation groups.

Note that the statement of Example 3.24 acknowledges that the trial development team are aware of potential updates of the Declaration of Helsinki. This will also be the case for any of the other regulatory and other codes of practice that may pertain, as these too are continually being revised to meet new circumstances. However, if regulatory changes are made, they may or may not be invoked for ongoing protocols that have current approval status.

> **Example 3.24 Protocol PRESSURE (2000): Pressure relieving support surfaces: a randomised evaluation**
>
> The study will be conducted in accordance with the Declaration of Helsinki in its latest form. The study will be submitted to and approved by a Regional Multicentre Research Ethics Committee (MREC) and the local Research Ethics Committee (LREC) of each participating centre prior to entering patients into the study. The NYCTRU will provide the LREC with a copy of the final protocol, patient information sheets and consent forms.
>
> The conduct of the trial will be monitored by a Trial Steering Committee consisting of an independent Chair and two independent advisors as well as the project team (Appendix H).

A major ethical requirement is to ensure that the potential participants in trials understand that participation is voluntary. They are free to withdraw their consent at any time and, in doing so, will not in any way compromise the future treatment that they will receive.

> **Example 3.25 Protocol SQGL02 (1999): Brimonidine as a neuroprotective agent in acute angle closure glaucoma**
>
> The right of the patient to refuse to participate without giving reasons must be respected. After the patient has entered the trial, the clinician must remain free to give alternative treatment to that specified in the protocol at any stage if he/she feels it to be in the patient's best interest. However, the reasons for doing so should be recorded and the patient will undergo an early termination visit for the purpose of follow-up and data analysis. Similarly, the patient must remain free to withdraw at any time from protocol treatment without giving reasons and without prejudicing his/her further treatment.

3.11.2 Informed consent

Before any trial can take place individual subjects have to be identified, and formal processes for their consent will have to be instituted. The precise details will depend on the type of trial contemplated, for example, whether it involves an invasive procedure, concerns primary intervention or has therapeutic intent. If it involves participants such as children, the very elderly, healthy volunteers, the terminally sick or women of fertile age, then this may raise particular issues (e.g. requiring proxy consent or reassurance that the trial drugs will not compromise subsequent fertility).

Importantly, the patient should understand that no-one knows in advance which therapy will be allocated, and that they should be willing to accept the allocation whatever that may be. If they are unwilling, they should decline to be recruited to the trial.

The ideal is that each patient or volunteer gives fully informed and written consent. However, departures from this will be appropriate in specific circumstances. For example, such departures may concern patients that are unconscious at admission to hospital, patients with hand burns that are so severe that they affect their ability to provide their signature, very young children or those mentally compromised. In these cases, a proxy may consent for them or, in the case of those with severe burns, witnessed verbal consent may be substituted.

Example 3.26   Protocol SQGL02 (1999): Brimonidine as a neuroprotective agent in acute angle closure glaucoma

Before entering patients on the study, clinicians must ensure that the protocol has received clearance from their local Ethics Committees. The patient's consent to participate in this trial should be obtained after full explanation has been given of the treatment options, including the conventional and generally accepted methods of treatment, and the manner of treatment allocation.

All the possible options on trial should be explained impartially to the patients concerned. This explanation must be provided before the randomization is effected as knowledge of the assignment may influence the way in which an investigator explains the alternatives. A key feature of the informed consent process is to explain the randomization procedure and to emphasize that participation is completely voluntary and that the patients can withdraw from the protocol at any time.

An example of a combined consent form and information sheet as used in protocol SQOLP01 (1999) describing a randomized trial in patients with oral lichen planus is shown later in Section 3.15. This form satisfied the local regulations and was used concurrently with verbal explanation as required.

3.12   Protocol – organizational structure

The contents of this section will depend to a large extent on the size and complexity of the design of the trial. For example, protocol SQCP01 (2000) involves only two clinical centres but different countries with very different first languages, and which are geographically quite distant. Because this trial is organizationally complex, and involves many clinical disciplines, specialists in surgery, orthodontics and speech therapy must be recruited. Since each specialist would have a role to play over a very long period of 17 or more years, keeping track of the individuals concerned is a major challenge. However, each centre has experience of dealing with such complex issues. The protocol runs with four named craniofacial/plastic surgeons, four orthodontic coordinators, three speech therapy coordinators and two research coordinators. At the statistical centre, a medical statistician and clinical project coordinator are designated to the trial. The protocol contains full names, addresses, telephone and fax numbers and e-mail addresses of these individuals. As may be imagined, the actual individuals concerned will no doubt change as the trial progresses forward in time.

In contrast, the SQNP01 (1997) was conducted within a single centre and three clinical coordinators were identified, one representing radiation oncology and the other two medical oncology. The conduct of this trial reflected the day-to-day management practices of the centre concerned. At the statistical centre, a medical statistician was designated and the shared nurse coordinator had responsibilities for the trial within the cancer centre recruiting the patients and the trial office. The protocol contains full names, addresses, telephone and fax numbers and e-mail addresses of these individuals.

In situations where the demands of a trial are somewhere between these two extremes, the protocol development team must ensure that the necessary organizational structure is in place and each component thereof knows of their individual responsibilities. One important role of the trial office is to maintain this functionality throughout the life of the trial.

If at all possible, the protocol should fit as closely as possible within the confines of current practice in the centres concerned, with the proviso that the aims of the trial are not compromised by doing so. This facilitates acceptance of what is new in the protocol from the local team and should help with the smooth running of the trial and hopefully maximize recruitment rates.

3.13   Protocol – publication policy

There will inevitably be several members of the team in most clinical trial groups, and should the trial be multicentre then the collaborating team may be numerous. It is useful to have stipulated a clear policy as to who the authors of the final publication will be and in what order they appear on the title page. Provided this is clear and agreed by all concerned (including latecomers to the trial once it is ongoing), this need not be included in the protocol itself. If a large number of collaborators are involved, then it may be more sensible to publish under a group name with a full list of the investigators included as an appendix to the report. Again, this should have been discussed and agreed from the outset.

Example 3.27   Protocol SQOLP01: Comparison of steroid with cyclosporine for the topical treatment of oral lichen planus

Publication Policy

The results from the different centres will be analysed together and published as soon as possible. Individual clinicians must not publish data concerning their patients which are directly relevant to the questions posed by the trial until the main report is published. This report will be published under the name of the *Asian Lichen Planus Collaborative Study Group* listing all members of the group and any others contributing patients.

In the event, the editor of the journal publishing the eventual report of Poon, Goh, Kim, *et al.* (2006) refused publication under a group name, although a full list of contributors was permitted. Collaborative groups may therefore need to verify the policy of the target journals before stipulating a formal policy in this respect.

The panel also underlines an important requirement that individual groups should 'not publish data concerning their patients which are directly relevant to the questions posed by the trial until the main report is published'. An important reason for this is that such publication can only (at best) refer to a subgroup of the total number of patients recruited to the trial. This number is consequently less than that stipulated by the design and so any analysis will be under-powered for the hypotheses under test. For example, such an analysis may report 'no statistical difference' in situations where the whole trial data may conclude the opposite. Premature publication by an individual group may also jeopardize the acceptance for publication of a report of the full trial.

3.14   Protocol – trial forms

Since recording the patient data is integral to successful trial conduct, inclusion of the trial forms into the protocol itself is often desirable even when they are quite simple in structure. We give some examples in Chapter 4.

The forms should be developed in parallel with the protocol, and may (depending on local regulations) have to be submitted for approval with the trial protocol itself in any event. The number, structure and complexity of the forms required for a trial will be very trial specific. As a minimum, there will be forms containing subject-specific information relevant to the registration and randomization process including the intervention assigned, those encapsulating eligibility and other baseline characteristics of those recruited, as well as a form for the endpoint assessment. In almost all circumstances there will be many more than this; most trials will include special forms for recording details of, for example, any surgical procedures undertaken or adverse events should they arise.

In general terms, the forms for the clinical trial should focus on essential detail that is necessary to answer the question(s) posed by the design and should not be cluttered with irrelevant items. This focus keeps the clinical teams aware of the key issues and reduces the time spent recording inessential details. Consequently, there are likely to be fewer errors. The completed form also becomes easier to check if there are fewer items, reducing the data management processes. This also speeds up the checking process so that any problems remaining can be fed back to the clinical teams more rapidly (which again reduces the workload at the clinical centre). The briefer the forms, and indeed the simpler the trial procedures, the easier it becomes for collaborators and the more rapidly they are likely to recruit the patients required. This must be balanced against the need to ensure that the forms *do* contain all the necessary information that will be required for the analysis. However, the experience of many groups indicates that most trials collect far too much information that is never analyzed or reported.

Forms may need to include patient management details, such as the date of the next follow-up visit, or to confirm if an action has been taken such as the despatch of a laboratory specimen or the completion by the patient of a quality-of-life questionnaire.

It is best if these are kept to a minimum and located in a distinct part of the form (perhaps the last items). This implies that when the forms are received for processing at the trials office, these items can easily be distinguished from variables that must be included in the trial database.

3.15 Protocol – appendices

As often as not, a protocol will almost certainly have to contain Appendices. For example, in many cancer clinical trials, toxicity is a major concern so that the criteria for reporting adverse events as recommended by the National Cancer Institute (2003) will often be reproduced.

APPENDIX IV   *SQOLP01*

PATIENT INFORMATION AND CONSENT FORM - SAMPLE

A Randomised Controlled Trial To Compare Steroid With Cyclocporine
For The Topical Treatment Of Oral Lichen Planus

Patient's Name   : _____

NRIC/Passport No : _____

Dr. _____ has fully explained to me the nature and purpose of the study in which I have been asked to participate. I have been told that I will be allocated at random to one of two treatments: I will need to apply either a steroid paste or a cyclosporine solution, to the affected areas as instructed. I have also been told that both medications can cause a transient burning sensation immediately after application. Cyclosporine, when administered orally or by intravenous route, has been known to cause increased hair growth, tremor, fatigue, gum swelling, gastrointestinal disturbances, high blood pressure, impaired liver and kidney function. However, I am told that when applied topically it is generally safe with little or no side effects. Moreover I understand that I will be monitored by blood tests to ensure that I am not suffering from any side effects of the medication. I understand that I am free to withdraw my consent and discontinue treatment at any time without prejudice to me or effect on my medical care.

I have been given the opportunity to ask questions concerning the drugs and the study. I have also consented to photographs to be taken of the affected areas at the start and end of the study. I understand that blood tests will be required prior to, during and at the end of treatment with cyclosporine.

I freely agree to participate in this study.

Patient's signature   : _____   Date : _____

Name in block letters   : _____

Doctor's signature   : _____   Date : _____

Name in block letters   : _____

Witness's signature   : _____   Date : _____

Name in block letters   : _____

Figure 3.2 Combined consent form and information sheet utilized in a multinational clinical trial in patients with symptomatic oral lichen planus (SQOLP01, 1999)

Appendix E   **Assent by Relative Consent Form - Pressure Trial**
(Form to be on headed paper)

Centre Number:
Study Number:
Patient Identification Number : Initials and Date of Birth

CONSENT FORM –ASSENT BY RELATIVE
Title of Project: Pressure Trial – A study of Mattresses for Pressure Sore Prevention and Treatment

Name of Researcher: Research Nurse

Please initial box

1. I confirm that I have read and understand the information sheet dated ....

    (version ....) for the above study and have had the opportunity to ask questions.

2. I understand that my relative's participation is voluntary and that I am free to withdraw them at any time,

    without giving any reason, without their medical care or legal rights being affected.

3. I understand that sections of any of my relative's medical notes may be looked at by responsible

    individuals from [NHS Trust] or from regulatory authorities where it is relevant to them
    taking part in research. I give permission for these individuals to have access to my relative's
    records.

4. I agree for my relative to take part in the above study.

Name of Patient	Name of Next of Kin	Relationship to Patient
	Date	Signature of Next of Kin
Research Nurse	Date	Signature

1 for patient; 1 for researcher; 1 to be kept with hospital notes
Version 2 August 2000

Figure 3.3   Section of a consent form designed to obtain assent from a relative (with permission from protocol PRESSURE, 2000)

As informed consent is such a critical process, reviewing committees will almost certainly wish to see the proposed patient information sheets and the consent forms to be used. We have included two examples here. Figure 3.2 from protocol SQOLP01 (1999) combines information and consent, while the form from PRESSURE (2000) of Figure 3.3 is designed for proxy consent, in this case by a relative who gives assent.

3.16   Regulatory requirements

3.16.1   Protocol amendments

Although great care should be taken in preparing the trial protocol, once the approved trial has opened for patient recruitment and is in progress, unforeseen circumstances may impact on the contents of the protocol. Such circumstances could range from the relatively trivial to the very serious. At one extreme, perhaps the packaging of a study drug is changed by the supplying pharmaceutical company without change to the potency or any significant aspects. At the opposite extreme, perhaps unanticipated and serious reactions in some patients occur, raising concerns about whether the trial medication is safe and consequently impacting on whether or not the trial should continue as originally planned. The consequences of the latter might, for example, either result in restricting the trial entry criteria by identifying those who are likely to be vulnerable and making them no longer eligible, or reducing the dose should the anticipated reaction occur. Both of these represent an important change to the protocol. The protocol would then have to go through a reapproval process. In contrast, the major change in packaging may only require informing the authorities of this fact. In this instance, if the protocol has to be changed for any other major reasons, then it would of course be prudent to make these minor changes at the same time.

Since protocol modifications are not infrequent, it is wise to keep the protocol as concise as possible: exclude all irrelevant detail; ensure main sections start on new pages; ensure page breaks do not break paragraphs (perhaps not important in the background but may be critical if describing details of an intervention); and number sections, tables and figures in such a way as to minimize the need for future renumbering or repagination of the protocol. Without such precautions, there can be severe consequences if any additions or modifications happen to occur in sections from the early pages of the protocol.

3.17   Guidelines

As we have indicated, GCP (ICH E6 R1 1996) will dictate in full the items that are mandatory for such a protocol. It is particularly important, and especially for clinical trials seeking formal registration of a new product, that investigators check local, national and even international requirements for what has to be included in the protocol itself. The definition given by Day (2007) and slightly amended in our Glossary includes the phrase 'important details', so it is imperative to check the current status of exactly what these are. For example, the ICH E6 R1 (1996, section 6) specifies for protocols sections on: direct access to source data/documents; quality control and quality assurance; data handling and record keeping; and financing and insurance which we do not include in Figure 3.1. ICH E6 R1 (1996, section 8) also includes: before the clinical phase of the trial commences; during the conduct of the trial; and after completion or termination of the trial. Although these sections may be more appropriate to trials for products seeking regulatory approval, they contain many items pertinent in a wider context. As we indicated in Chapter 1, a useful booklet is provided by the Institute of Clinical Research (2008) while Day (2007, appendix 1) lists eighteen ICH 'Efficacy' Guidelines. The latest updates of these can be obtained from the ICH official web site: www.ich.org

3.18   Protocols

AHCC01 (1997) Randomised trial of tamoxifen versus placebo for the treatment of inoperable hepatocellular carcinoma, Clinical Trials and Epidemiology Research Unit, Singapore.

ENSG5 (1990) Comparison of high dose rapid schedule with conventional schedule chemotherapy for stage 4 neuroblastoma over the age of one year. UKCCSG, Leicester, UK.

PRESSURE (2000) Pressure relieving support surfaces: a randomised evaluation. University of York, York and Northern and Yorkshire Clinical Trials Research Unit, Leeds, UK.

SQCP01 (2006) A randomised controlled trial comparing speech and growth outcomes between 2 different techniques and 2 different timings of surgery in the management of clefts of the secondary palate. KK Women's & Children Hospital, Singapore and Chang Gung Memorial Hospital, Taiwan.

SQGL02 (1999) Brimonidine as a neuroprotective agent in acute angle closure glaucoma. Clinical Trials and Epidemiology Research Unit, Singapore.

SQNP01 (1997) Standard radiotherapy versus concurrent chemo-radiotherapy followed by adjuvant chemotherapy for locally advanced (non-metastatic) nasopharyngeal cancer. National Medical Research Council, Singapore.

SQOLP01 (1999) A randomised controlled trial to compare steroid with cyclosporine for the topical treatment of oral lichen planus. Clinical Trials and Epidemiology Research Unit, Singapore.

UKW3 (1992) Trial of preoperative chemotherapy in biopsy proven Wilms' tumour versus immediate nephrectomy. UKCCSG, Leicester, UK.

CHAPTER 4

Measurement and Data Capture

This chapter emphasizes the essential requirement of all trials of taking appropriate measurements. The importance of clearly defining those measurements needed to determine the endpoint(s) and how, when and by whom they are to be taken is highlighted. The particular value of masked assessment is stressed as is the necessity to make the observations with sufficient precision, avoiding bias and recording the data in a suitable medium. Examples of different endpoint types and problems associated with their determination are described. We stress that it is vital that all forms on which to record data are clear, easy to complete and readily transferable to the trial database.

4.1 Introduction

In every clinical trial information will have to be collected on the subjects included, their progress through the trial and the determined endpoint(s). An important aspect of trial design is therefore the choice of measurements to be made and observations to be recorded. Once identified, details of how and when these measures are to be taken also have to be specified. Some of these measures may be straightforward to determine, such as gender or date of birth, while others may require detailed and invasive clinical examination followed by laboratory assessments before they can be finally determined. Once available, the data collected need to be recorded in a logical and consistent manner. We will assume for didactic reasons that these will be on previously designed paper forms which will be entered onto a computerized and interactive trials database.

At an early stage, it is important to distinguish between several classes of data. There are those that are collected for purely descriptive purposes, to characterize the patients in the trial, and which are either weakly or not at all related to the outcome measures. There are those that are known to be prognostic for outcome and possibly used when allocating subjects to the interventions for stratification purposes or may need to be taken account of when assessing the trial results. There are those which may be important for purely management purposes, for example, the date a pathology specimen was centrally reviewed (in this case the review panel outcome may be vitally important but not the date the review was undertaken). There may be data related to the safety of the patient, so the date of the unanticipated event plus details of the event

Randomized Clinical Trials: Design, Practice and Reporting David Machin and Peter M Fayers
© 2010 John Wiley & Sons, Ltd

itself will both be essential. Most important of all will be the intervention allocated at randomization and the endpoint variable(s) which are to be used for the comparison of these interventions. Crucial to these are the date of randomization and the date(s) at which the endpoint variables are determined.

It should be emphasized that the class for a specific variable, for example age of the participants, is not determined by the nature of the variable itself but rather by its use in the trial synthesis. Age may therefore be purely descriptive in the context of one clinical trial in which it has no prognostic influence whereas it will be prognostic in another where age is known to be an important determinant of outcome. For example, in children with neuroblastoma, age is a very strong predictor for ultimate event-free survival time.

The data collected in a clinical trial setting should not contain extraneous information which is not essential for progressing the trial or for its final synthesis. There is often a temptation to record 'interesting' information collected as an aside from the main thrust of the trial. The relevance of any such information must be weighed by the design team before the trial commences and, if not vital, it should not be recorded.

In addition, in the data checking and verification processes the relative importance of variables should always be appreciated. For example, if the date of the pathology review examination is missing yet the outcome recorded, sensible judgement has to be made as to whether the actual date needs to be found. Even if not considered important for trial analysis purposes, the missing date may be a requirement of Good Clinical Practice (GCP) and perhaps those responsible for the omission have to be contacted to provide it.

As we have indicated, it is also important to distinguish variables which are to be used for descriptive and which for more analytical purposes. Comparisons between the intervention groups of the former will only be descriptive (as the variables themselves are) in nature while one (or more) analytical variables will be necessary to determine the endpoint. Others will be used statistically in the comparisons made between the intervention groups. Further, although we will give some details of analysis in Chapter 8 and some general expressions for trial size in Chapter 9, these will have to be selected and/or modified depending on the type of measure involved (defined in Section 4.5).

4.2   Measures and endpoints

In general, a typical trial report will include information on a range of different variables including demographic, prognostic and endpoint. An illustration of some of these is given in Table 4.1, extracted from a report of a randomized trial comparing two treatments for elderly patients with multiple myeloma conducted by Palumbo, Bringhen, Caravita, *et al.* (2006).

In this example, it was not immediately clear whether stage, creatinine clearance, age or β_2-microglobulin were merely descriptive or of prognostic importance. However, the *Statistical analysis* section of the published report indicates that age, as perhaps expected in an elderly group of patients, and β_2-microglobulin are indeed regarded as

Table 4.1 Selected baseline, adverse event and endpoint results from a trial in patients with multiple myeloma treated by melphalan and prednisone (MP) alone or with the addition of thalidomide (MPT) (selected from Palumbo, Bringhen, Caravita, *et al.*, 2006, Table 1)

		MPT	MP		
Number of patients		129	126		
Baseline					
Stage	IIA	50 (39%)	49 (39%)		
	IIB	4 (3%)	3 (2%)		
	IIIA	64 (50%)	62(490%)		
	IIIB	11 (8%)	12 (10%)		
Creatinine (mg/L)	Median	8	8		
	Range	5.6–102	6–68		
Prognostic					
Age (years)	Median	72	72		
	<65	4 (3%)	3 (2%)		
	65–70	49 (38%)	51 (41%)		
	71–75	44 (34%)	37 (29%)		
	76–80	26 (20%)	28 (22%)		
	>80	6 (5%)	7 (6%)		
β_2-microglobulin	Median	3.7	3.7		
(mg/L)	Range	0.36–40.0	0.2–37.5		
	≤3.5	53 (41%)	53 (42%)		
	>3.5	63 (49%)	57 (45%)		
	Missing	13 (10%)	16 (13%)		
Adverse events				*p*-value	
Haematological	Grade 3-4	29 (22%)	32 (25%)	0.59	
Gastrointestinal	Grade 3-4	8 (6%)	1 (1%)	0.036	
Endpoints				Difference	95% *CI*
Response at 6 months	Complete or partial	98 (76.0%)	60 (47.6%)	28.3%	16.5 to 39.1%
				HR	95% *CI*
Event-free survival	Progression, relapse or death	42 (33%)	62 (49%)	0.51	0.35 to 0.75 *p*-value = 0.0006
	2-year	54%	27%		

prognostic factors. In this case, it is unfortunate that the latter measure is missing for 11% (29/255) of patients. When it is known that a particular variable is to be used for prognostic purposes, in that it will be taken account of in the intervention comparison, it is vital that the investigators are made fully aware of its importance. The management team must do all they can to ensure the variable is recorded. In practice, this is not as easy as it may sound, particularly in the context of this trial which involved 54 different centres spread over a wide geographical area.

Table 4.1 also includes the Grade 3-4 events of two of the ten toxicity types reported. Each of these, although not the primary outcome variables, is compared statistically in the format shown.

Endpoint variables included response, as defined by the European Group for Blood and Transplantation/International Bone Marrow Transplant Registry and described by Bladé, Samson, Reece, *et al.* (1998), and event-free survival (EFS), defined as the time from diagnosis until the date of progression, relapse or death from any cause or the date the patient was last known to be in remission. Response rates were compared and the hazard ratio (HR) calculated, with both endpoint summaries suggesting an advantage to melphalan, prednisone and thalidomide (MPT).

4.2.1   Assessments

In any trial, some of the assessments made may focus on aspects of the day-to-day care of the patient while others may focus more on those measures that are necessary to determine the trial endpoint(s) for each subject. It is important that these assessments are well defined and that endpoints are unambiguously defined so that they can be determined for each patient recruited. There will rarely be difficulty in determining or recording a date of death but, even with everyday clinical measures, it may be necessary to define carefully how these are to be taken. For example, a physician may only need to know for diagnostic purposes if the temperature of the patient is elevated, say beyond 37.5°C. In a trial, it may be important to record the temperature precisely as the trial may be investigating the change in these values following a specific intervention. In addition, it will be important to specify meticulously how (and when) the measure is to be taken, for example, the particular type of thermometer and whether by oral, aural or rectal readings.

If blood, urine or other samples are to be taken, once again 'when' will need to be specified but the exact manner in which these are to be handled, stored and tested will also need to be detailed. If specimens are analyzed by a reference laboratory then their procedures also have to satisfy the trial requirements.

It is particularly important to assess carefully the implications of those measures which initiate a course of action if their value attains a certain level. For example, in a clinical trial of patients with burns, one may state that: 'patients are expected to be discharged from the hospital burns unit once their wound has healed to a *sufficient degree*'. However, how is 'sufficient degree' defined so that it can be unambiguously applied to each patient? In practice, it may also depend more on the support available 'at home' for the patient once discharged than on the intrinsic condition of the burn wounds themselves. In which case, this definition may lead to early discharge of the patient, preventing assessment of the wound for the purposes of a clinical trial to determine the relative efficacy of alternative treatments for wound healing.

4.2.2   Endpoints

The protocol for every trial should detail the assessments to be made, and it is essential to identify and carefully define which of the measures taken are indeed regarded as the major endpoints of the trial. The trial question and hence the objectives determine the endpoint or endpoints to be used in assessing the results. Such endpoints clearly depend on the type of trial concerned. They may range from birth weight of babies born in their own home, standard clinical measures such as systolic blood pressure (SBP) or diastolic blood pressure (DBP), the response rate in elderly patients with multiple myeloma or the date of death of patients with cystic fibrosis to relatively complex measures defined as any of: cardiac death, Q-wave myocardial infarction or target lesion revascularization for patients with single de novo lesions in the native coronary artery trial of Example 1.12 by Erbel, Di Mario, Bartunek, *et al.* (2007). Another complex measure is that of Comi, Pulizzi, Rovaris, *et al.* (2008) who, in the report of their trial of the effect of laquinimod on MRI-monitored disease activity in patients with relapsing–remitting multiple sclerosis, state:

> Their primary efficacy outcome measure was the cumulative number of GdE lesion on week 24, 28, 32 and 36 scans (i.e. the last four scans).

The endpoints will have been considered when determining trial size, and they will be the main focus for the final evaluation and reporting. They therefore need to be assessed with particular care and objectivity.

In some trials, a single measure may be sufficient to determine the endpoint in each subject, for example, the patient response at 6 months post diagnosis in Table 4.1, from which the response rate in each intervention group can be calculated and compared. Essentially, those who respond are termed successes and those that do not failures. In this case, the groups will be summarized by the proportion of responders and compared using the difference between these or the odds ratio (OR). Alternatively, again as in Table 4.1, the endpoint event-free survival (EFS) may be defined as the time from randomization to the allocated intervention until the time when the patient experiences the first of the components of what is termed the event. In this situation, repeated assessments over the time of disease status (to detect progression or relapse should they occur) and their current survival status (to record death should it occur) will be made. The endpoint 'event' is the first of these to occur. The interval between the date of randomization and the date of recording the 'event' is the endpoint (survival) measure of interest. In this case, the groups will be summarized by, for example, their median survival times and compared using the HR.

4.2.2.1 Multiple measures

In certain circumstances, there may be more than one possible location for the measure within a subject. For example, in determining whether or not a subject has glaucoma, the left, the right or both eyes may have the disease. Similarly, there may be evidence of failure in the left, the right or both kidneys. An extreme example is whether or not each individual tooth is affected by caries. In many cases, these may be reduced to a single primary measure such as the number of teeth with caries or an ordered categorical variable, indicating that 0, 1 or 2 eyes have evidence of glaucoma.

On the other hand, it may be advantageous to keep these aspects as distinct. For example, if we were concerned with the resolution of eczema, in 'moderate-to-severe' cases there is likely to be more than a single (distinct) site concerned. Monitoring the progress of all sites may lead to a more efficient statistical design, but at the analysis stage it is essential to make allowance for multiple sites being monitored within each patient; it would be a mistake to regard these observations as independent as they come from the same individual.

4.2.2.2 Repeated measures

In a trial taking repeated temperature assessments, these may be recorded in order to determine a single outcome – 'time for the temperature to drop below 37.5°C'. In other situations, all the successive values of body temperature themselves may be utilized in making the formal comparisons. If the number of observations made on each subject is the same, and the intervals between successive observations is also the same for all subjects, then the analysis may be relatively straightforward. On the other hand, if the number of observations recorded varies, if the intervals between successive observations differ from patient to patient or if there is occasional missing data, then the summary and analysis of such data may be quite complex. Such complexities of data structure often arise in trials using a health-related quality of life (HRQoL) outcome in patients who, for example, are terminally ill.

4.2.2.3 Several endpoints

If there are many endpoints defined, the multiplicity of comparisons made at the analysis stage may result in spurious statistical significance. This is a major concern if endpoints for HRQoL and health economic evaluations are additional to the already defined, more clinical, endpoints. For design purposes it is essential to focus on the major (and few) key endpoints and it is these same endpoints that provide the focus at the analysis and interpretation stages once the trial is complete. Any secondary level endpoints should be identified as such at the planning stage and the manner in which they are to be summarized and reported indicated. Often less formal statistical comparisons will be made of these than for the principle endpoints.

4.2.2.4 Objective criteria

In certain situations, there is not necessarily an obvious measure to take. For example, although one may regard tumour shrinkage as a desirable property of a cytotoxic drug when given to a patient, it is not immediately apparent how this is to be measured. If every tumour were of a regular spherical shape, the direction in which it is measured is irrelevant. Furthermore the diameter, a single dimension, would lead immediately to the volume of the tumour. However, no real tumour will comply with this ideal geometrical configuration. This has led to measures such as the product of the two largest (perpendicular) diameters to describe the initial tumour, and a specified reduction in this product to indicate response following treatment.

The response measure, used as a secondary endpoint in the context of the trial conducted by Palumbo, Bringhen, Caravita, *et al.* (2006), is detailed by Bladé, Samson, Reece, *et al.* (1998). This offers the necessary guidelines to encourage uniform reporting of outcomes in the context of blood and marrow transplants. Investigators of trials may argue about the fine details (and no doubt these guidelines will need revision in time), but they would be foolish to ignore these recommendations when conducting and subsequently reporting their trial.

If there are justifiable reasons why other criteria should be used or the recommendations cannot be followed for whatever reason, then these should be reviewed by the investigating team before the trial commences. There is no point in conducting a trial using measures not acceptable to other groups, including the referees for the clinical journals, as the results will not be seriously considered. The best option is to follow the guidelines for the primary endpoint as close as possible, and using the other measures for secondary reporting and contrasting the two in any discussion.

Example 4.1   (Subjective) skin assessment to identify bed sores

Brown, McElvenny, Nixon, *et al.* (2000) described some practical issues arising during the conduct of a trial of post-operative pressure sore prevention. They indicated that the inclusion of the category for reactive hyperaemia in the skin assessment scale of Figure 4.1, which they were using as the endpoint measure, was subject to some debate. The committee monitoring the trial became concerned that a subjective endpoint measure had been chosen.

Grade	Description of skin	
0	No discolouration	
1	Redness to skin – blanching occurs	Reactive
2a	Redness to skin – non-blanching area	hyperaemia
2b	Superficial damage to epidermis broken or blistered	
3	Ulceration progressed through the dermis	
4	Ulceration extends into subcutaneous fat	
5	Necrosis penetrates the deep fascia and extends to muscle	

Figure 4.1 Skin assessment scale used for the grading of pressure sores (after Table II of Brown, McElvenny, Nixon, *et al.*, 2000)

In some situations, less than optimal measures may have to be used. For example, although precise levels of pain experienced may be measured in the laboratory, such methodology may not be practical when levels need to be assessed at the bedside. A practical method of recording pain, or variables such as strength of feeling, is by means of a visual analogue score (VAS). A patient completes a visual analogue scale by making a mark on either a horizontal or vertical line to provide, once measured, an apparently continuous scale. It is useful for measuring aspects that may be difficult to put into words when used to assess pain. In this context, VAS behaves as if it is approximately linear (in the sense that a score of say 4 is twice as much pain as a score of 2). Also, because individuals tend to be internally consistent, VAS is good when measuring change within individuals; it is not so good when comparing across individuals.

Example 4.2   VAS – Pain assessment

In their clinical trial of patients with severe burns, Ang, Lee, Gan, *et al.* (2003) (see also Example 2.2) used a VAS to assess the pain levels experienced by the patients. It may be that the patients make such assessments themselves, marking their pain level experienced on a 10 cm VAS. However, when designing the trial, the authors anticipated that some patients would have burns which affect their ability to write easily, some would be too ill to complete the task and others would have language and literacy issues. As a consequence, for this trial, the responsible nurse used when necessary the less-refined verbal alternative administered in a local language or dialect familiar to the patient, and assisted the patient to mark the scale when needed. It is clear from this example that the trial design team were aware of the difficulties involved and made adjustment to their methodology in light of these.

4.2.2.5   Surrogates

There are times when it may be that the true endpoint of interest in a clinical trial is difficult to assess for some reason. In this case, a 'surrogate' may be sought. For example, when investigating the possibilities of a novel marker for prognosis it may be tempting to use EFS as a surrogate endpoint for the overall survival (OS) time of patients with the cancer concerned. An advantage is that, for many cancers, relapse occurs well before death and so the evaluation of the marker can occur earlier than would be the case if OS was to be observed.

A formal definition of a surrogate endpoint is: a biomarker (or other indicator) which is intended to substitute for a clinical endpoint and predict its behaviour. If a surrogate is to be used, then there is a real need to ensure that it is an appropriate surrogate for the endpoint of concern. In most phase III trials, the relevant endpoint will be an outcome that patients also perceive as being relevant, despite some investigators being keen to establish efficacy by using more sensitive biomarkers that can detect changes not reflected by clinically important benefits.

A distinction is made between 'intermediate' and 'surrogate' endpoints by Parmar, Barthel, Sydes, *et al.* (2008), who discuss design options for speeding up the evaluation of new agents in cancer. Such an outcome (they use disease-free survival or DFS) is required to be related to the primary outcome measure but does not have to be a true surrogate. It can also be argued that the time experiencing DFS is highly relevant to patients, as time spent in progression when the disease has returned is more likely to be associated with suffering.

4.2.3   Patient-reported outcomes

Most randomized controlled trials are primarily intended to address simple endpoint questions of efficacy. However, sometimes other objectives such as HRQoL or other patient-reported outcomes (PROs) are particularly important, for example, in patients with chronic conditions who are terminally ill. The measurement process is then by means of one or more HRQoL instruments, perhaps applied repeatedly over time.

If a single domain of a single HRQoL instrument (measured at one time point) is to be used for intervention comparison purposes, then no new principles are required either for trial design purposes or analysis. On the other hand, and more usually, there may be several aspects of the instrument that need to be compared between interventions; these features will usually be assessed over time. This is further complicated by often unequal numbers of assessments available from each patient, caused by missing assessments that may, for example, arise for reasons related to a patients' changing health status (termed informative missing) or may be missing at random.

Although design principles may not change to a large degree, logistical problems are magnified. These include determining the schedule for when the HRQoL assessments are to be made and by whom (the patient or the carer – this may also be instrument specific), checking that all questions are completed and dealing with the large quantity of data at the analytical and reporting stages.

These instruments are developed according to a very strict series of procedures and, in general, cannot be quickly developed just for the trial in hand. Fayers and Machin (2007) discuss these and other features of HRQoL data in some detail.

4.2.4   Economic evaluation

As with HRQoL, there may be circumstances where an economic evaluation of the relative merits of two treatments is required. This may be particularly important if non-inferiority is to be demonstrated or if the relative costs associated with particular modalities are difficult to quantify. If we were to design a trial primarily to compare costs associated with different treatments, we would follow the basic ideas of blinding and randomization and then record subsequent costs incurred by the patient and the health provider. A very careful protocol would be necessary to define which costs are being considered, so that these are measured consistently for all patients.

However, most trials are aimed primarily at assessing efficacy and a limitation of investigating costs in a clinical trial is that the schedule (and frequency) of visits by the patient to the physician may be very different to what they would be in routine clinical practice. Typically patients are monitored more frequently and more intensely in a trial setting than in routine clinical practice. The costs recorded in a clinical trial may well be different (probably greater) than in clinical practice.

4.3   Making the observations

4.3.1   Masking

4.3.1.1   Open

The majority of measures taken on the subjects recruited to a clinical trial will be made with full knowledge of the specific intervention allocated. However, in a trial, basic demographic variables should be recorded and eligibility verified before the subject is randomized and so these assessments cannot be biased in any way by the eventual allocation. At this stage, the clinical assessor and corresponding participant are essentially masked. Such masking is very important if a baseline (before randomization) measure of the endpoint is to be used in the evaluation. For example, in the trial conducted by Meggitt, Gray and Reynolds (2006), the SASSAD score of the patients with eczema was determined before randomization and this was repeated at 12 weeks post-randomization. The actual endpoint was defined as the percentage reduction in 12-week score from that recorded at baseline. However, the desirable feature of masked assessment no longer automatically applies once the intervention has been allocated (unless specific steps are taken). Indeed, in this case, all assessments were made by a single investigator who was 'trained and skilled in measuring SASSAD'; assessment may be regarded as 'open' alternatively termed or 'non-blinded' or 'non-masked' in this case.

In studies that assess HRQoL, it is usual to ensure that a baseline assessment of HRQoL is made before randomization. This value can then be used when analyzing subsequent measurements of HRQoL after the intervention is applied.

Prognostic or predictive variables are also generally assessed before randomization, while the allocation is therefore still unknown. This is particularly important if these variables are to be used when analyzing the trial outcome measures.

4.3.1.2   *Extent of blinding or masking*

Any investigator deeply involved in a trial, of whatever type, will be aware of the hypothesis under investigation and knowledge of the intervention allocated to a patient may influence (however unintentionally) the recordings made. Consequently, if at all possible, assessments should be made by persons, or by some means, with no knowledge of which intervention has been given. The observers are then 'blinded' or 'masked' in these circumstances.

If the recipient of the intervention can be blinded to the actual intervention given, for example, in a randomized placebo controlled trial, then whoever makes the assessment cannot be informed of the specific treatment by the subject. If both the participant and the observer are blind to the therapy, then the measure is taken in a 'double-blind' way.

The concept of blinding can be extended. For example, in circumstances where the patient and the nurse who takes the blood sample are blind to the intervention, it is desirable that the blood sample taken and sent to the laboratory should be assessed there blindly. Once at the laboratory for analysis, there may be no difficulty in ensuring the objectivity of the measurement process. However, if the sample is labelled in such a way as to indicate the values of the measures anticipated, then the measurement and recording process could be biased in some way.

The ideal situation is that the subject, the treating physician and nurses and the assessors are blinded to an appropriate extent. The extent of the blinding depends on the particular trial concerned; a desirable goal is to make assessment double-blind as far as is possible. For a laboratory sample, this may be easy to achieve while in other circumstances (such as taking the pain assessment in patients with burns) this may not be possible. In this latter case the treatments (two types of dressing) cannot be disguised from the patient or the nurse. However, swabs taken from the wounds to assess the presence of methicillin-resistant *staphylococcus aureus* (MRSA) can be sent to the laboratory for testing in a coded format to ensure objectivity at that level.

We stated in Chapter 1, as indicated in Figure 1.1, that the double-blind randomized controlled trial when suitably designed, conducted and reported, provides the strongest evidence possible when comparing alternative interventions. We emphasize again that, wherever possible, this type of trial should be implemented.

4.3.2 Which observer

In certain circumstances, it has to be made very clear who can be classified as an appropriate observer. If a HRQoL instrument is being used to assess patients, there are clear guidelines that have been published by Young, de Haes, Curran, *et al.* (1999) for the clinical trials of the European Organization for the Research and Treatment of Cancer (EORTC). These describe the manner and circumstances in which the instruments should be completed. For example, the patient is the 'observer' and is responsible for completing the instrument, in this case the EORTC QLQ-C30. Only in specific circumstances can a proxy be used for this purpose, and this must be recorded in the trial documentation.

4.3.3 Precision

A question often arises as to whether a continuous variable should or should not be recorded as a categorical variable for data recording and so future analysis. For example, is it better to classify the variable SBP into three separate categories say, hypo-tension (SBP <110 mmHg), normo-tension and hyper-tension (SBP > 160 mmHg) rather than bother with individual blood pressures? The difficulty here is that, despite the relative ease of coding, the categories are not so intuitive if recorded as 1, 2 or 3 (say) and this may increase the risk of a recording error. In addition, we are stuck with the definitions used at the onset. Should they be required to change (perhaps others have used a different categorization), then comparisons between trials will be difficult. It is usually best to record the variable as precisely as is reasonable. Most individuals know their date of birth and the experimenter knows the date of the enquiry so that age can be easily computed at a later stage. It could then be rounded to convenient categories by creating a new variable within the database, while preserving the two dates indicated. However, when describing an endpoint variable, the direct use of the continuous variables themselves (rather than the same variable categorized) is statistically more efficient. The effect of grouping data is that the design will require more subjects than would be the case if the endpoint variable is utilized in its continuous form.

If the underlying variable is continuous, then the precision with which this is to be measured has to be defined. This will depend on the 'ruler' available for the measuring process. Furthermore, it is common to find that observers show digit preference, such that the last digit of a particular measure tends to be rounded to a 'nice' number such as 0 or 5. A useful solution is to ask all observers to record results to 1 decimal place further than the trial actually requires, and leave the rounding process until the computational stage.

4.4   Baseline measures

There are three kinds of baseline assessments that might be made and recorded on a pre-treatment pre-randomization form. These are the baseline (descriptive) characteristics of the patients themselves, together with relevant prognostic factors. In addition, there may be a single baseline assessment of what are one or more endpoint(s) variables. Such a single baseline assessment is very frequently made for any outcome that is subsequently assessed on a repeated basis post-randomization. An example is the baseline assessment of HRQoL, using a patient-completed pre-randomization HRQoL questionnaire. Finally, a run-in series of outcome measurements may be made up to and including the baseline (immediately prior to randomization) measure.

As in the example of a pre-randomization assessment of SASSAD score in patients with eczema (Example 1.2), the variable which is identified as the endpoint of concern may be assessed not just at a single time point but on several occasions. In some circumstances, there may be several pre- and several post-randomization series of measures. The first series represents a run-in period prior to the active intervention, which is quite common in the cross-over trials described in Chapter 12. This information may be used to assess the degree of within-subject variation or more usually to define a (pre-intervention) level which can be compared to that achieved post-intervention. There are several ways in which the baseline measures may be used as indicators of the effect of the intervention: one is to calculate the percentage change as used by Meggitt, Gary and Reynolds (2006) and illustrated in Figure 1.1, and a second is to use the difference in scores for each patient as the unit for analysis. However, these methods are statistically sub-optimal and not to be recommended. The most efficient approach is to use the baseline measure to extend the model of Equation (2.1) and use a regression approach to analysis.

4.5   Types of measures

4.5.1   Qualitative data

4.5.1.1   Nominal or unordered categorical

Nominal data are data that can be named; they are not measured but simply counted. They often consist of binary or dichotomous 'Yes' or 'No' type observations, for example: Dead or Alive; Male or Female; diagnosis of Sudden Acute Respiratory Symptoms (SARS). The corresponding summary statistic is the proportion (or percentage) of subjects within each category, often denoted by p, and the difference between two groups is p_2-p_1. In this list, Dead or Alive may well be an endpoint variable while the others may be mainly descriptive of the type of patients to be recruited or characteristics of such patients. Nominal data can have more than two categories, for example: country of origin, ethnicity or blood group (O, A, B or AB). All of these are unlikely endpoints. In clinical trials binary endpoints are frequent, as in success/failure and cured/not cured, but unordered categorical data is rarely an endpoint. However, this latter type quite frequently arises, for example when histology (cell type) is used as a prognostic indicator for survival in cancer trials, or marital status as an indicator for time to discharge from hospital in trials concerned with care of the elderly.

4.5.1.2 *Ordered categorical or ranked*

If there are more than two categories it may be possible to order them in some way. For example, after treatment patients may be either improved, the same or worse; the diagnosis of SARS may be suspected, probable or definite, while Meggitt, Gary and Reynolds (2006) categorize patients at the end of the treatment period as: worse, no change, slight improvement, moderate improvement, striking improvement or complete resolution of the eczema. In this situation, it may be appropriate to assign ranks and to utilize these as numerical values. Similarly, patients with rheumatoid arthritis may be asked to order their preference for four dressing aids. Although numbers representing the order may be assigned to each aid, they cannot necessarily be treated as numerical values.

4.5.2 Numerical or quantitative data

Numerical discrete data are counts such as 0, 1, 2 and so on, for example the number of episodes of migraine in a patient in a fixed period (say, 4 weeks) following the start of treatment. Depending on the distribution of the resulting trial data, the mean and standard deviation (SD) or the median and range might be used as summary statistics. In practice, a reduction in migraine episodes may be regarded as a partial success, but the percentage of patients with zero episodes might be considered as the most important single summary statistic.

   In contrast, numerical continuous data are measurements that can, in theory at least, take any value within a given range. Examples are the descriptive variable maternal age (year) at conception, and the endpoint variable the weight of the baby (gm) at delivery. The corresponding summary statistics are often the mean $\bar{x}$ and the corresponding standard deviations.

4.5.3 Time-to-event

In many disease areas, survival is the most obvious and most important endpoint. This has led to event-time analysis being loosely called survival analysis. In general, a time-to-event measure is the interval from randomization until the patient experiences a particular event, for example, the healing of their burn wound in the trial of Example 2.2. The key follow-up information will be that which is necessary to determine healing. For example, burn healing might be defined as the final closing of all damaged body surface area. To establish this, the burn area may have to be monitored on a daily basis to determine exactly when this final closure is achieved.

For those patients for whom healing occurs, the time from randomization to healing can be determined in days by calculating the difference t between the date of complete healing and the date of randomization. For those whose wound does not heal with medical treatment, but have to be excised or amputated, the time from randomization to this can be assessed but not their healing time. Their data are therefore classified as *censored* at the time of operation. The time from the date of randomization to this censoring date is termed $T+$. The eventual analysis of these 'survival' times involves either a t or a $T+$ for every patient.

4.5.4 Practice

The eventual design of the trial depends crucially (among other things) on the type of endpoint(s) chosen, as this determines the type of statistical analysis that will be required. This then influences the number of subjects that need to be recruited to the planned trial. The required trial size (discussed in Chapter 9) will usually be far greater for binary data compared to continuous, and so it is better for example to assess pain on a NRS-11 scale 0 to 10 rather than merely classify patients into pain requiring (or not requiring) analgesia. Similarly, analysis of survival data may require observations of many events (for example deaths) per group, so that trials involving hundreds of patients are often necessary. Thus a vital component when considering design options is the type of measurement(s) to be undertaken.

4.6 Data recording

4.6.1 Forms

The number and types of forms required will depend on the particular features of the trial, but will usually consist of those to record: (i) baseline information concerned with patient description and eligibility; (ii) details necessary for the randomization to be affected and the actual allocation made; (iii) information while the intervention is being administered; (iv) details following the completion of the intervention; and (v) endpoint information. Forms are generally of two broad types – single and repeated. A single form may be that describing the 'On trial' characteristics of the participants while a repeated form may be completed on several occasions during the active treatment period, perhaps every 4 weeks after each course of treatment is completed. In this latter case, it is clear that a key component of this information is the date upon which the patient is examined in order to furnish the specific entries into the form. Recording the respective endpoint variables for the trial is clearly vital; but so too is other information such as that concerned with determining the eligibility criteria.

Forms are used to record factual information such as a subject's age, blood pressure or treatment group. They are commonly used in clinical trials to follow a patient's progress and are often completed by the investigating team. For forms, the main requirement is that each form is clearly laid out and all investigators are familiar with it. However, even if all the data are to be collected by a single investigator, it is still important that this is carried out in a clear and unambiguous way. Clarity of the experimental record with respect to the observations taken is becoming a routine feature of GCP that must be adhered to in clinical trials for regulatory purposes (ICH, 1996). Variables, and their names, will need to be included in a database for further analysis. Forms therefore provide a good *aide memoire* for a trial conducted some time ago.

4.6.1.1 Layout

A balance between a cramped and cluttered layout and a well spaced but bulky series of forms has to be made. Each form should contain clear instructions about how to respond to each question. Sometimes more than one response to a question is possible. It is important to make clear whether a single answer is expected, or whether multiple responses are acceptable. It may seem obvious, but questions and possible answers should be kept together; one should avoid having the question on one page and the response options on another.

Example 4.3   Form design – Randomized trial in colorectal cancer

Tang, Eu, Tai, *et al.* (2001) used the (single) form of Figure 4.2 to register and randomize patients to their clinical trial of open *versus* laparoscopically assisted colectomy in patients with colorectal cancer. The top sections of the form were completed by the clinical team before contacting the central randomization office who, once details were confirmed, provided the trial number (unique for each patient) and the allocated treatment.

4.6.1.2 Closed question

Closed questions can be answered by completing the answer in a relevant box or, as for the patient eligibility questions in Figure 4.2, ticking confirmation. When constructing responses to closed questions it is important to provide a clear range of replies. For example, this form provides a single box for the (closed) response to the question concerning 'Allocated Treatment'; with permitted responses of either 'O' or 'L' corresponding to Open or Laparoscopically assisted surgery. If this form were administered on a computer screen, entry procedures could be designed to prevent anything but an O or an L being entered in this space. This cannot be achieved using a paper-based system.

NMRC
National Medical Research Council

CLASICC TRIAL

REGISTRATION FORM

Conventional versus Laparoscopic-Assisted Surgery In Colorectal Cancer

Please return this form, by post or fax, immediately after randomisation to:
NMRC Clinical Trials Office, #02-14 Bowyer Block, Singapore General Hospital, Singapore 169608. Fax: 225 3584

A patient sticker with the following information may be used for this section if available:

Patient Name_____   NRIC_____

Hospital_____   Surgeon_____

Date of birth: ☐☐ ☐☐ ☐☐
              day   month   year

Eligibility: Please tick the boxes to confirm the following:

☐ The patient has colorectal cancer.

☐ Informed consent, according to local practice, has been obtained.

What is the patient's WHO performance status? ☐
(for definition see overleaf)

NOW TELEPHONE THE NMRC CLINICAL TRIALS OFFICE (222-7632) TO RANDOMISE
(Monday-Friday 8.30am-5.30pm, Saturday 8.30am-12.30pm)

Trial number ☐☐☐☐   Date of randomisation: ☐☐ ☐☐ ☐☐
                                                    day   month   year

Allocated Treatment: ☐   O. Open Surgery   L. Laparoscopic-Assisted Surgery

Signed_____   Date_____

Figure 4.2   Registration form (utilized in the trial by Tang, Eu, Tai, *et al.*, 2001)

Forms may require a numerical answer so that in the (single) form of Figure 4.3, also part of the trial documentation of Tang, Eu, Tai, *et al.* (2001), the responses are 1 (for No) or 2 (for Yes) to, for example, the question: 'Abdominal bladder injury?' However, it is not totally clear how the boxes for 'Trocar injury' and 'Instrumentation injury' are to be completed. Alternatively, we might either have to tick boxes or circle the appropriate Yes/No response, since asking the clinical teams to translate into numerical codes may be inviting errors. It is easier for data entry staff to focus on the coding and, if scanning/optical reading forms are used, it is also common to use ticks in boxes.

On the form of Figure 4.3, the closed question for 'Volume of blood lost' provides the unit of measure (here ml) required and an appropriate number of boxes for the

NMRC
National Medical Research Council

CLASICC TRIAL   SURGERY AND INTRA-
OPERATIVE COMPLICATIONS FORM

Conventional versus Laparoscopic-Assisted Surgery In Colorectal Cancer
Please return this form, following surgery, to:
NMRC Clinical Trials Office, #02-14 Bowyer Block, Singapore General Hospital, Singapore 169608
A patient sticker with the following information may be used for this section if available:

Patient's name_____   Trial Number □□□□

Hospital_____   NRIC_____

To be completed by the surgeon as soon after surgery as possible

Has a liver ultrasound been carried out less than 30 days before planned surgery?   □   1. No
                                                                                        2. Yes

If yes, date of liver ultrasound: □□ □□ □□   Liver metastases present?   □   1. No
                                 day month year   2. Yes

Did the patient experience any of the following complications during operation?

Gross faecal contamination   □ 1. No   Ureteric injury   □ 1. No
                                2. Yes   2. Yes

Duodenal injury   □ 1. No   Cardiac insufficiency/dysrhythmia □ 1. No
                                2. Yes   2. Yes

Pulmonary insufficiency   □ 1. No   Surgical emphysema   □ 1. No
(from pneumoperitoneum)   2. Yes   2. Yes

Significant intra-operative haemorrhage   □ 1. No
(ie haemorrhage that requires   2. Yes   Volume of blood lost: □□□□ ml
peri-operative transfusion)

Other complications (please specify)   □ 1. No
                                          2. Yes   Specify_____
                                                    Trocar injury   Instrumentation injury

Abdominal bladder injury   □ 1. No   □   □
                              2. Yes

Small bowel injury   □ 1. No   □   □
                              2. Yes

Major vessel injury   □ 1. No   □   □
                              2. Yes
                                                    PLEASE TURN OVER

Figure 4.3 Surgical complications form (utilized in the trial by Tang, Eu, Tai, *et al.*, 2001)

numerical value to be recorded. If the variable to be recorded requires two decimal places, then a style of boxes on the form such as: □□□●□□ is a convenient reminder of this.

Dates will also frequently need to be recorded and, because of the different conventions used and the transition over the millennium, it is important to indicate clearly the requisite (boxes) for day, month and year by, for example: dd.mm.yyyy. In the example shown, however, the layout with respect to day-month-year is not of this format and would also have been better located closer to the boxes concerned.

SQNP01: FOLLOW FORM

Radiotherapy versus Concurrent Chemoradiotherapy Followed by Adjuvant Chemotherapy for Locally Advanced Non-Metastatic Nasopharyngeal Cancer

Patients are required to be followed-up 4 monthly for the first year, 6 monthly for 2 years, and annually thereafter, the anniversary date of follow-up being taken as the last day of RT.
Please return this form immediately after each follow-up to:
NMRC Clinical Trials & Epidemiology Research Unit, 10 College Road, Singapore 169851. Fax: (65) 220 1485

Patient Name__________ Trial Number ☐☐☐☐

NRIC__________ Hospital__________

Section A

Date of follow-up ☐☐ ☐☐ ☐☐ (day month year)

Clinical Status (please circle)

1. Primary NED / Static / Equivocal / Prog*
2. Neck NED / Static / Equivocal / Prog*
3. Distant NED / Static / Equivocal / Prog*

*If progression please fill in a relapse form

Section B (To be filled at *4 months and annually after the last date of RT)

*CT Scan PNS ☐☐ ☐☐ ☐☐ (day month year) Chest X-ray ☐☐ ☐☐ ☐☐ (day month year)

Findings__________ Findings__________

Section C

If the patient has died:

Date of death ☐☐ ☐☐ ☐☐ (day month year)

Cause (please tick):

Disease related ☐ Treatment related ☐ Other ☐ Specify:__________

Signed__________ Date__________

Figure 4.4 Follow-up form (utilized in the trial by Wee, Tan, Tai, *et al.*, 2005)

4.6.1.3 Open questions

In an open question, respondents are asked to reply in their own words. For example, in Figure 4.2 there is also an open question: 'Other complications (please specify)'. In the context of this clinical trial, any responses would be expected to be of only one or two words from the investigating team, whereas in other circumstances a full description may be expected. In clinical trials, open questions are generally best avoided or at least kept to a minimum.

4.6.1.4 Follow-up or repeat forms

Any form that has to be completed a repeated number of times for every subject within the trial by the clinical team, perhaps over an extended period and at infrequent intervals, needs special attention given to its design. Not only must the form clearly demark the variables it wishes to capture, it must also make very clear the precise scheduling of the patient examinations that are necessary. The follow-up form of Figure 4.4, used by Wee, Tan, Tai, *et al.* (2005) in their trial which recruited patients with nasopharyngeal cancer, specifies in the header the following instructions:

> 'Patients are required to be followed-up 4 monthly for the first year, 6 monthly for 2 years, and annually thereafter, the anniversary date of follow-up being the last date of RT.'

Although this schedule is clear, there is nevertheless some ambiguity over what is intended with respect to the schedule for the two components of Section B.

4.6.2 Questionnaires

In certain situations, a form may be in the format of a questionnaire to be completed by a subject recruited to the trial. The distinction between a form and a questionnaire is that a questionnaire is an 'instrument' for measuring something, perhaps the HRQoL status of a patient, whereas a form is merely for recording information. In practice, a questionnaire may contain form-like questions such as asking for gender and date of birth as well as the instrument variables themselves. A questionnaire may try to measure personal attributes such as attitudes, emotional states and levels of pain or HRQoL, and is often completed by the individual concerned.

A convenient distinction between forms and questionnaires (although not always the case) is that the investigating team completes forms while the trial participants themselves complete questionnaires. Forms can therefore be short and snappy, and any ambiguities explained among the investigators. In contrast, questionnaires need to be very carefully designed, particularly with respect to the choice of language they use to pose the questions. For example, technical jargon such as that scattered throughout the form of Figure 4.3, is suitable for a specialist surgical team but should be avoided in a questionnaire.

4.6.2.1 Layout

As with forms, the questionnaire should have clear instructions and an attractive layout. It helps to reduce bulk by copying on both sides of a page, and reducing the size of text to fit a booklet format. However, if those completing the questionnaire are older with poorer eyesight or have to complete the form in an area of inadequate lighting, it may be necessary to increase the size of the text.

It is generally believed that shorter questionnaires achieve better response rates than longer questionnaires. However, it is difficult to define what is 'too long'. Piloting of what is intended before the trial commences may be advisable to determine how burdensome the questionnaire is likely to be for the trial patients.

For questionnaires, particularly those trying to evaluate something such as HRQoL, the pragmatic advice is do not design your own but (if possible) use an already established questionnaire. There are a number of reasons for this apparently negative advice. First, use of a standardized format means that results should be comparable between trials. Secondly, it is a difficult and time-consuming process to obtain a satisfactory questionnaire. Thirdly, standard instruments will usually have been developed by a team that includes researchers from a wide range of disciplines, and the instrument should have undergone a lengthy validation process.

Example 4.4   Question layout – Sexual function

Jensen, Klee, Thranov and Groenvold (2004) developed a questionnaire to evaluate sexual function in women following treatment for a gynaecological malignancy as a preliminary to a longitudinal study. Part of their final questionnaire, developed from the process described by Sprangers, Cull and Groenvold (1998), is reproduced in Figure 4.5.

Physical contact and sexual relations can be an important part of many people's lives. People who suffer from illnesses involving their pelvic region may experience changes in their sex life.

The questions below refer to this. The information you provide will remain strictly confidential.

Please answer all the questions yourself by circling the number that best applies to you

4.8.1 Part 1

During the past month:

		Not at all	A little	Quite a bit	Very much
1.	Have you been interested in close physical contact (a kiss and a cuddle)?	1	2	3	4
2.	Have you had close physical contact with your family and close friends?	1	2	3	4
3.	Have you had any interest in sexual relations?	1	2	3	4
		Yes	No		
4.	Do you have a partner? (If not, please continue to **question 8**)	1	2		

Figure 4.5 Part of the questionnaire (SVQ) for self-assessment of sexual function and vaginal changes after gynaecological cancer (from Jensen, Klee, Thranov and Groenvold, 2004)

4.6.2.2 Closed questions

Although a questionnaire may include some form-like closed questions such as asking for the gender of the participant, there may be others eliciting less directly measurable information.

> ### Example 4.5 Closed question – Sexual function after gynaecological cancer
>
> Jensen, Klee, Thranov and Groenvold (2004) ask on the SVQ: 'Have you had close physical contact with your family and close friends?' For this closed question the response options are: (i) not at all; (ii) a little; (iii) quite a bit; and (iv) very much. However, a trial participant may object to being forced into a particular category, and simply not answer the question as a result. Patients may be very elderly, and it is not clear how someone should respond if all their family and close friends are deceased.

One type of closed question, termed a Likert scale, is one that makes a statement and then asks how much the respondent agrees or disagrees.

> ### Example 4.6 Likert scale – SF-36
>
> Ware, Snow, Kosinski and Gandek (1993) use Likert-type questions in the general health section of their SF-36 quality of life instrument, as shown in Figure 4.5.

11. How TRUE or FALSE is each of the following statements for you?	Definitely true	Mostly true	Don't know	Mostly false	Definitely false
a) I seem to get sick a little easier than other people	○	○	○	○	○
b) I am as healthy as anybody I know	○	○	○	○	○
c) I expect my health to get worse	○	○	○	○	○
d) My health is excellent	○	○	○	○	○

Figure 4.6 General health question from SF-36 (after Ware, Snow, Kosinski and Gandek, 1993)

This format has the advantage of being compact, and there is little chance of people filling in the wrong bubble. However, some questionnaires avoid central categories such as the 'don't know' of the SF-36.

4.6.2.3 Open questions

Just as with forms, open questions pose difficulties. Although they allow the participant to freely explain their response, this brings problems of data summary for the investigating team if the number of participants is more than a few.

4.6.2.4   *Response bias*

One problem associated with asking questions is to know the extent to which the answers provided by respondents are valid. In other words, do their responses truly reflect their experiences or attitudes? If they do not, what are the causes of bias? Response bias can arise in any one of a variety of ways. One such bias is 'social desirability bias' and this arises particularly regarding questions on sensitive topics. It occurs when respondents conceal their true behaviour or attitudes and instead give an answer that shows them in a good light, or is perceived to be socially acceptable. Respondents' answers may also differ according to who is asking the questions. 'Recall bias' affects questions involving recall of past events or behaviour, and may result in omission of information or misplacing an event in time. Biases can also arise from the respondent mishearing or misunderstanding the question or accompanying instructions.

Questionnaire wording and design can also induce response bias, for example through question sequencing effects (where the response given to a particular question differs according to the placement of that question relative to others) and the labelling and ordering of response categories.

4.7   Technical notes

Just as we utilized Equation (2.1) to represent the model underlying structure for design purposes, we can describe aspects of the measurement process in a similar way. We can therefore express the measurement we are making as follows:

$$x = X + \eta. \tag{4.1}$$

Here X is the true value of the reading that we are about to take on a trial participant. After we have made the measurement we record the value of X as x. We know that with most measurements made we will not record the true value but one that we hope is close enough to this for our purposes. We also hope, over the series of measurements we take (one from each participant), that the residual (or our error) $\eta = x - X$ of Equation (4.1) will average out to be small. In which case, any errors we make will have little impact on the final conclusions.

However, if there is something systematically wrong with what we are doing (possibly something of which we are quite unaware), then the model we are concerned with becomes

$$x = B + X + \eta. \tag{4.2}$$

This second model implies that even if we average out η to be close to zero over the course of the trial, we are left with a consistent difference B between the true value X and that actually recorded, x. This is termed the bias. When taking measurements, we should therefore try from the outset to ensure that $B = 0$.

4.8   Guidelines

ICH E6 (R1) (1996) *Guideline for Good Clinical Practice*, EMEA, Canary Wharf, London, www.emea.eu.int

Of particular relevance to this chapter is Section 5.5 Trial management, data handling and record keeping.

ICH E9 (1998) *Statistical Principles for Clinical Trials*, CPMP/ICH/363/96. EMEA, Canary Wharf, London, www.emea.eu.int. Section 2.2.6 comments on the use of surrogate variables.

ICH E9 Expert Working Group (1999) Statistical principles for clinical trials: ICH harmonised tripartite guideline, *Statistics in Medicine*, **18**, 1905–1942.

Young, T., de Haes, J.C.J.M. Curran, D., Fayers, P.M. and Bradberg, Y. (1999) *Guidelines for Assessing Quality of Life in EORTC Trials*, EORTC, Brussels.

This is a very practical guide, the value of which is not confined to those conducting clinical trials in cancer.

CHAPTER 5

Randomization

The method of choosing which intervention is assigned to a particular subject is an essential feature for maximizing the useful information from a clinical trial. We provide the rationale for why a random element to the choice is desirable and describe how random numbers may be used to assist the implementation of this. We describe how interventions may be grouped into randomized blocks such that the balance between interventions set by the design is maintained. Situations where there may be a gain in recruiting a larger number of patients to one group than the other are introduced.

5.1   Introduction

As we indicated in Chapter 2, in any clinical trial where we intervene in the natural course of events, a decision has to be taken as to which intervention is given to which individual. In general, whatever the basic design, we should choose the structure of the design to answer the question posed and then make the choice of intervention as 'random' as possible.

A key reason to randomize the alternative interventions to patients is to ensure that the particular one chosen for the individual patient is not predictable. The trial protocol will therefore describe in careful detail the type of subjects eligible for the trial and, for example, the options under test. Only subjects for whom *all* stated options are appropriate should be entered into the trial. If one option appears to be less favourable for the subject being assessed for recruitment, then he or she should not be entered into the trial. Consequently, if the intervention intended is known in advance (or at least thought to be predictable) by the assessment team, then this knowledge may (perhaps subconsciously) influence the clinical team's decision to include (or exclude) that individual from the trial. They might not judge fairly whether each of the options is appropriate for the particular subject under consideration.

Any prior knowledge or accurate predictions of the intervention to be given may also compromise the informed consent procedure. The knowledge may lead the assessment team to a more selective description of the options available within the trial setting, thereby focusing more on the intervention that they anticipate will be given and less on the alternative(s). It is therefore important that the investigating team are not aware of

Randomized Clinical Trials: Design, Practice and Reporting   David Machin and Peter M Fayers
© 2010 John Wiley & Sons, Ltd

the treatment to be allocated to the next patient. If the particular treatment intended is known by the patient, for example it may be the 'new' therapy, a patient may more readily volunteer because *that* is the treatment that he or she will receive. On the other hand, if the patient knows they are to get the standard or traditional approach, they may be more reluctant to consent to enter the trial.

Any prior knowledge of the allocation by either the clinical team or the patient can therefore introduce selection bias into the allocation process, and this will lead to unreliable conclusions with regard to relative efficacy of the interventions under test.

In the randomized-controlled trial, patients are usually recruited one at a time and over a prolonged period. Allocation to the intervention therefore has to be made sequentially in time and then usually patient-by-patient. The randomization process will therefore continue until the last patient is recruited. There will be very few occasions in which all the patients are recruited to a clinical trial on the same day. As we have indicated in Section 2.7, it is best if the randomization is made as soon as possible after consent has been given and that the intervention commences immediately thereafter.

5.2 Rationale

In essence, the purpose of any experiment is to estimate the parameters of a model analogous to that of Equation (2.1). We therefore collect data with this purpose in mind. We would like to believe that the estimates we obtain in some way reflect the 'true' or population parameter values. In principle, if we repeated the trial many times, then we would anticipate that these estimates would form a distribution that is centred on the true parameter value. If this is the case, our method of estimation is without *bias*. For example, in a clinical trial comparing two treatments, the parameter β_1 (termed β_{Treat} in some later sections of the book) corresponds to the true difference (if any) in efficacy between them, and the object of the trial is to obtain an unbiased estimate of this. While taking due account of the trial design, the method of selecting which of the eligible patients are to be included in the trial does not effect this, but the way in which those patients who are recruited to the trial are then allocated to a particular treatment does. Of fundamental importance here is the random allocation of subjects to the alternative treatments. Randomization also provides a sound basis for testing the underlying null hypothesis, effectively testing if $\beta_1 = 0$ in Equation (2.1) by use of a statistical test of significance.

5.3 Mechanics

5.3.1 Simple randomization

5.3.1.1 *Random numbers*

The simplest randomization device is a coin which, if tossed, will land with a particular face upward with probability one-half. Repeated tossing generates a sequence of heads

(H) and tails (T), such as *HHTHH TTHTH*. These can be converted to a binary sequence 00100 11001 by replacing *H* by 0 and *T* by 1. An alternative method would be to roll a six-sided dice and allocate a 0 for faces 1, 2 and 3 and a 1 for faces 4, 5 and 6.

To avoid using a dice for randomization, we can produce a computer-generated table of random numbers such as Table T5, based on the principle of throwing a ten-sided dice with faces marked 0–9 on many occasions. Each digit is equally likely to appear and cannot be predicted from any combination of other digits. The random numbers in Table T5 are grouped in columns of 5 digits for ease of reading. The table is used by first choosing a point of entry haphazardly, perhaps with a pin, but deciding in advance of this the direction of movement along the rows or down the columns. Suppose the pin chooses the entry in the 10th row and 13th column and it had been decided to move along the rows, then the first 10 digits give the sequence 534 55425 67 (highlighted in bold in Table T5).

5.3.1.2 Simple random allocation

The first step in the simplest form of randomization for a parallel two-group comparative trial is to assign one intervention *A* to even numbers (0 is regarded as even) and the other intervention *B* to odd. The next step is to use the random numbers of Table T5 to generate the sequence of length $N = 2m$, where *m* is the planned number of recruits for each group. For example, using the previously chosen sequence 53455 42567 generates *BBA BBAAB AB*. The first 10 recruits involved will therefore receive the interventions in this order, and once this is complete 4 individuals will have received *A* and 6 individuals *B*.

We cannot emphasize too strongly that the person producing such a randomization list MUST conceal the list from the participating clinicians. Each allocation must only be disclosed AFTER a patient has been recruited and registered into the trial. The whole merit of randomization is otherwise lost because the next allocation is known (see Section 5.5).

Example 5.1   Simple randomization – Chronic gastro-oesophageal reflux

Csendes, Burdiles, Korn, *et al.* (2002) recruited 164 patients with chronic gastro-oesophageal reflux to their clinical trial using simple random allocation on a 1 : 1 basis to each treatment. This resulted in 76 randomized to receive fundoplication but 88 to calibration of the cardia. The achieved allocation ratio was therefore 1 : 1.158, which is quite a disparity from that intended.

5.3.2 Blocks

As we have just seen, simple randomization will not guarantee equal numbers in the different intervention groups. To ensure equal numbers, balanced arrangements can be introduced. This leads to various 'restricted randomization' schemes. One way to achieve balance is by generating short 'blocks' that contain the combinations of the interventions, as follows.

The block size is taken as a convenient multiple of the number of interventions under investigation. For example, a two-group design with a 1 : 1 allocation may have block sizes 2, 4, 6 or 8, whereas for a three-group design blocks of size 3, 6 or 9 would be appropriate. In addition, the actual block size is often also chosen as a convenient divisor of the planned trial size N. For example, if $N = 64$ and with two interventions planned, a block size of 4 or 8 would be preferable to one of 6, since 4 and 8 are divisors of 64 but 6 is not. Blocks are usually chosen as neither too small nor too large so that for two intervention groups, block sizes of 4 or 6 are often used.

Suppose that equal numbers are to be allocated to A and B for successive blocks of 4 subjects. To do this we first identify, among all the 16 possible combinations or permutations of A and B in blocks of 4, those that contain two As and two Bs. Here we ignore those permutations with unequal allocation, such as $AAAA$ and $AAAB$. The six acceptable permutations are summarized in Table 5.1.

These permutated blocks are then allocated the numbers 1 to 6 and the randomization table used to generate a sequence of digits. Suppose this sequence was again 53455 42567; then reading from left to right we generate for the first 24 recruits the allocations *BAAB ABBA BABA BAAB BAAB* and *BABA*.

We note that, within this sequence, *BAAB* is repeated three times and *BABA* twice while, for example, *AABB* is not used. To avoid this imbalance of sequences, a particular digit for the sequences of Table T5 would not be used a second time until all other relevant individual digits had first been used. In this case, the sequence ignores the repeated digits and any outside the range of 1 to 6 and becomes, in effect, 534-- -2-6-. This generates *BAAB ABBA BABA* as previously, but is now followed by Permutations 2 and 6 of Table 5.1, which are *ABAB* and *BBAA*. Finally we note that Permutation 1 has not been used so that *AABB* completes the full 24-unit allocation sequence.

Such a blocking device ensures that for every 4 successive recruits included in the trial, a balance between A and B is maintained. Once we have recruited 24 individuals, 12 will therefore receive A and 12 will receive B. In the event that recruitment has to cease before all 24 units are allocated then, at whatever point this occurs, there will be approximately equal numbers in each intervention group.

If the design specifies that 48 individuals are required to be randomized, then the sequences of Table 5.1 are randomized again using the next digits from Table T5, which are: **170 67937 88962 49992** and so on. Working along this sequence results in the permutations 1, 6, 3, 2 and 4, and then 5 is taken to complete the set.

In some circumstances it may be desirable to avoid runs of the same treatment in successive patients. For example, there could be resource implications if different medical teams are responsible for the different treatments. Thus, if Permutation 1 of Table 5.1 is followed by Permutation 6 then we have *AABB BBAA*. This sequence comprises a subsequence within it of 4 consecutive patients all assigned to B. To avoid

Table 5.1 All possible permutations of length 4 for two treatments A and B each occurring only twice

1	AABB	4	BABA
2	ABAB	5	BAAB
3	ABBA	6	BBAA

this happening, if Permutation 1 is selected, then Permutation 6 may be excluded as a possibility for the next block to be chosen. One possibility is first to generate all the possible sequences of the 6 permutations and then screen all of these and remove those with runs of either *AAAA* or *BBBB*. From the reduced list, select one at random to be the sequence used for the first (in our case) 24 individuals.

As can be imagined, the randomization process can become very tedious and so it is usual to use a computer program for this. Such programs should generally enable the particular options, for example the number of interventions and the block size specified for the planned trial, to be accommodated.

5.3.2.1 Randomized block designs (RBD)

If Table 5.1 is reformatted into that of Table 5.2, then the so-called randomized block design (RBD) structure for the first 24 units randomized becomes more apparent. The contents of the blocks 1 to 6 are formed by randomizing the 6 permutations as described.

The basic structure of Table 5.2 can be extended to fit the needs of any trial design. For example, if $N = 48$ then, as we have illustrated, the RBD is replicated a second time but with the permutations randomized again for this second time.

Equally, the basic structure can be adjusted to the numbers of interventions concerned. Table 5.3 therefore includes a RBD for $t = 3$ interventions A, B and C conducted in blocks of size $b = 3$, but over 18 units. This design includes all possible 6 permutations of size 3. The eventual assignment of these permutations to the corresponding $r = 6$ replicate blocks will be made at random.

5.3.2.2 Variable block size

The investigating clinical team, especially those members concerned with identifying suitable patients, should not be aware of the block size. If they come to know the block

Table 5.2 Randomized block design (RBD) for 24 units comprising 2 interventions (A, B) in blocks of size 4

Block	1	2	3	4	5	6
Permutation	5	3	4	2	6	1
	B	A	B	A	B	A
	A	B	A	B	B	A
	A	B	B	A	A	B
	B	A	A	B	A	B

Table 5.3 Randomized block design (RBD) for 18 units comprising three interventions (A, B, C) in blocks of size 3

Block	1	2	3	4	5	6
	A	B	C	A	B	C
	B	C	A	C	A	B
	C	A	B	B	C	A

size, then guessing the next treatment to be allocated as each block of patients nears completion may lead to subconscious inclusion or exclusion of certain patients from the trial. In fact, simple permuted blocks are rarely used but a number of subterfuges can be applied to make the scheme less apparent to the clinical teams. The potential difficulty referred to can therefore be avoided by (randomly) changing the block size as recruitment continues to reduce the possibility of a pattern being detected by the investigation team. Clearly this may not be an issue in double-blind trials, where neither the attending physician nor patient knows of the actual treatment given to earlier patients. However, it could become an issue if, for any reason, the blinding is not fully effective: for example, if one particular (although blinded) treatment produces a specific reaction in the patient but this is not observed with the others. So even here a variable block size might be a wise precautionary strategy. Other possibilities for concealing future allocations include adding random components to the final element in each block and to the avoidance of runs. Even so, some argue that simple randomization, despite its disadvantage in terms of not ensuring perfect balance, is the only way to fully conceal the randomization.

5.3.2.3   Allocation ratio

We have implicitly assumed that, for two interventions, a 1 : 1 randomization will take place. However, the particular context may suggest other ratios. For example, if the clinical trial patients are limited for whatever reason, the design team may then argue that they should obtain more information within the trial from (say) the test intervention group T rather than from the well-known control or standard S. In such circumstances, a randomization ratio of say 2 : 3 or 1 : 2 in favour of the test intervention may be decided. The first could be realized by use of a dice with sides 1 and 2 allocated to S, 3, 4 and 5 allocated to T and 6 neglected. The latter ratio could be obtained also by using a dice but with sides 1, 2 for S and 3, 4, 5 and 6 for T. However, moving from a 1 : 1 ratio involves an increase in trial size (Chapter 9), and this increase should be quantified before a decision on the final allocation ratio is made.

If an allocation ratio of 2 : 3 for S and T is chosen, then this implies a minimum block size of 5 with each block comprising one of the permutations given in Table 5.4.

If a design for a trial comprised $N = 25$ subjects, then the first sequence of random numbers that we used (**534 55425 67**) generates, using Table 5.4, the 5 blocks with the permutations *TSSTT*, *STTST*, *STTTS*, *STSTT* and *TSTST*. The next block of 5 would then randomize the order of the unused permutations (0, 1, 7, 8, 9) of Table 5.4 using

Table 5.4   All possible permutations of length 5 for two interventions S and T allocated in the ratio 2 : 3

1	SSTTT	6	TSTST
2	STSTT	7	TSTTS
3	STTST	8	TTSST
4	STTTS	9	TTSTS
5	TSSTT	0*	TTTSS

*Note that 0 replaces 10 to facilitate the use of random number tables.

Example 5.2   Unequal allocation – Hepatocellular carcinoma

In a double-blind trial conducted by Chow, Tai, Tan, *et al.* (2002), three doses of tamoxifen (0 Placebo, 75 and 150 mg/m^2) used the allocation ratios of 2 : 1 : 2. Consequently, the patients were stratified by the 10 recruiting centres and randomized within each centre using a fixed block size of $b = 5$.

(say) the sequence **170** 6797 889**62** 49992 to obtain *SSTTT, TSTTS, TTTSS, TTSTS* and finally the unused permutation 8, *TTSST*, would be added to complete the sequence.

5.3.2.4   *Stratified randomization*

As in the trial conducted by Poon, Goh, Kim, *et al.* (2006) of Example 2.1, trials often involve more than one clinical centre. In this case, there were single centres from India, Korea, Singapore and Thailand. In such multicentre circumstances it is usually desirable to maintain the design-balance between treatments for each centre involved, whether 1 : 1 or in a different but defined ratio. This implies producing a distinct randomization list for each centre. In this way, the relative experience of treating patients with the trial options is shared by all centres concerned.

Example 5.3   Stratified randomization by recruiting centre – Treatment of uncomplicated falciparum malaria

In the report of the trial conducted by Zongo, Dorsey, Rouamba, *et al.* (2007), the authors state:

> Nurses were responsible for treatment allocation, on the basis of computer-generated randomisation lists, which were stratified by the three clinic sites. These lists were provided by an off-site investigator who did not participate in administration of the trial.

A generic term equivalent to 'centres' in the above example is 'strata'; this general concept of strata can be extended to other situations. For example, in children with neuroblastoma those with metastatic disease are known to do less well (are more likely to relapse following treatment) than those without. Consequently, if both metastatic and non-metastatic patients are recruited to a randomized trial then, although the balance between treatments using randomized blocks may be maintained overall, there is no guarantee of balance within each of the distinct disease groups. This can be rectified by using metastatic disease status (absent or present) as strata and then randomizing treatment within each of these. In this way, balance is maintained within each metastatic group as well as for the trial as a whole.

Further, if this trial is multicentre then, for each centre involved, the randomization to treatment can be conducted within each metastatic disease group, thereby ensuring the protocol specified allocation ratio of the interventions is closely maintained within each strata and also within the centre. This process can, at least in theory, be extended to more and more strata but this may not be sensible. The principal reason for stratifying by centre is to give each centre a similar experience, whereas the reason for stratifying by presence or absence of metastatic disease is because the disease status of the patient is a very important determinant of outcome. Should the balance of patient metastatic status be different in the two intervention groups, this may distort the final treatment comparison.

To give an extreme example, suppose by chance *all* the metastatic patients happened to receive the same treatment, say A, and none received B. Then the true effect of A versus B will be compromised – in fact, B may appear to have a clear advantage in terms of survival over A. However, had half the metastatic patients been included in B and half in A, then group A would improve over the previous situation while B worsens so that difference between those receiving A and B would be less extreme.

In our example of neuroblastoma in children, there are other factors (apart from treatment itself and metastatic status) which affect outcome, such as stage of the disease and age at diagnosis. However, further stratification makes the randomization process more difficult and, as the potential numbers of strata becomes large, there is a distinct possibility of only a few patients falling into some of the strata subgroups. Thus if four centres were involved, with strata for metastatic status with two levels and (say) stage with three levels, this creates $4 \times 2 \times 3 = 24$ substrata. The number of patients per treatment within the substrata (assuming equal numbers in each level occur within strata, although this is unlikely to be the case) is $N/48$, which is clearly less than an average of 10 patients unless the trial size is 480 or more. Stratified randomization as a method of achieving balance can therefore become unworkable if there are too many stratification variables.

For continuous prognostic variables such as age, stratification can only be carried out when these variables are divided into categories. There is then the difficult decision of what cut-off value of age to use. Although age (or some other continuous variable) may be prognostic for outcome, it is usually preferable not to stratify for this but to record the information for each patient and take account of this in a retrospective sense at the analysis stage.

If there are several potential variables for stratification, these should all be variables that are known or are believed to be influential on outcome in a substantial way. The choice is then to decide which will be the design strata that are taken account of at the randomization stage, and which can be viewed as retrospective strata (to be recorded at the patient eligibility stage and then adjusted for in the final analysis). Centre will usually be added to the former group while continuous variables are usually best left for the latter. In whichever category the variables fall, it is also important (at the planning stage) to judge if the subsequent analysis taking account of these will be sufficiently robust. In broad terms, are there enough subjects in the trial to ensure that the appropriate statistical models can be estimated with reasonable precision?

5.3.3 Dynamic allocation by minimization

Stratification only works when the number of strata is few. As a consequence, a number of dynamic methods have been developed, of which the simplest is 'minimization'. Dynamic methods are used to replace the randomization process with a largely deterministic method that is based on the characteristics of the patients already in the trial and the characteristics of the patient about to be allocated to an intervention.

Example 5.4   Stratified randomization – cranberry or apple juice for urinary symptoms

Campbell, Pickles and D'yachkova (2003) used a simple 1:1 randomization, within each of 4 substrata, to assign treatment either by cranberry or apple juice to alleviate urinary symptoms during external beam radiation for prostate cancer. Their allocation into the 2×2 stratification groups of previous transurethral resection of the prostate (TURP) (negative or positive) and International Prostate Symptom Score (IPSS) (<6 or ≥ 6) for each randomized treatment (cranberry or apple juice) are given in Table 5.5.

Table 5.5 Stratification groups for a trial for alleviating urinary symptoms (from Campbell, Pickles and D'yachkova, 2003)

Juice	TURP IPSS	Negative <6	≥ 6	Positive <6	≥ 6	Total
Apple		17	27	6	7	57
Cranberry		14	27	6	8	55
	Total	32	54	12	15	112

In this trial, approximately equal numbers are randomized to apple and cranberry juice with achieved allocation ratio 57/55 or 1.036 : 1, which is very close to the design specification of equal allocation. It should be noted that the proportions TURP negative (86/112 or 77%) and TURP positive (24%) are far from equal, as are the numbers IPSS < 6 (39%) and IPSS ≥ 6 (62%). There are also reasonable numbers within the cells of the TURP negative group, but they are small within those that are TURP positive.

To demonstrate how minimization works, suppose that we wish to recruit an additional patient to the trial of Campbell, Pickles and D'yachkova (2003). We therefore suppose we wish to allocate apple or cranberry, once eligibility has been confirmed and consent obtained, to Patient 113 who is TURP negative with IPSS < 6. First we have to construct Table 5.6, which gives the distribution of the first 112 patients recruited of Table 5.5 by each covariate (TURP and IPSS) and treatment allocation.

The minimization method counts the numbers in Table 5.6 with each of these two prognostic characteristics (TURP negative or positive; IPSS <6 or ≥ 6), in each treatment group separately. Note that patients are counted more than once (here, twice). In the apple group, this count comes to $A = 44 + 23 = 67$ and in the cranberry group $C = 41 + 20 = 61$. The method then allocates the new patient to the group with the lower total. In this case, Patient 113 receives cranberry juice since 61 is less than 67. The effect of the allocation of this patient to cranberry juice is to bring the actual allocation ratio 57/56 or 1.018 : 1 closer to the design specification of 1 : 1.

Table 5.6   Distribution of patients with prostate cancer according to TURP and IPSS stratification groups in a clinical trial for alleviating urinary symptoms (data from Campbell, Pickles and D'yachkova, 2003)

		Treatment Juice	
Prognostic factor		Apple (A)	Cranberry (C)
TURP	Negative	44	41
	Positive	13	14
IPSS	<6	23	20
	≥6	34	35
Total randomized		57	55

Scott, McPherson, Ramsay and Campbell (2002) came to the conclusion that:

> ...minimization is an effective method for allocating participants to treatment groups within a randomized controlled trial. In the majority of cases, minimization has been shown to outperform simple randomization in achieving balanced groups; this greater performance is particularly marked when trial sizes are small. Minimization has also been shown to be advantageous compared to stratified randomization methods, as it has the ability to incorporate more prognostic factors.

They advocate wider adoption of the technique within clinical trials. However, the Conference on Harmonisation (ICH) E9 Expert Working Group (1999) (*Statistical Principles for Clinical Trials*) recommended that a random element should be incorporated into dynamic allocation procedures. This could be carried out in the worked example above once the totals $A = 67$ and $C = 61$ had been derived. Rather than automatically allocating Patient 113 to C, we could toss a biased coin which favours C in the ratio of $67/(67 + 61) = 0.52$. This would of course be carried out in practice by a computer program. This procedure favours C at this stage, but does not guarantee that it will be chosen – hence the desirable random element is introduced.

Despite all this, the advantage of simple randomization is that it is the easiest to operate, preserves the lack of predictability and ensures greater validity for the statistical tests.

Example 5.5   Trastuzumab for HER2-positive breast cancer

Smith, Procter, Gelber, *et al.* (2007) (Example 1.8), used a minimization procedure to allocate patients to treatment, taking into account region of the world, age, nodal status, prior (neo)adjuvant chemotherapy and hormone receptor status, together with the intention to use endocrine therapy. There were therefore six factors as well as the three different treatment groups to be allocated. However, since their trial planned to recruit upwards of 5000 patients with HER2-positive patients with breast cancer, the numerous strata could be accommodated. This number of strata would not be sensible for trials of a more modest size.

5.4 Application

As we have continually stressed, randomization is a key element of the design implementation for clinical trials and, as we have indicated, the randomized trial is considered the 'gold' standard against which alternative trial designs are compared.

Randomization ensures (in the long run) balance between the groups in known and *unknown* prognostic factors. We have shown how balance for prognostic factors that are known to be important can be achieved by stratification, but there is no other way except by randomization to ensure long-run balance of *unknown* prognostic factors.

Clinical trials may require large numbers of patients and seldom will all these patients be available at the opening of the trial. Instead, they will first present as and when their illness or condition appears and so will only become available for treatment or intervention, and hence the trial, at unpredictable intervals. The intervals between patients may be lengthy if the incidence of the condition in question is low. We cannot allocate patients to the interventions before the trial is started, although the 'process' for randomization needs to be established before the first patient has consented to recruitment.

Further, although simple randomization gives equal probability for each participant to receive A or B, it does not ensure that by the end of recruitment to the trial equal numbers received A and B. In fact, even in relatively large trials, the discrepancy from the desired equal numbers of participants per intervention group can be quite large. The same applies if the allocation ratio is not equal, in which case there is no guarantee that the chosen ratio will be closely preserved once all participants are randomized.

As we have indicated, the use of blocks is open to abuse with the potential for some investigators to go to extreme lengths to guess the treatment allocation when they may be nearing the end of a block. This knowledge could potentially lead to choosing the patient for the treatment allocated, rather than allocating the treatment to the patient. However, even if this is the case, any selection bias is likely to be small provided the patient eligibility decisions and subsequent request for randomization are not always determined by a single investigator. This argues both for multicentre trials involving several investigating teams and, more importantly, a trials office providing the randomization and functioning independently of their clinical colleagues. The risk of selection bias can be further reduced if block lengths vary and investigators are not given details of any stratifying factors. The latter may not be so easy to conceal since stratifying factors (preferably only 1 or 2) should be chosen to be strongly prognostic for outcome. Most clinical teams within the specialty concerned will know what these are, and have to provide this information when contacting the trials office for the patient randomized allocation.

The contrary argument to the use of blocks is to advocate simple randomization, and use analytic methods to adjust the estimate of the final treatment comparison for any chance imbalance in prognostic factors in the various treatment groups concerned. However, we would advocate the use of the variable block system over the simple randomization methods, so that large imbalances between participant numbers in each of the allocated groups are avoided.

The advantages and disadvantages of the different options for randomization are given in Table 5.7.

Table 5.7 Advantages and disadvantages of different types of randomization

Type	Advantages	Disadvantages
Simple	Easy to implement	May result in imbalance in design allocation numbers per intervention group
	Unpredictable	There may be a chance imbalance of prognostic factors
Blocked	Ensures (almost) design allocation numbers in each group even if the trial stops early	There may be a chance imbalance of prognostic factors
		Slightly predictable but this can be reduced by randomizing the block size
Stratified and blocked	Ensures (almost) design allocation numbers and balances prognostic factors in each group	Can only balance a few prognostic factors
		Slightly predictable although this can be minimized by randomizing the block size
Minimization	Can balance a number of prognostic factors	Requires all information on the strata factors of previous patients to be available
		Potentially predictable, not strictly random although the method can be modified to be random to some extent

5.5   Carrying out randomization

5.5.1   Design

The full planning team will usually be involved in discussing aspects of the randomization processes, such as identifying the type of randomization to implement or relevant strata. However, a neutral party (in the sense of not being involved in any way with patient care or management), usually the statistician assigned to the trial, would work out the final details without revealing these to the other members of the team. These confidential details would include, for example, the choice of block size and the process by which the randomization of the allocation is generated. All these details should remain confidential (but fully documented, securely recorded and stored) until the trial is complete. In most circumstances, it is best if the list (or a dynamically generated equivalent) is retained in an appropriate trial office that can be contacted by the responsible investigator once patient eligibility and their consent are obtained. However, even within the confines of a trials office, it is best if the random allocation is revealed only one-at-a-time to whoever receives the call from the investigator wishing to randomize. This usually implies that a secure password-protected computer-based entry system is needed for feeding in key details of the new patient and supplying the associated randomization.

5.5.2 Preparing the list

In principle, the randomization can be conducted as each eligible patient is identified, for example, by tossing a coin and assigning the patient whichever intervention is indicated by a head or tail. Alternatively, we can prepare in advance a numbered list against which a particular randomized intervention is listed. Once recruitment begins, successive patients are given a sequential study number beginning with the first and are then assigned the associated intervention from the list. This removes the possibility of the clinical team using unacceptable methods for assigning the interventions and also allows the imbalances from the desired allocation ratio arising from the use of a simple randomization device to be avoided.

It will usually be more efficient if the list can be computer generated, particularly in situations with unequal allocation ratios and/or variable block sizes. This method is more reliable in ensuring the protocol specifications are maintained, and furthermore the list can be reproduced if, for any reason, it is lost or as required for regulatory purposes. It is important that this list is generated by, and remains confidential to, the statistical group. Although broad details will be agreed by the full protocol development team, specific details such as block size are not revealed to the clinical colleagues involved with recruiting the trial subjects. However, once the trial is closed to recruitment, these details will form a part of the ensuing reports and publications.

One device for allocating the randomization, which is certainly useful in small-scale trials, is to prepare sequentially numbered sealed envelopes that contain the appropriate intervention inside. These can be of an opaque 'salary-slip' format, which cannot be opened without destroying part of the envelope. The responsible collaborator only prepares to open the envelope once he or she has verified that the patient concerned is eligible and has consented to enter the trial. The process begins by writing the name of the patient (or a code for unique but confidential identification) on the exterior of the envelope, then tearing the envelope open to reveal the allocation. Once this is complete, the envelope and 'salary-slip' should be stored carefully and these, and any unused envelopes, retained as a check on the integrity of the randomization process. Intrinsically, there is nothing wrong with this system but, because of the potential for abuse as envelopes can be opened and switched or disregarded, it is not regarded as entirely satisfactory. However, in some circumstances it will be unavoidable; perhaps a trial is being conducted in a remote area with poor communications. In such cases, every precaution should be taken to ensure that the process sytem is not compromised. One simple way is to have the envelopes kept out of the clinic itself and held by someone who can give the randomization over the telephone. The physician rings the number, gives the necessary patient details (perhaps confirming the protocol entry criteria), and is told which treatment to give or, in a double-blind trial, a code number identifying the particular drug package to be given to that patient.

5.5.3 Double-blind trials

Many potential problems in trials of an 'open' design are avoided in double-blind clinical trials, in which both the attending clinician and the patient are blinded to the intervention allocated. In a double-blind trial of a drug against placebo, the alternatives have to be identical in appearance, weight, texture, smell and taste, and packaged in identical but suitably labelled containers. In this situation, the randomization list is generated ensuring that the required allocation ratio between the active and placebo is maintained. The appropriate packages (active or placebo) are then consecutively labelled beginning with the first number of the sequence (possibly listed within each recruiting centre and corresponding strata). The intervention is therefore randomized before the first patient is recruited. Once trial recruitment begins, the first eligible and consenting patient is randomized by giving that patient Package 1, the second Package 2 and so on, which might be stored in the pharmacy. At that stage, to avoid obvious difficulties, the patient's name would usually be added to the package exterior by the prescribing pharmacist.

In these circumstances, it is very important to ensure that the randomization is activated with the utmost care and that no mistakes are made in labelling which of the identical packages are placebo and which are active. Further, it is vital that additional and secure copies of the randomization list are produced so that, should the working copy be lost or damaged, the trial remains uncompromised.

Key steps in preparing the randomization list for a parallel group trial include the following:

establish the number of options under test;

if the trial is multicentre, is stratification by centre appropriate?

identify any key stratifying prognostic factors;

establish the total number of subjects to be allocated;

establish whether an allocation ratio other than 1 : 1 is to be used;

determine an appropriate block size – is a variable size advisable?

in trials with 'one-at-a-time' recruitment consider randomization by minimization;

consider how the randomization is going to be implemented;

once generated, ensure the randomization list cannot be compromised.

Example 5.6   Prevention of pain and bruising following hand surgery

For the randomized double-blind, placebo-controlled trial to compare placebo with homeopathic arnica 6C and arnica 30C of Stevinson, Devaraj, Fountain-Barber, et al. (2003) of Example 1.9:

> Medication bottles were labelled with study numbers derived from a computer-generated randomization list in blocks of three by an individual not involved with running the trial. The randomization list was kept in a sealed envelope in a locked drawer until the end of the trial. All patients and investigators, including the surgeon, physiotherapists and data analysts, remain blinded to the treatment allocation until after data analysis.

Example 5.6 *(Continued)*

In practice, and as we note in the Glossary, the degree of blinding implied by the use of terms such as double-blind are not consistent and vary somewhat between trial reports. The reader therefore needs to establish the full implications of the use of these terms. Stevinson, Devaraj, Fountain-Barber, *et al.* (2003) therefore use the term double-blind, yet their method may be more accurately referred to as triple-blind.

5.5.4 Breaking the code

If a trial is double-blind then, by definition, neither the patient nor the responsible clinician knows what treatment is actually being taken. However, should an untoward event occur and the responsible physician feels that knowledge of what is being given is imperative for appropriate clinical management of the patient, provision for code break has to be in place. Indeed, this is likely to be a requirement set as part of the formal trial approval processes. It is usual that only the chief investigator has the authority to approve a code-break, so it is essential to ensure that the communication processes are clear to the whole investigation team. Once a code-break is authorized, it is important to record the reasons for it and to document the consequences for the patient concerned. For example, this information may initiate a serious adverse event (SAE) notification to the relevant authorities but, at the very minimum, should be reported in the subsequent trial findings.

5.5.5 Computer-based systems

Whatever form that the randomization takes, it is usually best to have a computer-based system which can cover the full range from generating the randomization list to recording and verifying key information when a subject is to be randomized, allocating the intervention, informing all concerned (such as the responsible clinical teams) and updating the trial database.

5.6 Documentation

If a clinical trial is being conducted with a view to submission for (say) drug registration, then there may be specific regulatory requirements such as the ICH E6 (R1) (1996) Guideline for Good Clinical Practice and ICH E9 (1998) that need to be adhered to. These concern, in part, documentation of the processes involved in the trial conduct. In this respect, it is particularly important that the method of generating the randomization is recorded carefully and that, if there is a list, it can be regenerated. It is additionally useful should the list get lost, although this contingency should be covered by a second copy of the list held in another but secure location. As we have seen, this makes very practical sense in the context of the randomization for a double-blind trial, in which the alternatives are packaged in such a way as to be indistinguishable.

Although tossing a coin is a perfectly good means of obtaining random numbers, any list obtained by such a method is not reproducible. That is, repeating the tossing will not generate the same list. This implies that the randomization procedure cannot be verified if circumstances arise that make it necessary to check, for example, that the intervention issued by the trial office was that which was actually allocated at the participating centre. Consequently, the trial of Lo, Luo, Tan, *et al.* (2006) (Example 1.5), comparing types of root restorations, may no longer comply with current standards:

> We tossed a coin to allocate the selected lesions randomly to receive one of the two study treatments: restorations placed by the conventional or by the ART approach.

The results of this simple randomization process for 162 restorations led to 78 teeth assigned to ART (Atraumatic Restorative Treatment) and 84 assigned to conventional treatment in 103 elderly patients with a mean age of almost 80 years.

If a computer program is utilized to generate the list, this too must be verifiable. This usually means recording carefully the process actually used and, in particular, the choice of 'seed' to begin the randomization process. Once again, this is particularly important for trials which are of a double-blind nature.

5.7   Unacceptable methods

Any allocation method that is not 'random' should be avoided. Pseudo-methods for the allocation process have been used, such as giving successive patients the alternate treatments. This method is not random since, at least after the first patient, it is totally predictable so that the clinical team will know the intervention planned 'before' they see the patient. As we have noted, this knowledge may bias the final comparison. Similarly, if allocation is made on the basis of, for example, date of birth, it will always be clear which treatment is planned for which patient. Examples of these quite unacceptable methods continue to occur, but the corresponding trials would not be accepted for publication in reputable clinical journals as they contravene the CONSORT Guidelines described by Moher, Schultz, Altman, *et al.* (2001). Experience has also shown that comparisons of treatments made by comparing non-randomized groups of patients given the alternatives under test are often very misleading. This does not preclude the possibility of making non-randomized comparisons in certain situations, but is a reminder that they are intrinsically unreliable.

5.8   Software

A directory of randomization software and services for clinical trials, including both simple do-it-yourself software and 24-hour telephone randomization services, is provided by M. Bland, University of York. It is intended to help people planning and seeking funding for clinical trials. It is available at www-users.york.ac.uk/~mb55/guide/randsery.htm.

5.9 Guidelines

ICH E6 (R1) (1996). *Guideline for Good Clinical Practice.* CPMP/ICH/135/95. EMEA, Canary Wharf, London.

ICH E9 (1998). *Statistical Principles for Clinical Trials.* CPMP/ICH/363/96. EMEA, Canary Wharf, London.

ICH E9 Expert Working Group (1999). ICH Harmonised Tripartite Guideline: Statistical principles for clinical trials. *Statistics in Medicine,* 18, 1905–1942.

ICH E9 specifically refers to aspects of randomisation in Section 2.3.2.

CHAPTER 6

Trial Initiation

However important a question the clinical trial poses and however well designed it is it is imperative that the mechanisms for implementing the trial are in place. In this chapter we describe some of the necessary prerequisites that need to be established to ensure the trial is successfully launched, conducted, completed and reported. We stress the need for a dedicated trials office which can act independently from the clinical teams entering and dealing with trial participants, whether or not they are patients. We also emphasize the need to check local regulations with respect to ethical clearance of trials, informed consent processes for those receiving the interventions and the requirement to formally register each trial before it commences.

6.1   Introduction

Designing a clinical trial of any size is a major undertaking. It is vital to bring together a skilled multidisciplinary team to ensure that an optimal design is chosen and that the mechanisms are in place to ensure it is successfully completed. Although the design of the trial will be the main focus at the early stages of planning, it is important to keep in mind that the eventual trial protocol developed must be implemented. Members of the protocol development and implementation teams should therefore include representatives of, for example, the diagnostic clinic, pharmacy, hospital ward, data management and statistical office.

The size and composition of such teams will depend critically on the trial of concern and therefore may range from a very small tightly knit group within a single centre to a complex (even multinational) membership encompassing many components. We will use a multicentre trial of modest size and complexity as the basis for this chapter. Whatever the requirements there will usually be a common core. For the purposes of our explanation, the core can be described as having two major components: clinical (including all those concerned with aspects of patient care) and statistical (including data management in its widest sense), with seamless links between them to ensure they act and react in unison.

Randomized Clinical Trials: Design, Practice and Reporting   David Machin and Peter M Fayers
© 2010 John Wiley & Sons, Ltd

6.2   Trial organization

6.2.1   Trial steering committee

Developing a randomized clinical trial is usually an evolutionary process, beginning with the germ of an idea and gradually expanding over time to become a reality. At some stage of this process, the skeleton of the eventual trial steering committee (TSC) will be formulated, a principal investigator identified and the necessary expertise and resources gradually ascertained and assembled. For example, on the more clinical side, it would be natural for the extended TSC membership to include those from relevant medical specialities who will eventually be delivering the interventions under consideration. These members will, for example, provide major input into refining the interventions themselves including dosage or scheduling, the appropriate patients to include and their assessment and care. The extended TSC will also debate the size of the anticipated clinical benefit (the difference between the Test and the Standard intervention, say) which the trial will be designed to detect.

The TSC will be responsible for overseeing the trial from launch to completion of follow-up, and also for ensuring that as many patients as possible enter the trial. All members should be convinced that the trial is appropriate and necessary. They should be committed to its successful completion, and therefore willing to invest energy and enthusiasm to this end.

6.2.2   Identifying the tasks

Parallel to the stages outlined in the trial schema of Figure 2.1, which concentrates on the path for a potential trial participant, the components of Figure 6.1 indicate some of the key stages that the TSC will need to go through before the trial can begin.

Once the trial is underway, then the sequence illustrated in Figure 2.1 should be adhered to with every successive patient. In contrast, when planning the trial, the sequencing of Figure 6.1 is much more flexible. This will usually depend on trial-specific issues, although the penultimate step will often be receiving ethical approval for the go-ahead. For example, identifying the potential centres may well be part of the early assessment of feasibility. Even though the trial question has been identified and refined to suit the purpose intended, it may have to be refined again following submission to external scientific review or ethics committees, who may have concerns with respect to the design that the trial team had not anticipated. Also, once a trial is up and running, some of these issues may re-emerge if unforeseen circumstances arise.

6.2.3   Trials office

The necessary arrangements will differ from trial to trial, but whatever the circumstances a trial office will be required. How big, how complex or where located will again depend on circumstances. Even if the office is virtual (in that all trial office activities are not confined to a single location), access to key personnel and facilities are required.

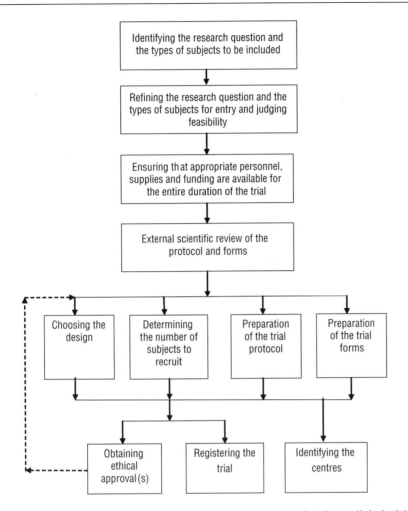

Figure 6.1 Schematic representation of some stages involved when planning a clinical trial

For purposes of exposition we will assume the trials office is in one location and that the personnel include, as a minimum, a trial statistician and a trial coordinator, backed up with good information technology (IT) and administrative support. Although we may not give so much attention to these latter groups in this book, no modern organization can run without skilled IT and appropriate levels of administrative support. Setting such an organization in place for a single trial is time consuming and expensive. If only limited funds are available, it might not be possible to assemble an experienced team; this does not auger well for the successful completion of the trial. It is important not to underestimate the importance of establishing the trials office team.

There are many tasks to perform in developing the trial protocol itself but, as shown in Figure 6.1, even before it is finally approved for activation there are many other functions to oversee before recruiting the first patient. It is important that someone has the overall responsibility of coordinating this activity. This is usually best done by a member of the trials office staff rather than by (say) the principal (clinical) investigator. These activities will include:

- arranging meetings of the protocol development team;
- ensuring the protocol contains all the elements necessary and is of appropriate clarity for such an important document;
- coordinating the production of the final protocol;
- collating the paperwork necessary to obtain ethical approval.

The role of the statistician involves providing advice on:

- key information with respect to the suitability and ranking in priority of endpoint measures including their frequency and method of assessment;
- choice of trial design;
- the sample size required;
- the ultimate analytical approach to analysis;
- devising a suitable randomization strategy including, for example, the allocation ratio for the interventions, stratification groups, block sizes and how the randomization process will be activated.

These activities provide key reasons why the trials office team should be able to act independently of the remainder of the TSC members with respect to certain features of the trial planning processes.

Importantly, the trials office will take the lead in designing the corresponding forms for data capture, while collaborating with the other members of the protocol development team to ensure the forms are consistent with the needs of the trial protocol and that their content imposes minimum burden on the trial participants – be it patients, clinical colleagues or themselves at the data checking and processing stages. They will make sure what has to be done is done, for example registering the clinical trial appropriately. The trials office will also design the data base, and plan the checking and verification processes for the eventual data as it accumulates once the trial opens.

6.2.4   Protocol and form production

We have described in detail the development of a clinical trial protocol and the design and the content of forms for data recording. It is also important that they are produced and printed to a high standard. The clinical and other teams involved with trial implementation need to be able to readily identify the component sections of the protocol and the forms as a patient progresses through the relevant stages, whether these details relate to: specific aspects of the treatment to be given; patient samples that need to be taken and laboratory tests requested; or the date of death of a patient who has died. Once content of both the protocol and forms have been determined, then issues such as layout should be discussed by the development team and the trials office commissioned to implement these. Layout issues may range from apparently trivial concerns such as font size and colour for headings, to more substantial issues of ensuring distinct sections are not divided on recto-verso pages that make it difficult for the clinical or other teams to follow what is intended.

All sections of the protocol need careful phrasing; experience suggests that terms such as 'off study', 'off protocol' and 'patient withdrawn' often lead to confusion. Clearly any subject recruited to a clinical trial can withdraw consent to participate at any time and, in such a case, it may be that no more than the data already collected will ever become available for such a patient. In contrast, 'off study' or 'off protocol' may just mean the patient did not receive the intended therapy: possibly they were too ill, simply refused or it was felt no longer advisable by the clinical team. In these circumstances, the patient is still in the trial. As much documentation as is relevant should continue to be completed by the responsible clinical teams. To give a specific example, if a cancer patient refuses more chemotherapy then, despite this, the actual date of his or her subsequent follow-up visits (and ultimate death) should, if local regulations permit, continue to be returned to the trial office.

One should also bear in mind that, despite careful planning, once the trial is activated the accruing experience with the trail patients and their associated care may reveal points within the protocol that require amendment. For example, if untoward toxicity occurs then treatment doses may have to be modified or delayed. Good practice dictates that all those involved with treating patients need to be made aware of unexpected serious adverse events (SAEs). These events will usually necessitate informing the committee(s) concerned with approving the trial of their occurrence and possibly result in amendments to the protocol documentation. These amendments may only involve a few added lines to the original protocol so, as we advised in Chapter 3, use of suitable blank space within the protocol document may leave the pagination unaffected. This allows the protocol to be revised with a minimum of work and delay, retaining the current format although it must be made very clear that a change has been made.

Considerable care with respect to the clarity and quality of the data forms for the trial is required, especially if these are to be completed on a one-screen-at-a-time data entry system within the clinic environment. Wherever possible, the data fields should follow a logical and practical sequence so that whoever is responsible for completing the form does not need to go back and forth (or up and down on the computer screen) at the data entry stage. Just as the protocol may have sections relevant to several disciplines within the medical teams, so there may be information requested on the forms which has to be completed by a specific team. In which case, the form should be split into sensible sections or, as is often the case, separate forms produced for each component. For example, if surgical procedures are necessary then a Surgical Form can be designed to be distinct from the Pathology Form, on which the outcome of histological review of the resected specimen is recorded. It is usually better to have more but targeted forms, rather than long forms that are passed from one clinical group to an other as the patient progresses through the trial. This format enables completed forms to be forwarded more rapidly to the trials office. In this way, the patient information recorded in the database is kept as current as is reasonably possible.

Before the trial commences, it is important to ascertain whether any of the forms are difficult to complete because of layout or phrasing of questions. One approach is for members of the TSC to take the forms to their own centre or department and attempting to complete them with information from comparable patients currently under their care. They could also check with, for example, the local laboratory staff to verify whether the trial form requests are in a suitable format for their purposes.

6.2.5   Obtaining approval

A critical stage in the trial development process is the formal submission to the relevant authorities for their approval for the trial to be conducted. The TSC should ensure, well in advance of the intended submission date, that they are fully aware of the processes concerned and the stipulated requirements. Failure to obtain approval on a bureaucratic detail is irritating for everyone and extends the approval process unnecessarily. We have emphasized the need for a high-quality protocol both in content and appearance, designed in such a way to facilitate reading and understanding. This not only assists the clinical and other teams involved directly in the trial itself, but also members of the approval and ethics committees whose membership will often include lay individuals. A document which is easy to read, albeit technical in nature, will help such members to better understand the purpose of the intended trial. Experience suggests that these lay members may be particularly concerned about the information provided for patients and the consent process. A major concern for all should be patient safety. If concerns are raised by the approval authorities then the TSC should try to answer these in as timely and as complete a manner as possible. Once approval has been obtained, the potential collaborating groups should be informed so that local mechanisms can be set in place. The aim is to launch the trial in every centre concerned with the minimum of delay.

6.2.6   Trial registration

An important criticism made by the teams conducting systematic reviews (see Chapter 14) of clinical trials is that the relevant trial results are not always published. This may be because the trial was never completed, resulted in equivocal or negative results or perhaps due to mere indolence on the part of the investigating team. Nevertheless, systematic overviews seek out those trials that are unpublished as well as those that are published in the medical literature. There is evidence that those unpublished trials may represent the more negative of trials conducted so that, if an overview is made without them included, the associated meta-analysis may provide an unduly optimistic view of the (new) therapy under test.

   To overcome some of these difficulties, Dickersin and Rennie (2003) argue, as have many others previously, that an important first step in the trial development and conduct process would be to formally register trial protocols. This registration should be completed *before* the trial begins. Each trial should be given a unique identifier so that there can be no ambiguity at a later date. This unique identifier will, for example, have to be quoted to the relevant journal editor when submitting the clinical results for publication. It allows those conducting systematic reviews to be sure that *all* relevant trials are included in their review. Some of the details that may be required for satisfactory

Identifying Information	Name of organisation conducting the trial Name of trial sponsor Protocol number
Trial details	Purpose All interventions Title and acronym Disease or condition Eligibility criteria Design Planned trial size Locations where recruitment takes place
Funding	Full details of all funding with associated reference numbers
Contact	Lead principal investigator and other key personnel.
Conduct	Date first patient entered Recruitment status Date of last patient entered

Figure 6.2 Suggested details necessary for trial registration purposes (adapted from Dickersin and Rennie, 2003)

registration purposes are listed in Figure 6.2. Many of the items should be easily provided as they form part of the key information that will be included in all good clinical trial protocols. It is somewhat more difficult to specify all the locations where the trial may eventually take place. This tends to suggest that the registration will have to be updated as the trial progresses but, provided the information required is not too extensive, this should not be too large a burden for a well-organized investigating team.

It is important to note that the International Committee of Medical Journal Editors, as reported by De Angelis, Drazen, Frizelle, *et al.* (2004), gave notice that the clinical journals which it embraces will only consider a clinical trial for publication if it has been registered in an appropriate registry. Some problems associated with the possibility of trials being registered in duplicate are raised by Grobler, Siegfried, Askie, *et al.* (2008). They describe the situation of a multinational trial in which ethics insists that the trial be registered in each country's national register. If indeed this has to be done, then it is vital that the TSC are aware of this requirement so that the registration procedures and the trial reference numbers given become part of the trial documentation held by the trials office. The problem with duplicate registration is that anyone searching for information on trials may be misled into thinking that many trials are ongoing within their area of concern whereas the opposite may be the case. Grobler, Siegfried, Askie, *et al.* (2008) indicate mechanisms as to how the WHO (2008) registry platform may help to overcome this problem.

Registration should take place immediately when the trial is approved for activation by the appropriate authorities. Section 6.7 lists some sources for registries of trials.

6.2.7 Establishing the network

Although the TSC itself will often have representatives of some of the centres involved, frequently this group does not include representatives of all the key specialities and locations concerned. It is therefore important that a communications network is established. Initially this may just contain the names and details of all concerned who can then all be contacted electronically (as a group or subgroups) whenever the need arises. It is almost inevitable that some urgent message may need to be sent to all – for example, the trial has completed recruitment – so it is important that the trials office keep this list up to date. As the trial progresses through its stages, updates to all participants, notices of meetings and other trial-related information could also be provided in this way.

6.2.8   Mechanisms – supplies

6.2.8.1   The protocol

Once the protocol has been formally approved for launching, the potential participant centres, which should have been identified to some extent during the development and feasibility stages of the protocol, will need to be informed of the successful completion of the approval processes. They will also need the associated trial documentation comprising the protocol and forms, plus any other information such as copies of patient information sheets and consent forms. The recruiting centre(s) should receive sufficient copies of protocols to ensure key members of the associated medical teams have their personal copy and that spares are held at the centre to cater for any contingencies.

6.2.8.2   Supplies

If the trial requires special supplies, such as a double-blind packaged drug, then sufficient and appropriate storage space will be required at a location where it can easily be dispensed for use whether in the hospital ward or the outpatient clinic. Situations may arise in double-blind trials that necessitate the attending medical team (perhaps in an emergency situation, for patient safety) knowing which of the blinded drugs the patient has received. The TSC must therefore establish careful procedures for any such eventuality. Perhaps a 24-hour hotline needs to be in place so that a rapid decision can be made to authorize breaking the blind and rapidly feeding the relevant information back to the patient care team. In such cases, a careful record of the reasons for the code break, the actual drug prescribed, and details of the eventual outcome for the patient concerned will have to be made. Before the trial is opened to patient entry, the investigating teams need to be made aware of these emergency procedures and a test of the practicability of these procedures should be instituted.

If patients are required to complete forms for quality of life or other patient-reported outcomes then sufficient supplies of the instrument, mechanisms for distributing to the patients, manpower to provide assistance where necessary and checking processes to make sure they are indeed fully completed need to be in place.

6.2.8.3 *Training*

Each participating centre, perhaps with the assistance of members of the TSC, should rehearse the protocol implementation within their own centre to ensure that the procedures so outlined can be followed, assessments made as required and the information returned to the coordinating centre in a timely manner. It is also important that training on case record form completion is also provided as, despite care in their preparation, ambiguities may still remain. Further, within each centre, we may often need to clarify where some particular items of information can be obtained.

Everyone also needs to be aware of the schedule for form completion and how it may vary from patient to patient, and what to do if circumstances arise for which the forms do not allow for this contingency. All participating staff should be made aware of the need to complete the forms in a timely manner and to dispatch the information as rapidly as possible to the coordinating centre. They should be made particularly aware of special requirements such as the reporting of SAEs which may (often for legal reasons) have to be fast-tracked to the data centre and possibly to the regulatory authorities concerned.

6.2.9 Registering and randomization of patients

Registration of all patients into the trial will usually be an integral part of the randomization process and it is customary for careful attention to be made to this point. Indeed, the reporting requirements of the clinical journals and the regulatory authorities make it explicit that registration is required, especially if the results are to be part of a product license application.

In the case of a double-blind trial, the randomization is completed before the drugs are despatched to the collaborating centres so that, once an eligible patient is identified, the next package (individually numbered) among the batch will be allocated to the patient. Thus, as the drugs are available locally, extra care has to be taken by the recruiting team to ensure that the central trials office is immediately notified of every allocation by registering the patient onto the trial. This contrasts with the situation for open trials, where the recruiting centre has no option but to contact the central office for randomization and thereby be notified of the particular intervention the patient will receive.

6.3 Data collection and processing

6.3.1 Data forms and their scheduling

Patient-specific details – ranging from assessments made when determining eligibility, the randomized intervention actually allocated and details of progress during the active intervention phase to possibly long term follow-up information – will be recorded on the case record forms. The precise items for these records will have been discussed in parallel with the protocol development so that implications, one for the other, can be reviewed by the trial development team as they arise. The contents of the forms should be focused on answering the questions the trial is established to answer so that any redundant or tangential information should be kept to a minimum.

In addition, the distinct types of forms will be identified and the precise scheduling for their completion will be determined and recorded within the protocol itself, but also indicated on the different form types.

6.3.2   Missing forms and data

An important logistical requirement of the trials office is to track the timely arrival of completed data forms. Once a patient is registered and randomized onto a trial, a corresponding timetable for receipt of forms should be established for that patient. Not only should late arrival of a form initiate action by the trials office, to remind the recruiting centre of its absence, but rather the system should anticipate the arrival of a form and remind the clinical teams that it is due. It is better to be proactive rather than reactive in this respect, if at all possible. Despite this careful process, there will be forms for which no schedule can be anticipated: for example, should a patient experience a SAE the clinical teams may have a responsibility to notify this, or if a patient relapses then details of their relapse will be required. In anticipation of such situations, the trials office may send routine reminders to the participating centres indicating that 'should such an event occur' then the trials office should be informed immediately by return of the corresponding case record form.

Of course, even although a form may have been received on schedule, it may not have been fully completed so that pertinent information is missing. It is therefore important that procedures for prompt detection of missing items are in place so that a rapid request for further details can be made. However, this request should not be issued until all other (non-missing) items on the form are first checked and verified so that all problems identified may be dealt with simultaneously.

The investigating team need to be aware that missing or incorrect data, particularly that related to the endpoint variables concerned, may compromise the eventual conclusions drawn at the analysis stage of the trial. A major cause for concern is that the lack of these data may result in bias, and that the apparent results of a clinical trial will then not reflect the true situation. We will not know if the difference we observe (or lack thereof) between treatments is a truly reliable estimate of the real difference. Also the precision of the estimated difference will be less than that anticipated by the design. If the proportion of missing data is small then, providing the data are analyzed appropriately, we can be confident that little bias will result. However, if the proportion of missing data is not small, it is a matter of judgement as to whether this will impact seriously on the conclusions drawn. It is best that every effort is made at the trial initiation stage to anticipate the missing eventualities and to set in place mechanisms to keep these to a minimum.

The satisfactory flow of data obtained from every recruited patient and the checking of such data are vital components to the successful completion of a clinical trial.

6.3.3   Database

Although the choice of an optimal database will depend to some extent on the complexity of the trial planned, it is important that it is reasonably easy to establish (preferably with minimal assistance from the IT team). In particular, the variables and their type should be simple to define, make data entry and editing easy and, once entered, safe and secure. The data so entered should then be easy to access, extract, manipulate and transfer to a statistical package for analysis and the statistical package chosen must be capable of the analysis intended by the design. It is now often mandatory to require, certainly for trials seeking regulatory approval, that the database has the facility to store audit trails, that is, the ability to record all changes made to individual data items following their first entry to the database. For example, this implies that if a correction is made to an earlier item, the old value is still retained and suitably tagged in the database together with details of when and by whom that change has been made. A list of any changes made can then be produced should this be required by the regulatory authorities.

6.3.4 Checking

Although there is an increasing trend towards electronic data capture, much of the data in medical trials is still captured on paper-based forms. The advantage of electronic forms is that range and cross-checks (checking the consistency of the new data with itself and with that already in the database) can be instantly applied. In addition, missing values can be immediately queried and irrelevant questions avoided. For example, following a question on whether or not a patient has relapsed, if the answer is NO then questions pertaining to details of the relapse (although necessarily on the paper form) can be automatically skipped. However, paper forms are often used for practical reasons and may be the first choice for trials of a modest size.

Despite all precautions taken in the trial protocol to ensure that measurements are made according to carefully documented procedures, mistakes do occur in the recording of these values. Some of these errors may be detected by a quick check of the form on which the result has been recorded, while others may be missed and passed to the data file. At this stage, range and cross-checks, easy programming of which needs to be an integral feature of the database, may help to identify such problems. If problems are found, these can be checked against case records for correction of any erroneous values identified. In some cases, this will provide confirmation that the apparent error is not an error at all. Some outlier values may not be identified by range checks alone, but by reference to previous or subsequent data on the same subject or by comparison with data from other subjects in the total dataset. It is important that data validation occurs as soon as possible after the data item is collected, so that the possibility of making any correction that may be necessary is maximized. It is always a bad idea to leave such checking until the trial is closed and no more new data are anticipated. Any problems identified should be tagged within the database until resolved. Once resolved, only the residual yet unresolved problems remain and these can readily be listed should the need arise.

However, these data capture and checking procedures need to be in place before the first patient is recruited onto the trial. Experience with trials, perhaps in the same or a related condition, may enable the trials office to anticipate many of the problems that will arise. Discussions during the protocol development stages will also have identified specific items that require particular attention. However, once the trial gets underway, it is almost inevitable that further items for careful checking will arise. It is therefore important that the preliminary work done in the early stages allows for some operational flexibility once the trial becomes live.

6.4   Data monitoring

6.4.1   Internal

Although data checking and validation procedures are an integral part of good trial conduct, the trial office should also be active in monitoring the information provided by the trial data and not just be a passive recipient who, although ensuring the data are complete and correct, takes no positive action. Some of the different aspects of a trial that require such monitoring are listed in Figure 6.3.

The trial office also has a responsibility to monitor these data in a scientific sense. This is particularly important for survival studies, especially when testing new procedures or new treatments about which little is known. Such scrutiny is essential in a multicentre setting. For example, single untoward events may occur in several centres which, although noticed, may cause no particular concern but once collated together within the trial office may be sufficient to trigger some (perhaps remedial) action to avoid future cases by the TSC. The duty of the trials office is therefore not only to report on trial progress on a regular basis, but also to act on suspicious or unusual circumstances as the trial data accumulates. It is difficult to plan in advance for all contingencies, except to remind the trial office staff that this is an important part of their responsibilities and that they should be vigilant.

The content of routine reports to the TSC (and those for the wider group of collaborators) should be established. These reports need to be informative and provide, for example: the latest recruitment figures; some basic tabulations describing the patients entered; and a summary of the flow of the data forms (comparing what is anticipated with what has been received). However, it is essential to studiously avoid details which may give any hint of the relative efficacy of the interventions under test, which could thereby compromise the ethical equipoise of those involved in treating individual patients.

The rate of recruitment of patients and whether all centres are contributing patients as anticipated
Ensuring appropriate supplies are available
Monitoring each patient schedule for form receipt
Identifying and resolving data errors or omissions on the forms received
Detecting ambiguities or other needs for modifying forms
Monitoring for protocol violations
Monitoring for toxicity and similar events
Monitoring for SAEs
Looking for the unanticipated – particularly excess failure or death rates

Figure 6.3   Aspects of the progress of a trial that require monitoring by the responsible trial office

6.4.2 External data monitoring committee

In addition to the internal monitoring by the trial office and the overview of the trial progress provided by the TSC group itself, there may still be concerns that a more independent overview of issues, particularly those of safety, should be provided. Should data from the incomplete trial indicate, for example, a clear benefit to one group over the other, then it may not be desirable to continue to recruit to the trial. This would then enable the findings to be brought into clinical practice sooner and thereby bring the 'proven' benefits into patients more rapidly.

Although not listed specifically in the major components of a clinical trial protocol in Figure 3.1, many trials, especially those with patient survival as an endpoint or trials that could result in adverse consequences for the patients, will also have an independent data monitoring committee (DMC). On behalf of the TSC the DMC will, with the full collaboration of the trials office, review the progress of the trial. It is a fundamental requirement of good trial practice that the clinical teams recruiting patients should remain uninfluenced by the accumulating evidence on the relative efficacy of the interventions concerned, both during the active recruitment and ensuing treatment schedule stages of the trial. The object is to maintain their equipoise, so that they can continue to obtain informed consent in an objective manner and hence continue to randomize patients until the number specified by the protocol are recruited. It is not difficult to imagine that keeping the clinical teams in ignorance of the accumulating situation is not without problems, as it is only natural for them to be concerned to do their best for the patients in their care. As a consequence, members of the DMC are independent of the TSC and of any colleagues who are responsible for recruiting patients. They are empowered to review the trial data and provide reassurance that the best interests of patients continue to be safeguarded. They are expected to be cognisant of results from rival trials, which may affect the relevance of the trial they are responsible for.

An important aspect of pre-trial launch activities is therefore to identify the potential members of the DMC and to establish the corresponding terms of reference. Although specifics may change, the broad terms of reference for a DMC are indicated in Figure 6.4 and these would be discussed and reviewed with the eventual members to ensure relevant issues are all included.

It is usual to have at least three members of such a committee, one of whom should be a clinical trials statistician, and to define their role as advisory to the TSC. Of particular importance here is ensuring the rapid feedback to the TSC of any recommendations. Appropriate administrative support should therefore be provided to the DMC to ensure their report is completed before the close of the meeting. In an ideal setting, this report might be provided in three parts: a note for further information and action by the trials office team, a confidential statement to the TSC (perhaps raising issues that require review and response to the DMC) and a short summary which could be suitable for wider dissemination to all those involved with the trial. Only in extreme situations would the latter two comment upon the relative efficacy of the interventions concerned. However, they may contain statements indicating, for example, concerns that recruitment is falling below that anticipated; there are no safety issues and provide answers to specific points which the TSC may have asked the committee to address.

| To review the accumulating trial data as it relates to treatment effects, adverse events, trial performance and any other matters that may be of concern |
| In particular to ensure that the trial is safe, and warrants continuation. |
| Review patient recruitment, and the continuing feasibility of the trial. |
| Advise the Trial Steering Committee (TSC) with regards to further conduct and to make clear recommendations (as appropriate) to continue the trial as currently planned, suggest some modification to the trial protocol on minor but important detail (perhaps widening the eligibility criteria or suggesting dose modification if untoward toxicity occurs) but not the fundamental structure of the interventions themselves, or terminate the trial. |
| Respond to concerns or issues raised by the TSC. |
| Report back fully, and confidentially, the results of their review to the trial office responsible for producing the DMC report. |
| Provide an in progress report that can be issued to the TSC without compromising confidentiality. Suggest which aspects of this report (perhaps all) may be disseminated to all investigating teams concerned. |
| To recommend when the next DMC should meet if this departs from the schedule envisaged in the protocol itself. |
| Request the trials office to respond to specific queries by the DMC arising from their meeting. For example, these may concern a query raised in the meeting itself that could not be resolved on the day or that there was an early indication of a potential difficulty for which additional information on particular patients may be needed. |
| Advise on analysis and publication schedules. |

Figure 6.4   Key aspects concerning the role of an independent data monitoring committee (DMC) for a trial

Further initial steps to establish how often the DMC will convene (depending on circumstances these may be teleconference rather than physical meetings), the information that will be provided and how it will be presented should be taken. It should also be made clear that the central trials office statistician and coordinator responsible for the protocol will prepare the reports and attend the DMC meetings. However, it is usually appropriate for the TSC chair, or another designated member of the clinical team, to be available (perhaps at the end of a telephone) to clarify clinical or practical aspects of the trial concerned. They will only be called upon to provide information, and must not be present while the DMC debate the confidential information about accumulating results of the trial. The DMC should also be free to have a closed discussion, perhaps to enable them to have a collective view on the quality of the report provided by the trials office staff and agree any action that needs to be taken in this respect.

Some trials specify in the trial protocol that formal interim statistical analyses of the accumulating data will include 'stopping rules' with respect to decisions on trial continuation. Although the precise details will depend on the specific needs of the trial in question, usually these should not be planned for more than one or two occasions during the recruitment stage (although we describe in Chapter 14 sequential trials where a much greater frequency would in general be required). The DMC will be aware of this (as they will have copies of the protocol) and may have to make recommendations to the TSC to continue or stop the trial subsequent to the findings of such analyses. We comment in Chapter 7 on specific details of the statistical aspects of interim analyses for DMC purposes, and give an example where a DMC recommended continuing a trial even although a first interim analysis suggested that the trial might close. A key role of the statistician member of the DMC will be to provide technical help with the interpretation of such analyses.

In the early stages of a trial, the focus of the DMC may be more on safety concerns and the patient recruitment rate than effectiveness of the different interventions under test. Hopefully any such concerns should then be resolved at this early stage so that, although safety monitoring should continue, the emphasis would move away from such issues.

6.5 Ethical and regulatory requirements

6.5.1 Routine reporting

When conducting a clinical trial there may be external considerations, beyond the immediate control of the investigators themselves, which impact on the daily work of the trials office. For example, funding agencies or the committees giving approval for the protocol to commence may need routine reports on progress, perhaps annually, until such time as all patients have been recruited and their trial endpoints been evaluated. It is therefore important that systems are in place for these to be produced and that the material and data for their content has been identified so that the process can be activated without undue difficulties once the trial has started.

6.5.2 Serious adverse events

Of particular concern here may be the requirement to report any SAEs in a timely manner to the relevant authorities. The trial protocol should therefore contain a definition of how these are identified and, should they occur in practice, the consequent action required by the responsible clinical team described. This may, for example, involve direct notification to the authorities themselves or immediate notification to the trials office, who will then report to the relevant authorities. Should the clinical teams be required to inform the authorities directly, then the mechanisms in this respect should require that the trials office is informed simultaneously. A total picture can therefore be immediately accumulated and perhaps then fed to the DMC, should this be necessary.

6.6 Launching the trial

Aspects of all this preparatory work are being activated, hopefully at an increasing pace, as the protocol approaches the stage for formal approval. It may then be tempting to await approval before making further progress. However, any such delays (although natural to understand) are likely to increase the interval between the receipt of the approval and recruitment of the first patients. The trial cannot be opened until such approval is obtained, but the plan for the trial launch should be in place for activation as soon as the go-ahead has been given. The TSC should therefore develop a strategy which gives the new trial a high profile and invigorates the teams concerned, who may have been exhausted by the (long) process of protocol development and approval. They should be reminded of the importance of the question posed, and how rapid recruitment is vital to ensuring the answers are provided in as short a time frame as is possible.

6.7   Trial registries

A number of international, national and pharmaceutical company trial registers exist, including the following. Many countries do not maintain their own registers but actively participate in those that are international.

6.7.1   International

International Standard Randomized Controlled Trial Number Register www. controlled-trials.com/isrctn

WHO International Clinical Trials Registry Platform: Universal Trial Reference Number (UTRN). www.who.int/ictrp/utrn/en/index.html

6.7.2   National

Australia and New Zealand Registry (ANZCTR): www.ANZCTR.org.au
China: www.chictr.org/Site/English/Index.htm
Germany: www.germanctr.de/
Hong Kong: www.hkclinicaltrials.com
India: www.ctri.in:8080/Clinicaltrials/trials_jsp/index.jsp
Japan: rctportal.niph.qo.jp/link.html
South Africa: www.sanctr.gov.za/
United States of America: US National Institutes of Health register www.clinicaltrials.gov/

6.7.3   Industrial

Glaxo Smith Klyne (GSK): www.gsk-clinicalstudyregister.com/
Roche: www.roche-trials.com

6.8   Guidelines

The following guidelines are listed here, not to provide a detailed list of what must be done, but rather as pointers to issues to consider when initiating the *new* trial that is being developed. It is all too easy to overlook some key issues at this (and even later) stages so pointers about what to do are often very useful. A more comprehensive list is provided by Day (2007, p. 243).

ICH E2A (1994) Clinical Safety Data Management: Definitions and Standards for Expedited Reporting. CPMP/ICH/377/95.

ICH E2B (M) (2000) Note for Guidance on Clinical Safety Data Management: Data Elements for Transmission of Individual Case Safety Reports. CPMP/ICH/287/95.

ICH E3 (1995) Structure and Content of Clinical Study Reports. CPMP/ICH/137/95.

ICH E6 (R1) (1996) Guideline for Good Clinical Practice. CPMP/ICH/135/95.

ICH E8 (1997) General Considerations for Clinical Trials. CPMP/ICH/291/95.

ICH E9 (1998) Statistical Principles for Clinical Trials. CPMP/ICH/363/96.

ICH E10 (2000) Choice of Control Group in Clinical Trials. CPMP/ICH/364/96.

The above are available through the European Medicines Agency (EMEA), 7 Westferry Circus, Canary Wharf, London, E14 4HB, UK. or www.emea.europa.eu/htms/human/ich/background.htm

ICH E9 Expert Working Group (1999). Statistical principles for clinical trials: ICH Harmonised tripartate guideline. *Statistics in Medicine*, **18**, 1905–1942.

CHAPTER 7

Trial Conduct

Although the mechanisms to run a successful clinical trial should be in place before the launch, it will only be once the trial has started that these will be tested. This chapter gives practical hints on how problems might be dealt with or avoided. Emphasis is placed on ensuring the data flow mirrors the patient flow as closely as possible. The speedy resolution of queries arising, the provision of feed-back and encouragement to the medical and other personnel involved, the preparation of regular monitoring reports on progress; anticipating the final analysis and publication, and the planning of the next trial are also important.

7.1 Introduction

Once the protocol is approved and all the implementation procedures are complete, a trial opening date can be identified and recruitment can start. Following this opening date centres can enter, register and randomize their first patients and the trial is truly on its way. However, the systems put in place following the suggestions of Chapter 6 now have to be implemented. Some of these will be tested immediately, such as the randomization process, while others will only be tested as the trial progresses. It is important to monitor the processes closely so that should problems arise, they are detected as soon as is practicable and dealt with accordingly and with speed. However careful the advanced planning, the unforeseen will almost certainly arise so that the team needs to be ever vigilant and have the ability and flexibility to react to changing circumstances should such eventualities occur.

7.2 Regular feedback

7.2.1 Recruitment

The planning team will have identified key objectives for the trial so that, once in progress, these will need to be monitored. Amongst these will be the numbers of subjects actually recruited. The protocol will have specified the actual numbers

Randomized Clinical Trials: Design, Practice and Reporting   David Machin and Peter M Fayers
© 2010 John Wiley & Sons, Ltd

required and (usually) the feasibility of achieving this within a pre-specified timeframe. This permits the target accrual rate to be calculated, allowing the trial office to monitor recruitment and report progress to the trial steering committee (TSC) on a regular basis. Since protocol approval and clinical processes are of a very variable duration and the times for centres to come on stream may differ substantially, there should be updates to all concerned when a centre enters their first patient. As the trial progresses, the recruitment reality can be compared to that anticipated and, if necessary, appropriate action taken. This may imply finding extra centres, assisting with the protocol approval processes in others, identifying administrative hurdles or relaxing somewhat if anticipated targets are being met. Even if recruitment is on target or exceeds that anticipated, although this is more than satisfactory, any centres not yet recruiting or recruiting less than anticipated should be identified and remedial or support action taken if possible. It is important to maintain rates over the whole recruitment period as other centres may, at a later stage, experience difficulties that slow their recruitment rate. For example, change of personnel in a centre may alter previously satisfactory patient recruitment and data flow to that below acceptable standards. Depending on circumstances, a change in personnel may warrant a welcoming explanatory visit by a representative of the TSC.

If recruitment falls behind when the trial is well underway, then the TSC must seriously consider what remedial action to take. It may even be necessary to review whether the target desired is attainable. Clearly we will be looking for causes of the failure which may be multifaceted in nature. It is an easy option in such circumstances to give up, but the price of that is often very high – principally because the important question, which provided the rationale for the trial itself, will not be answered and so the investment in time and resources already expended will be wasted. At this stage, the TSC should search for more positive solutions: visit the centres, seek more centres, consider widening the eligibility criterion, reducing the number of assessments required, reimbursing the patients for their attendance, supplying free drugs or whatever may seem to offer a way forward.

7.2.2 Missing forms

As well as monitoring recruitment figures one also has to ensure that the data generated by the trial participants arrives at the data centre in a timely manner and as laid down by the protocol. If it does not then it may merely indicate some tardiness on the clinical teams involved or, more seriously, non-adherence to the protocol intervention schedule itself. Although the latter will be more critical for patient care, in both cases action needs to be taken to rectify the situation. Apart from the information on the patient recorded at randomization by the trials office itself, at the early stages of the trial only the first form (the on-study form) may be anticipated at the trials office. It is therefore easy to identify those patients whose form has not been returned on schedule and is (potentially) missing. The on-study form is also particularly important as it may contain information on details with respect to patient eligibility that need to be checked carefully. Often a reminder that particular forms are due can help ensure that return rates are high and on schedule.

As indicated in Chapter 6, keeping track of what forms are due is likely to be a complex administrative task. The number and type of forms expected will depend on the stage of the trial each participant has reached. Some follow-up (repeated) forms will have a specified schedule for completion, perhaps at monthly clinic visits. Other forms may be triggered when a specific event arises, for example, when a death or relapse occurs. In this case, some patients may have a single form for death or relapse. If missing forms are identified, whether they are regular follow-up forms or single forms, it is very important that the data centre actively pursues these by contacting the responsible clinical teams as soon as it becomes apparent that a form is missing.

Of particular importance in this process is ensuring that forms containing the end-point assessments are returned as, without this information, the patient is effectively lost to the final analysis. This is not only a waste of the resources used in recruiting and following the patient within the trial context, but may lead to a lack of statistical power due to reduced sample size and may even bias the eventual trial conclusions.

Some problems associated with missing case-record forms and data items are summarized below.

(1) Trials with a high proportion of missing forms may be unable to rule out the possibility of bias, especially if critics can argue that, for example, the patients with the poorest response tend to be associated with missing forms.

(2) Trials with a lot of missing data lose statistical power (essentially the effective sample size is reduced).

(3) Trials with a lot of missing data may become unpublishable.

(4) Forms for patient-reported outcomes or quality of life are frequently associated with a high rate of missing, and it should be anticipated that special measures will be necessary to counter this.

(5) A high rate of overdue forms is a sign of poor trial management, prevents timely checking of data and frequently leads to a high level of permanently missing data.

7.2.3 Validation

Once a form is received, whether on schedule or late, the items within each must be checked for completeness and any omitted items should be queried with the clinical teams immediately. Delays in form returns usually reduce the chance of correcting any aberrant or missing data items. Even if the data appear complete, there can still be errors within the form such as impossible answers to specific questions. This might for example occur if there is a list of numerically-coded response options for a particular measure and the investigator reports an out-of-range response. Continuous data, such as weight, height and many biochemical measures, may frequently be expected to lie within a range of valid values. The verification process can then apply range checks to detect values that are outside this pre-specified range. Consistency checks, which link several data items, may also indicate errors; for example, if a patient is marked as having died it would be inconsistent to have additional measurements dated as arising after this. Another example of a consistency check might be that a patient who is reported as having severe progressive disease would be expected to lose weight and show other indications of worsening status. Many errors or suspected errors can be detected and queried with the investigators who completed the forms. However, range checks or consistency checks may identify some apparent errors that are in reality valid yet unexpected recordings. Sometimes checks are expected to yield some false reports as, for example, when range limits for patients' weight are set at 95% limits of the normal range. However excessive levels of false errors may arise from checks having been inadequately or too rigorously specified by the computer programs, in which case the checks should then be adapted and revised. Alternatively, if a particular type of form is repeatedly found to contain true errors it may be indicative of a deficiency in the case record form itself, and therefore lead to essential modification. If this happens in respect of an important variable then the whole team may need to be informed and revised forms issued.

7.2.4 Basics

Throughout the trial there should be reports detailing information on recruitment levels, active and inactive centres, those awaiting approval and number and flow of data forms. Once the trial has recruited more than a few participants, the reports can also begin to describe those who have entered the trial, albeit in brief. For example, information on basic demographics and baseline clinical characteristics by randomized intervention can be given. This serves several purposes. It reassures the clinical collaborators that the data they have carefully recorded has indeed been received and can be processed. It can also reveal data errors or special features which may not have been detected in the validation and checking procedures. Further, these reports begin to give some idea of the case-mix of patients that are being recruited and may indicate that patients of a particular type, although eligible, do not appear to be appropriately represented. The reasons for this can then be explored to try and establish why this is so and to rectify or clarify the situation.

Importantly, such reports give the statistical and data management team and the eventual writing committee a realistic check on components necessary for the final reports that will be prepared once the trial is completed. However, in these reports we must be careful not to disclose information about the key endpoints as these details are reserved for the independent data monitoring committee (DMC) only. Revealing such information to the clinical teams recruiting patients may compromise the trial, in particular by disturbing the clinical equipoise that they have. In any event, it must be remembered that early data, which is by definition based on relatively few patients compared to the target recruitment, will have an unacceptably low precision and must be viewed and interpreted with extreme caution.

7.3 Publicity

7.3.1 Newsletters

There will often be many individuals involved in the successful conduct of a clinical trial and also many who, although not directly involved, may be very interested in the progress. For example, some of the patients with oral lichen planus in the trial conducted by Poon, Goh, Kim, *et al.* (2006) first presented at the national skin hospital but were then referred to the dental centre if they had an oral presentation of their condition. Such a centre, although not directly involved in treating the patients within the trial, was an important source of patients. The regular feedback through a newsletter enabled them to keep abreast of developments and provided a basis for informing potentially eligible patients about the trial. Such communications may stimulate less enthusiastic collaborators, and gives encouragement to everyone, including those who may not be part of the research team but are vital to the trial success. These may include clinicians, nurses, paramedical staff and other colleagues working in the centres involved. Similar information could be sent directly to patients for poster display at the clinics or sent to patient support groups. Birthday cards can also be used to stimulate patient cooperation.

7.3.2 Clinical journals

Another useful strategy is to describe the trial protocol in the medical journals. For example, Yeow, Lee, Cheng, *et al.* (2007) summarize the main objectives of their trial in children with cleft palette in the hope that other investigators may be interested to participate. Similarly the Systemic Therapy for Advancing or Metastatic Prostate Cancer (STAMPEDE) trial has been described in the clinical literature by James, Sydes, Clarke, *et al.* (2008) in the hope of encouraging a wider participation. These publications describe the rationale for the trial so that clinical colleagues responsible for similar patients, but who are not recruiting patients for the trial, are made aware that there is an important research question relevant to their patients. Because such articles will be subject to peer review and editorial approval, investigators who perhaps may be initially hesitant of a trials' clinical relevance may be persuaded of the value of the trial by the more objective nature of the information provided. In any event, even if such articles do not result in higher recruitment rates, they should sensitize clinical colleagues to the questions posed so that, once the results are available, they may more readily institute these within their own practices.

7.4 Data monitoring committees

7.4.1 Introduction

Once a clinical trial is under way, the responsible teams have much to do. In addition to recruiting and treating patients, often with a protocol which is more stringent than standard practice, they must monitor the accumulating data for safety and efficacy. Safety for the individual patients is not only of paramount concern; it is also the collective concern over many patients when determining whether a regimen is safe enough for use. If the regimen under test is found unsafe then this may lead to some modification or, in extreme circumstances, may justify premature closure of the trial. It is also possible that the early trial data indicates a real advantage (or disadvantage) to the new therapy under test, or that no clinically important difference between them is likely to be demonstrated. There may also be concern that the planned trial size is not sufficient for the design purposes.

As we have indicated in Chapter 6, it is best (and may even be mandatory) that an independent group monitors the trial progress although the individual clinical and statistical teams should always be on the lookout for the untoward. It is usual that this DMC is constituted of clinical members and a medical statistician, cognisant of the issues concerned but not participating in the trial itself. A proposed charter for clinical trial data monitoring committees has been proposed by the DAMOCLES Study Group (2005). Circumstances where such a DMC may not be essential are small trials, those comparing what are known to be safe alternatives, rapidly recruiting trials and those involving interventions of short duration. For the purposes of what follows we will assume a DMC has been established.

7.4.2   Interim data reviews

7.4.2.1   Safety

When the independent DMC come to review the trial data for the first time in the early stages of the trial, they may need to focus more on aspects of patient safety than other issues. However, as the trial progresses, and following earlier reassurances on safety concerns, efficacy then becomes more relevant. To assist the DMC with their tasks, the protocol itself may include sections which describe the interim analyses which will be presented at the meetings. The protocols of those trials that employ a stopping rule, and hereby effectively determining the sample size from the accumulating trial data as opposed to the more usual fixed sample size determined before the trial commences, should include a section about the role of the DMC when a 'stopping' rule is triggered.

Example 7.1   Monitoring for safety

The following text is taken from the draft of a protocol in which the role of the DMC was specified before the trial was activated. In this instance, the trial statistical office will only be responsible for monitoring the accumulating data and then convening a DMC review (should it be required).

> In order to monitor the possibility of an increased number of adverse events, the trial will be formally reviewed by an independent Data Monitoring Committee should the cumulative 1-year adverse event rate exceed 7.5% or the 1-year death rate exceed 1% at any time in either arm of the trial.

7.4.2.2   Trial size

Sometimes, the TSC might not feel entirely comfortable with the reliability of the sample size calculations of the trial about to be initiated. This could occur if there is a relatively large degree of uncertainty with respect to some of the basics required for sample size determination purposes (see Chapter 9). For example, there could be uncertainty about the survival rate associated with the standard approach or, if the endpoint is a continuous measure, they may be concerned with respect to value of the standard deviation used. In such a case the TSC may decide, while drafting the protocol, to ask a future DMC to review this aspect of the trial once a given fraction of the patients have been recruited and appropriate data accumulated.

In Protocol SQNP01 (1997) (Standard radiotherapy versus concurrent chemo-radiotherapy followed by adjuvant chemotherapy for locally advanced (non-metastatic) nasopharyngeal cancer), there were clear instructions to the DMC which implied they were not expected to suggest a reduction in sample size following their review, unless there were safety concerns which implied that they would recommend the trial should close immediately.

> With this initial target in mind and, in view of the uncertainty attached to the anticipated clinical response, disease free, distant metastases and overall survival rates, a DMC will be established to review the interim results of the trial once 100 patients have completed treatment. These data will be used as an internal pilot to review the appropriate trial recruitment target (Birkett and Day, 1994). The data for such a review will remain confidential to the DMC members who will report their recommendation to the Nasophryngeal Cancer (NPC) Work Group who will take the necessary action. Apart from reasons of safety, which may caution otherwise, the minimum trial size will remain as that initially planned, that is, 200.

This follows the guidance of Birkett and Day (1994) who, in describing a methodology for revising sample size, make it very clear that an 'internal pilot' should only examine whether the trial is *too small* for the purposes intended.

7.4.2.3 Superiority

Another scenario that a DMC might have to consider is whether to stop a trial if the data accumulated so far appears to suggest a larger, and therefore clinically extremely important, difference between treatments than that anticipated by the design team. Clearly if such an extreme benefit was truly present then it would seem important that the trial should stop immediately and the 'proven' treatment be immediately recommended for clinical use. In judging such a situation, the DMC will be aware that the uncertainty surrounding the potential benefit was high among the TSC at the planning stage of the trial, and that this uncertainty justified the trial question being posed in the first place. Further, this uncertainty provided the clinical equipoise to enable investigators to seek informed consent and randomize their patients. The DMC will also be aware that the purpose of conducting and completing the trial as planned is to reduce (we can never eliminate all) this uncertainly to such levels that the TSC would then be able to firmly recommend (say) the better treatment for clinical use. The DMC are therefore faced with the dilemma of whether to stop the trial early on the evidence from a relatively few patients or continue the trial and thereby potentially deprive some patients of the better option. If the trial concerns a life-threatening disease, rather than (say) a condition which will eventually resolve whatever the treatment given, then different decisions with respect to 'stopping' may be anticipated. In the latter situation, perhaps a DMC need not be established at all and provided safety is not an issue the only reason to stop early would be failure to recruit. Decisions with respect to recommending that a trial should stop might also differ if the Test intervention appears to be doing (much) worse than the Standard.

We should emphasize, however, that the role of a randomized controlled trial is to influence clinical practice, and that this means continuing a trial until there is sufficient evidence to convince even the most sceptical clinicians of the relative advantage of one intervention over the other. Experience suggests that trials are sometimes stopped too early and therefore may fail to convince reviewers, editors or readers of their findings. They are therefore a waste of resources and also fail to prevent future patients from being disadvantaged. The DMC must therefore consider these aspects of early stopping in their deliberations.

7.4.2.4   Futility

In some cases, as the evidence from the trial accumulates it may become quite clear that the options differ by less than what was considered by the design team as the minimal clinically important difference between them. The issue now concerns whether to continue, since it is unlikely that a useful benefit will become apparent. In contrast to the situation of 'superiority', we have that of possible 'futility'. If the alternative interventions are both of a particular type, perhaps easy to administer, no safety concerns, cheap and readily available, then one might argue that continuing until the planned end of the trial 'can do no harm', when a reliable estimate of the difference (however small) will then be obtained. On the other hand, if the Test differs markedly from the Standard in any of the respects just outlined this may persuade the DMC to recommend curtailing the current trial in this situation.

However, we are now in the situation of observing a difference which is much less than that envisaged by the TSC. Consequently, the DMC should consider whether there are any reasons why this should have occurred. One possibility could be that for some reason those receiving (say) the Test drug are less compliant than those on the Standard drug and so are perhaps receiving less of the drug than they should. This may be diluting the apparent difference between the two and hence the suggestion of the futility of continuing arises. In this case, rather than making a firm recommendation to stop the trial, the DMC might either suggest that the TSC should report back to them in more detail on the levels of compliance or perhaps suggest the dose given and/or scheduling of the Test might be reviewed since futility may arise if these are not optimal.

7.4.3   Stopping rules

In the scenarios discussed above, the trial data has at some stage(s) to be summarized by the statistical team and, if appropriate, presented to the DMC for their opinion. This was the case for safety monitoring in Example 7.1. However, in many instances the original trial protocol may indicate the schedule for such meetings and may also include full details of the (statistical) stopping rules that will be used to help guide the DMC decisions. Although we defer a technical discussion of the different types of stopping rules until Chapter 8, we give some examples here. We stress that any interim analysis will be based on fewer patients than that planned for the trial were it to complete recruitment. This increases the likelihood of drawing the wrong conclusions with respect to the relative efficacy of the interventions under test. This likelihood increases if multiple interim analyses are conducted on the accumulating trial data.

Example 7.2   Resectable hepatocellular carcinoma

The trial conducted by Lau, Leung, Ho, *et al.* (1999) which studies the use of adjuvant intra-arterial iodine-131-labelled lipiodol in resectable hepatocellular carcinoma stopped recruiting after 43 of potentially 120 patients, as the investigators conducted an interim analysis of their own results and found a very favourable reduction in recurrences in those receiving the lipiodol. In their paper they state:

> We planned one interim analysis when 30 patients (both groups together) had entered the study and had a median follow-up of 2 years. This analysis assessed the feasibility and tolerance of treatment. We used the Pocock group sequential methods for interim monitoring such that we would stop the trial early if the between-group difference in disease-free survival reached a significance of $p = 0.029$.

However, no independent DMC had been established to monitor the trial, although this was not unusual at the time the trial was initiated.

Their paper was published in the *Lancet* who also commissioned a commentary on the trial. The commentary of Pocock and White (1999) questioned the alleged benefit as 'too good to be true'. On this basis the confirmatory trial, Protocol AHCC03 (2001) was launched without the involvement of the initial investigating team, who felt they no longer had clinical equipoise in this situation. More recently Lau, Lai, Leung and Simon (2008) have published an update which substantiates their earlier findings. The results of the confirmatory trial AHCC03 (2001) are awaited.

In this example, there are two fundamentals that the investigators overlooked. One is that the data monitoring should be done by an *independent* group who then advise the TSC. The other is that statistical 'stopping' rules should only be used as guidelines by the DMC, who should also be mandated to weigh other evidence before making their recommendations.

7.5   Protocol modifications

We indicated in Chapter 6 that the TSC should be prepared for the possibility that important changes may need to be made to the protocol, either because of some direct experience with patients entered onto the trial itself or possibly external information. It is therefore important for the clinical teams and the trials office staff to monitor patient compliance with the interventions prescribed in the protocol. For example, the numbers of patients refusing treatment, withdrawing from the trial, or lost to follow-up may give a strong indication that one or more of the regimens under test may be in some sense unacceptable. If this is the case, changes to the precise nature of the interventions may be required. External information may arise from findings reported in the literature or may arise from further development work on (say) one of the drugs that is being tested within the trial itself. Whatever the reason, the need for such changes should first be quickly and thoroughly reviewed by the TSC and, once confirmed as necessary, speedily implemented. It is possible that the consequential changes may make it necessary to temporarily close recruitment to the trial and/or suggest remedial action for those patients currently receiving treatment.

7.6   Preparing the publication(s)

7.6.1   Preliminaries

As we have seen, while the trial is ongoing advance preparations should be made to expedite publication of the findings. The protocol itself will provide the basis, at least for a first draft, of the introduction, methods and reference sections of the manuscript. The routine reports to the TSC and the wider group of the investigators will supply much that is necessary for the CONSORT flow diagram (Section 10.5). The basic tabulations of demographics and other baseline features by randomized group will provide most of the information necessary for the opening paragraphs of the Results section. Further, if DMC reports are available then these may provide useful information in written text, tabular and graphical form which can be embedded into a preliminary draft. Together, these may also provide pointers as to what can then be presented in the results section. They may also give some guidance to literature searches that may be required to place the current trial results in context when drafting the Discussion. The more of this work that can be done while the trial is still in progress, the easier and more rapidly can the article be submitted for publication.

It is important to remember that the statistical and data centre teams are just as responsible for seeing the final publication produced as are the clinical leads. They should therefore not sit back and relax once the trial is closed to recruitment and their final report has been presented to the TSC.

7.6.2   Writing committee

Although at an early stage, the members of the writing committee will have been identified, it is important that the TSC keeps the membership under review so that, at the time of writing, all the committee members are able to fulfil their tasks in a timely manner. Important questions here are: Who holds the master copy? Who is actually going to submit the paper? In many instances these functions are best conducted by the trials office team, who may spend more time on clinical trial activities than the clinical investigators. These decisions are not to be confused with identifying who should be the first and subsequent authors. This too should have been resolved very early at the protocol development stage. However, this decision too may have to be reviewed by the TSC from time-to-time in view of possibly changing circumstances with respect to individuals concerned with the trial. It should not be overlooked, although it often is, that one important member of the writing committee is the person responsible for data management. In many cases, such an individual can give vital insight with regard to some fine details as they often have total familiarity with the data. They will certainly be responding to any patient-specific points raised while the publication is in preparation, perhaps having to contact centres to seek clarification with respect to some points of detail.

The writing committee will also have to decide in general terms how information about the trial will be disseminated. We have rather assumed that a paper will be prepared for an appropriate journal within the speciality covered by the topic of the randomized trial. However, there may also be the possibility of several publications of this type, perhaps addressing different endpoints or facets of the trial. For example if, in addition to the primary endpoint of survival time, quality of life had also been assessed (as in Protocol AHCC01), then one paper may be concerned mainly with the survival endpoint (perhaps mentioning only one aspect of the quality of life) and a second could summarize the treatment differences in a longitudinal manner using the full complement of quality of life data. For example, Ang, Lee, Gan, *et al.* (2001, 2003) published two papers on the results of their clinical trial, one comparing the burn wound healing of the two dressings under test and the second summarizing the associated pain levels experienced over the trial period.

In addition to journal publications, the writing committee should also consider presentations at relevant conferences, opportunities for invited talks and possibly meetings with patient groups. For the statistician, and possibly other members, there may be opportunities for spin-off papers describing issues arising from the trial which posed technical challenges of interest to a wider audience.

7.6.3 Practicalities

Following the preliminary work on preparing the publication (while the trial data is still accumulating), the time will come when the data on the database is frozen for purposes of final analysis. Depending on local facilities, sometimes this entails transferring a copy of the database to an analysis file which is then stored in another location on the computer system. The best time for doing this is always a difficult decision, unless the follow-up of randomized participants is of relatively short duration. In this case, the data should be complete shortly after the last patient recruited has been assessed for the relevant endpoint(s). However, even with this simple situation, once the final analysis is commenced it is almost bound to reveal some inconsistencies within the data (despite the careful checking and verification that has taken place) which will need to be resolved. There will often be other items that the writing committee might also wish to investigate in more detail. It may therefore be necessary to update the analysis file with supplementary data. For example, if a per protocol analysis is planned in addition to one using ITT, then two variables may be created within the analysis file which flag (or not) each patient for inclusion in the two distinct analyses. Other variables could be created to specifically identify those patients that are included in each of the spin-off publications or presentations planned.

Once the manuscript is complete and submitted for publication, then the associated frozen database and final version of the analysis file have to be preserved. It is likely that the journal referees will raise questions or seek clarification on certain issues. It is important that these can be addressed in a timely manner, using exactly the same database as for the initial analyses.

In trials with prolonged treatment regimens or extensive follow-up, when to freeze the database is not always entirely obvious. Additional information, including that arriving later than scheduled by the design, may be received at the trials centre on a daily basis. After freezing for analysis, there is only a short period when the database still contains the most up-to-date information. An extreme but very important situation is in trials with patient survival time as the endpoint, when deaths may occur at any time. In such cases, a strategy including several temporary freezes may be appropriate when preparing the trial for publication.

Following the CONSORT guidelines, the trial publication should contain information on the period of patient recruitment as well as the date that the database was closed for the purposes of the analysis presented. It is embarrassing for the authors, and may even prejudice the chances of the article being accepted, if there is a long delay between the date of closure and the date of submission of the article in question. Authors may have little control over the length of the editorial review period but should be ready to act quickly to revise the paper as suggested by the review process or resubmit the paper to another journal if rejected. Such delays, certainly if extensive, may provide the opportunity for the writing committee to move to a more current version of the database.

Once all the editorial processes are complete and the paper is accepted for publication, the database and analysis files that were used for preparing the manuscript should be permanently archived and stored. One reason for this is that, once published, the paper will hopefully stimulate wide interest and this may in turn generate comment in the correspondence column of the journal concerned. Critical or not, such correspondence usually demands a response from the authors and in preparing such a response it may be necessary to reproduce the published data and provide substantiating details from the archive.

7.6.4   New developments

Although the publications arising from the trial data should have been outlined in the trial protocol, the writing committee must also take note of any developments that have occurred in the interval between protocol preparation and completion of the trial. Such developments would be referred to in the corresponding Discussion section of the paper, but may also stimulate some additional examination and analyses of the trial data itself. Further, there may have been some statistical developments that suggest alternative approaches to data analysis and interpretation. It is important that the whole team remain vigilant for new developments that may influence what and how the trial results are reported.

7.6.5 Choice of journal(s)

It is likely that the TSC will have a journal or journals in mind for the eventual publication of the trial results. Since journals tend to have their own in-house rules with respect to many aspects of the publication process, the writing committee should ensure that an early decision is made on their choice of journal and the corresponding 'Instructions to Authors' carefully reviewed. This may lead to, for example, the regular reports from the trial office formatting tabulations as they would appear in the final publication, collating possible 'conflict of interest' statements from the investigating teams, preparing graphics in greyscale and adopting the required format for the reference list and method of citation. The instructions often contain limits for the numbers of words, tables and figures that can be included. Details of how the paper is to be (often electronically) submitted are outlined. Checking on these details will facilitate the preparation process and hence speed up the publication of the trial results.

7.7 The next trial?

Many first trials of collaborate groups often lead to a programme of further trials. This arises as a consequence of assembling the trial investigator teams, the statistical and data management office and the collaborative network which, once established, may be keen to pursue other research ideas arising directly from their first trial experience. An important role of the TSC, with the cooperation of the wider group, may be to identify the next question to follow from results of the current trial. Advance preparation of that anticipated new protocol would become part of the remit of the group. At this stage it is important to review 'what went right' and 'what went wrong' while conducting the current protocol, with the aim of both removing any deficiencies identified to avoid repeating the same mistakes, and learning from 'what went right' to see if even better results can be achieved in the next protocol.

   Ideally if a new protocol is ready to start as soon as the current protocol terminates recruitment, the interest of the collaborative group as a whole will be maintained. This will also enable some members of the support teams (e.g. the trial nurses and statistical teams) to be retained, so that the benefit of their collective experience can influence the successful conduct of the replacement trial.

7.8 Protocols

AHCC01 (1997): Randomised trial of tamoxifen versus placebo for the treatment of inoperable hepatocellular carcinoma. Clinical Trials and Epidemiology Research Unit, Singapore.

AHCC03 (2001). Randomised trial of adjuvant hepatic intra-arterial iodine-131-lipio-
    dol following curative resection of hepatocellular carcinoma. Clinical Trials and
    Epidemiology Research Unit, Singapore.
SQNP01 (1997): Standard radiotherapy versus concurrent chemo-radiotherapy fol-
    lowed by adjuvant chemotherapy for locally advanced (non-metastatic)
    nasopharyngeal cancer. National Medical Research Council, Singapore.

CHAPTER 8

Basics of Analysis

The main outcome of concern for a comparative trial is some measure of the difference between the various intervention groups with respect to the trial endpoint of interest. For a two-group randomized trial this 'effect size' may be the difference in the mean levels of some quantity measured on all participants within the groups, a difference in proportions or a measure of relative survival times. This chapter details the basic features of analysis with stress placed on estimating the effect size of primary concern and therefore providing an estimate of this together with a 95% confidence interval supplemented by a p-value.

8.1   Introduction

The key requirement at the design stage of any clinical trial is to identify the therapeutic question to be posed. The primary objective of participant recruitment is to provide the essential data and the first priority in any analysis is to answer this research question. For a two-arm parallel group trial, this essentially implies estimating the difference between the two treatment or intervention groups concerned. The statistic used for this difference will depend on the endpoint measure concerned. Depending on the situation it may be estimated by, for example, a difference between two group means or by a difference in proportions. We have reported on the results of several clinical trials in Chapter 1 and have highlighted there some summary measures and methods of analysis.

The focus of the analysis of a clinical trial is to estimate the difference between the intervention groups and to provide some measure of the uncertainty expressed through the corresponding confidence interval (CI). In most instances this analysis will be supplemented by the test of the corresponding null hypothesis, to provide a p-value from which statistical significance can be determined.

However, any analysis conducted must take full account of the design chosen. If the design chosen includes stratified randomization, or if several baseline (immediately before randomization) characteristics of the patients themselves strongly influence outcome irrespective of the intervention received, an efficient analysis will take the corresponding feature into account. This is particularly important if the baseline

Randomized Clinical Trials: Design, Practice and Reporting   David Machin and Peter M Fayers
© 2010 John Wiley & Sons, Ltd

measure is the same as that intended as the endpoint. In Example 1.2, the percentage of the body affected by atopic eczema was assessed at baseline and the aim of therapy was to reduce this measure; it was therefore assessed again once therapy had been completed. To account for this additional design feature, the corresponding analysis will require regression or model-based methods, some of which we describe.

To simplify the statistical issues relevant to analysis, we will again assume that we are planning a two-group trial in which participants are allocated at random to the alternative groups and that a single endpoint has been specified in advance. In doing so, we have also indicated how a computer package – in our case Stata (StataCorp, 2008) – would be used in the analytical processes. However, we have often modified the command terminology and the resultant output to make them more readily understandable to those not familiar with the package. We would also caution that statistical packages are continually being modified and improved so that the corresponding commands often change over time. What we describe will generally only give an indication of the precise commands needed for the statistical package used when analyzing a future trial.

8.2   Confidence intervals

From a statistical perspective, when conducting a clinical trial we are using a sample to estimate the true or underlying population values of particular parameters. Consider for the moment a study (as opposed to a trial) whose aim is to estimate the mean blood sugar levels of patients with diabetes receiving a particular form of treatment. Observations taken from these patients provide the summary statistic $\bar{x}$ (the arithmetic mean). We hope this value will be close to the true or population mean μ. As such a statistic is obtained from a sample, there is some uncertainty as to how close it is to the corresponding population value. This uncertainty is expressed by means of the standard error (SE) of the estimate and the associated confidence interval (CI).

Similarly, if a randomized trial had been conducted in such patients to compare a standard (S) with a test (T) therapy, then the trial results would provide two means, $\bar{x}_S$ and $\bar{x}_T$, which are estimates of the corresponding μ_S and μ_T. However, we are really interested in the 'estimated difference' between groups, which is $d = \bar{x}_T - \bar{x}_S$. This provides an estimate of the true difference between treatments, $\delta = \mu_T - \mu_S$.

Example 8.1   Difference in means – reduction in disease activity

One of the comparisons made by Meggitt, Gray and Reynolds (2006, Table 2) of Example 1.2 in their trial in patients with moderate-to-severe eczema is the difference in mean disease activity (SASSAD) reduction between the azathioprine (A) and placebo group (P). Hence the aim of their trial is to estimate the difference $\delta = \mu_A - \mu_P$. Once the trial is completed, the corresponding observed mean reductions in SASSAD are $\bar{x}_A$ and $\bar{x}_P$, respectively, while $d = \bar{x}_A - \bar{x}_P$ provides an estimate of the true difference δ.

In Example 8.1, and in many other situations, d will have an approximately Normal distribution. As a consequence, we can construct a confidence interval – a range of values in which we are confident δ will lie. Such an interval for the population difference δ is:

$$\text{(Estimated difference)} - z_{1-\alpha/2} \times SE(\text{Estimated difference})$$
$$\text{to} \tag{8.1}$$
$$\text{(Estimated difference)} + z_{1-\alpha/2} \times SE(\text{Estimated difference})$$

The values of $z_{1-\alpha/2}$ are found from Table T2. For example, for a 95% CI, $\alpha = 0.05$ and the corresponding value is $z_{0.975} = 1.9600$.

8.3 Statistical tests

8.3.1 Significance tests

Patients recruited to a comparative trial will vary in their basic characteristics and hence in their response to any intervention involved in a trial. Following completion of a trial, an apparent difference between groups may be observed but this may be entirely due to chance. In this case, such differences for one more extreme, do not indicate *real* differences between the groups being compared.

As a consequence of this chance, it is customary to use a 'significance test' to assess the weight of evidence for a real difference between groups. To do this, the probability that the observed difference for one more extreme, could in fact have arisen purely by chance is calculated. The results of the significance test are expressed through this *p*-value.

8.3.2 Null hypothesis

The first step in conducting the significance test is to identify the null hypothesis, termed H_0. This implies for the patients with eczema that $\mu_A = \mu_P$, that is, A and P are equally effective with respect to the mean in SASSAD reduction. Even when this null hypothesis is true, an observed value of d other than zero might well occur following completion of the trial in question. The probability of obtaining the observed difference d or a more extreme one, given that $\mu_A = \mu_P$ is true, can be calculated. If under this null hypothesis the probability (termed the *p*-value) is very small, then we would *reject* this null hypothesis. In such a case we then conclude, for example, that the two regimens (here A and P) do indeed differ in their effect.

The statistical test takes the form:

$$z = \frac{\text{(Statistic)} - \text{(Value of Statistic assuming Null hypothesis true)}}{\text{Standard Error of Statistic assuming Null hypothesis true}}. \tag{8.2}$$

Once the value of z has been obtained we refer this to Table T1 to obtain the total area in the two tails of the standard Normal distribution for the ordinate $|z|$, yielding the (two-sided) p-value. A p-value ≤ 0.05 would indicate that so extreme (or greater) an observed difference could only be expected to have arisen *only by chance* 5% of the time or less. Consequently, it is quite likely that a *real* difference between groups is present. On the other hand, the two-group comparative trial may result in a p-value > 0.05 and be declared 'not statistically significant'. However, such a statement may only indicate that there was insufficient weight of evidence to be able to declare that the observed difference between groups has *not* arisen by chance alone. It does not necessarily imply that there is no (true) difference between the groups.

However, if the sample size were too small the trial would be very unlikely to obtain a significant p-value even when a clinically relevant difference between the intervention groups is truly present. Also, if only a few subjects were included in the trial, then even if there is statistical significance indicating a real difference between groups, the results are likely to be less convincing than if a much larger number of participants had been assessed. The weight of evidence in favour of concluding that there is a clinically important effect will therefore be much less in a smaller trial compared to a larger trial.

8.4   Examples of analysis

8.4.1   Means

If we consider any one of the intervention groups in a clinical trial then, at the planning stage of the trial, the endpoint of concern is characterized by the corresponding values of the (so-called) population mean μ and population standard deviation (SD) of that group σ. Once the trial is complete, the data from m subjects $x_1, x_2, \ldots, x_m$ within one group is available. From these we obtain the estimated mean, $\bar{x}$ and SD s, of that group where

$$\bar{x} = \frac{\sum x_i}{m} \quad \text{and} \quad s = \sqrt{\frac{\sum (x_i - \bar{x})^2}{m - 1}}. \tag{8.3}$$

These summarize the knowledge we now have of the ultimate values of μ and σ which we will never know without an infinitely large trial. At the end of a parallel two-group trial, we have estimates from both intervention groups: $(\bar{x}_1, s_1)$ and $(\bar{x}_2, s_2)$. As we have already indicated, the difference between groups is calculated as $d = \bar{x}_2 - \bar{x}_1$ and this estimates the population difference $\delta = \mu_2 - \mu_1$. In a comparative trial we are usually more interested in estimating the value of δ than its individual components, μ_2 and μ_1.

Example 8.2   Patients with eczema — reduction in SASSAD

Figure 1.1 illustrated the variation in the reduction of SASSAD observed in the trial conducted by Meggitt, Gray and Reynolds (2006, Figure 2A) in 61 patients with moderate-to-severe eczema. Of these, 41 received azathioprine (A) with a mean reduction $\bar{x}_A = 12.93$ and standard deviation $SD_A = 9.30$, while 20 received placebo (P) with $\bar{x}_P = 6.65$ and $SD_P = 7.59$. The between treatments difference is estimated as $d = \bar{x}_A - \bar{x}_P = 12.93 - 6.65 = 6.28$.

To obtain a confidence interval, the standard error of the difference $SE(d)$ first has to be obtained. This is given by

$$SE(d) = \sqrt{\frac{SD_A^2}{m_A} + \frac{SD_P^2}{m_P}}. \tag{8.4}$$

Example 8.2   *(Continued)*

For this example equation (8.4) gives

$$SE(d) = \sqrt{\frac{9.30^2}{41} + \frac{7.59^2}{20}} = 2.2338$$

Using Equation (8.1), the 95% *CI* is $6.28 - 1.96 \times 2.2338$ to $6.28 + 1.96 \times 2.2338$ or 1.90% to 10.66%. This analysis indicates an advantage to A with a mean reduction of 6.28%, but with considerable uncertainty attached to it.

Hence, loosely speaking, we are 95% confident that the true population difference in mean SASSAD reduction between those receiving azathioprine as opposed to placebo for moderate-to-severe patients with eczema lies between 1.9 and 10.7%. Our best estimate is provided by the sample mean difference of 6.3%. These are not exactly the same as given by Meggitt, Gray and Reynolds (2006, Figure 2A) as we have extracted the data from the graphs and all are rounded to integer values.

Strictly speaking, in our description of the results of Example 8.2 it is incorrect to say that there is a probability of 0.95 that the population difference between mean SASSAD reduction lies between 1.9 and 10.7%, as the population difference is a fixed number and not a random variable which does not have a probability attached to it. The value of 0.95 is really the probability that the limits calculated from a random sample will include the population value. For 95% of calculated confidence intervals, it will be true to say that the population mean difference δ lies within this interval.

To calculate the corresponding statistical test, one assumption and several steps are needed. The first is to assume that both the *SD*s are essentially estimating the same population standard deviation, σ. Under this assumption, σ is estimated by

$$S_{Pool} = \sqrt{\frac{(m_A - 1) \times SD_A^2 + (m_P - 1) \times SD_P^2}{(m_A - 1) + (m_P - 1)}}. \tag{8.5}$$

Example 8.2   (Continued)

For this example, the pooled standard deviation is

$$s_{Pool} = \sqrt{\frac{(41-1) \times 9.30^2 + (20-1) \times 7.59^2}{(41-1) + (20-1)}} = 8.786.$$

The standard error takes the same form as Equation (8.4) but with s_{Pool} replacing both SD_A and SD_P. This gives

$$SE_0(d) = 8.786\sqrt{\left(\frac{1}{41} + \frac{1}{20}\right)} = 2.396.$$

The subscript 0 is added to SE to distinguish this situation from that of Equation (8.4).

The corresponding test of significance using Equation (8.2) gives

$$z = \frac{6.28 - 0}{2.396} = 2.62$$

and, from Table T1, p-value $= 2(1 - 0.9956) = 0.0088$. This implies a statistically significant advantage of A over P in these patients.

This analysis is best conducted by a standard statistical package by specifying the statistical test required (**ttest**), the endpoint variable of interest (**SASSAD**) and the groups (**Treat**) to compare. The actual data has to be in a suitable database which can be accessed by the package for this analysis. Edited commands and output for the analysis of SASSAD reduction in patients with eczema are shown in Figure 8.1. There we can identify some of the results of our earlier calculations (although quoted with more decimal places). Key features here are the estimate of the treatment difference (6.276829) and the p-value (0.0112), which are numerically close to those calculated previously.

Despite these similarities there are some differences. For example, the 95% CI of 1.48339 to 11.07027 is somewhat different as it is calculated using the standard error $SE_0(d)$ and not that of Equation (8.4). Further, $z = 2.62$ is replaced by $t = 2.6202$ here. This change of labelling, from z to t, is to indicate that this same command can be used whether sample sizes are large or small. In small samples, the Normal distribution is replaced by the Student's t-distribution (see Table T4), the shape of which depends on the degrees of freedom df. In this example, $m_A = 41$ and $m_P = 20$ so that $df = (m_A - 1) + (m_P - 1) = 59$. This is considered as large, in which case the Student and Normal distributions are very similar so that, for example, p-values obtained from either would numerically be

Example 8.2   *(Continued)*

Analysis command

```
ttest SASSAD, by(Treat)
```

Edited output

```
Two-sample t test with equal variances
-----------------------------------------------------------------------
   Group |   Obs        Mean    Std. Dev.  Std. Err. [95% Conf. Interval]
---------+-------------------------------------------------------------
Azathiop |    41    12.92683    9.296210
 Placebo |    20     6.65000    7.589986
---------+-------------------------------------------------------------
    diff |            6.276829              2.395528  1.48339 to 11.07027
-----------------------------------------------------------------------
    diff = mean(Azathiop) - mean(Placebo)                  t = 2.6202
Ho: diff = 0                              degrees of freedom = 59
                        Ha: diff ! = 0
                      Pr(|T| > |t|) = 0.0112
```

Figure 8.1   Edited commands and output for the analysis of SASSAD reduction in patients with eczema (after Meggit, Gray and Reynolds, 2006)

very close. This will not be the case if *df* is small. However in statistical packages the *t*-test is usually the default, in which case these considerations are automatically taken into account.

One problem with statistical packages is that the output often contains more than that required and so it needs to be examined carefully and superfluous output ignored. Fortunately, most commands and output can be cut-and-pasted into a report document and then suitably edited for the purpose intended, although perhaps still not in the format for submission to a clinical journal whose requirements may be very specific.

8.4.2   Medians

Although the difference between two means is estimated by calculating each separately and then subtracting one from the other, this is not the case when comparing medians. Thus there is a distinction between the 'median difference' and the 'difference of two medians'.

Suppose the observations from one of the groups are labelled $x_1, x_2, \ldots, x_m$ and those of the same endpoint variable from the other as $y_1, y_2, \ldots, y_n$, where m and n are the number of subjects in the respective groups. The median difference is estimated by the median of all the possible $m \times n$ differences $x_i - y_j$, for $i = 1$ to m and $j = 1$ to n.

The confidence interval for the median difference also uses the $m \times n$ differences and, for large samples, first involves calculating

$$K = \frac{mn}{2} - (z_{1-\alpha/2} \times SE_0) \qquad (8.6)$$

where

$$SE_0 = \sqrt{\frac{mn(m+n+1)}{12}}$$

The value of K obtained is then rounded up to the nearest integer value. The $100(1 - \alpha)\%$ CI is then obtained as the interval from the Kth smallest to the Kth largest of the $m \times n$ differences which have been calculated. Campbell and Gardner (2000) give details of what to do if sample sizes are small.

The test for statistical significance is somewhat easier to calculate. This is done by first combining the two sets of data and ranking them from 1 to $m + n$. If there are two or more subjects with the same rank these are called tied observations, in which case each should be given the same rank which is the average of the ranks assigned to each. The ranks are now apportioned among the treatment groups within each category and summed individually to obtain a rank sum W_m and W_n for each group. Note that $W_m + W_n = (m + n)(m + n + 1)/2$ is the sum of all the ranks. Finally the test statistic is

$$z = \frac{W_{Either} - W_0}{SE_0(W_{Either})} = \frac{W_{Either} - \dfrac{Either \times (m + n + 1)}{2}}{\sqrt{\dfrac{mn(m + n + 1)}{12}}}, \qquad (8.7)$$

where $Either$ is one of m or n.

This is in the same format as Equation (8.2) with the statistic as W_{Either} and the terms in the numerator and denominator corresponding to the null hypothesis values of W_{Either}, say

$$W_0 = \frac{Either \times (m + n + 1)}{2},$$

and the standard error (SE_0).

This test is known by two names: either the Wilcoxon rank-sum test or the Mann-Whitney U test. The two names arise from two different approaches to the calculation, which yield identical results.

Example 8.3 Patients with eczema – reduction in SASSAD

As discussed previously, Figure 1.1 illustrated the variation in the reduction of SASSAD observed in the trial conducted by Meggitt, Gray and Reynolds (2006, Figure 2A) in 61 patients with moderate-to-severe eczema. Supposing now we cannot assume that the distributions of SASSAD reductions are approximately Normal as we did when estimating their means. We therefore use the difference in medians to compare the treatments. However, with relatively large numbers $m = 41$ receiving Azathioprine and 20 receiving Placebo, there are therefore $mn = 41 \times 20 = 820$ differences and so the finding the median of these, although not difficult, is very tedious and prone to error. As a consequence, we have used a statistical program with the commands and output as given in Figure 8.2.

Analysis command

```
MTB > Mann-Whitney 95.0 'Azathioprine'   'Placebo';
SUBC > Alternative 0.
Mann-Whitney Test and CI: Azathioprine, Placebo
```

Output

```
                 N  Median
Azathioprine    41  14.000
Placebo         20   7.500

Point estimate for median difference A - P is 6.000
95.2 Percent CI for median difference is (1.002,11.001)
W = 1430.0
Test of null hypothesis is significant at 0.0149
The test is significant at 0.0148 (adjusted for ties)
```

Figure 8.2 Edited commands and output for the analysis of median SASSAD score reduction in patients with moderate-to-severe eczema treated by Azathioprine or Placebo (after Meggitt, Gray and Reynolds, 2006, Table 3)

The median reductions for Azathioprine and Placebo are 14.0 and 7.5%, respectively, and their median difference is estimated to be 6.0%, with 95% CI 1.0 to 11.0%. This contrasts with the difference of medians of $14.0 - 7.5 = 6.5$. The confidence interval excludes the null hypothesis of no difference between treatments. The corresponding output from the statistical test gives p-value $= 0.0149$ which is highly significant. There are several tied observations within the dataset, but taking account of these (as the statistical program does) only has a marginal influence; the p-value is essentially unaltered at 0.0148.

8.4.3 Proportions

In a similar way to the analysis comparing two means, a confidence interval can be derived for a difference in proportions. However if a response rate π rather than a mean

μ is to be estimated, then the *SD* in Equation (8.4) is replaced by $\sqrt{\pi(1-\pi)}$. In this case, the difference between the two proportions is $\delta = \pi_1 - \pi_2$, which has a standard error of

$$SE(d) = \sqrt{\frac{\pi_1(1-\pi_1)}{m_1} + \frac{\pi_2(1-\pi_2)}{m_2}} \tag{8.8}$$

These provide the necessary components for calculating the confidence interval from Equation (8.1).

Example 8.4   Oral lichen planus

In the randomized trial conducted by Poon, Tin, Kim, *et al.* (2006) of Example 2.1, one endpoint of concern was the clinical response at 4 weeks post-randomization to cyclosporine (C) or steroid (S). The observed response rates were $p_S = 37/71 = 0.5211$ and $p_C = 30/66 = 0.4545$, a difference $d = p_S - p_C = 0.0666$ or 6.7%. Thus, replacing π_S and π_C by their respective estimates in Equation (8.8) gives

$$SE(d) = \sqrt{\frac{0.5211(1-0.5211)}{71} + \frac{0.4545(1-0.4545)}{66}} = 0.0853$$

Using Equation (8.1), the 95% *CI* is $0.0666 - 1.96 \times 0.0853$ to $0.0666 + 1.96 \times 0.0853$ or approximately -10.1% to $+23.4\%$. This confidence interval is wide and covers the null hypothesis value $\delta = 0$, and so there is little evidence to suggest that the observed 6.7% advantage to steroid is established.

In Example 8.4 since neither of the response rates is close to 0 or 1, the large sample approximation for the confidence interval used here is likely to be reliable. If one or both of the rates were close to 0 or 1, then a more precise calculation using the recommended method suggested by Newcombe and Altman (2000) and described in Section 8.7 should be used. In this example, the recommended method gives -9.9% to $+22.7\%$ which is very close to the less precise calculations above. Although the approximate calculation gives a more intuitive feel of the processes involved, and so is presented here, the recommended method should always be used in practice.

Example 8.5   Patients with recurrent malaria – clearance of parasites

Zongo, Dorsey, Rouamba, *et al.* (2007, Table 2) of Example 1.7 quote a recurrent malaria parasite clearance rate (PCR) for $AQ + SP$ as $p_{AQ+SP} = 4/233 = 0.0172$ and for AL as $p_{AL} = 25/245 = 0.1020$. This gives $d = 0.0172 - 0.1020 = -0.0848$ or -8.48%. Further using Equation (8.8),

$$SE(d) = \sqrt{\frac{0.0172(1-0.0172)}{233} + \frac{0.1020(1-0.1020)}{245}} = 0.0211,$$

Example 8.5 *(Continued)*

and Equation (8.1) leads to a 95% *CI* for δ as –0.0848 – (1.96 × 0.0211) to –0.0848 + (1.96 × 0.0211) or –0.1262 to –0.0434. To avoid the negative values, the results are phrased as a *reduction* of 8.48% (95% CI 4.34 to 12.62%) in PCR with $AQ + SP$ as compared to *AL*.

In this example each PCR is small, that is, both are close to 0, so that the large-sample expression for the Confidence Interval of Equation (8.1) may not be so reliable. However, using the recommended method as described in Section 8.7, the 95% *CI* is 4.4 to 13.0% which is very similar.

An alternative way of expressing the result when comparing two treatments with a binary outcome is the use the number needed to treat (NNT). In a randomized trial comparing a new treatment with a standard (control), the NNT is the number of patients who need to be treated with the new treatment rather than the standard in order for one additional patient to benefit. The NNT is the reciprocal of the treatment difference. The corresponding confidence interval is obtained as the reciprocal of each confidence limit for the difference itself. In Example 8.5, NNT = $1/0.0848 = 11.8$ or approximately 12 patients, with 95% CI from $1/0.130 = 7.7$ to $1/0.044 = 22.7$ or 8 to 23.

To calculate the *p*-value from the significance test, the standard error has to be calculated under the assumption that the null hypothesis is true, that is, $\pi_{AQ+SP} = \pi_{AL}$, denoted SE_0. This results in

$$SE_0(d) = \sqrt{\overline{\pi}(1 - \overline{\pi})\left(\frac{1}{m_{AQ+SP}} + \frac{1}{m_{AL}}\right)}, \qquad (8.9)$$

where

$$\overline{\pi} = \frac{m_{AQ+SP}\pi_{AQ+SP} + m_{AL}\pi_{AL}}{m_{AQ+SP} + m_{AL}}.$$

The *p*-value is then obtained using Equation (8.2) with estimates provided by the data and referring the value of *z* to Table T1.

Example 8.6   Patients with recurrent malaria – clearance of parasites

For this example,

$$\overline{p} = \frac{m_{AQ+SP}p_{AQ+SP} + m_{AL}p_{AL}}{m_{AQ+SP} + m_{AL}} = \frac{4 + 25}{233 + 245} = 0.0607,$$

$SE_0(d) = 0.0218$ and $z = -0.0848/0.0218 = -3.89$. This is a large (far from zero) value and reference to Table T1 indicates the *p*-value < 0.001. In this example, the standard error under the assumption that the null hypothesis is true is very close

---

Example 8.6   *(Continued)*

to that calculated for the confidence interval; which one is used will have little impact on the interpretation of the results.

As in an earlier example, this analysis is best conducted by a statistical package. The corresponding statistical analysis command of Figure 8.3 is very brief and comprises two portions: the test to be performed (prtesti) followed by the data (233   4   245   25) to be compared and the data type (count).

Analysis command with data

prtesti 233 4 245 25, count

Edited Output

```
Two-sample test of proportion                                  x: Number of obs = 233
                                                               y: Number of obs = 245
------------------------------------------------------------------------------------
Variable |      Mean     Std. Err.     z      P>|z|         [95% Conf. Interval]
---------+--------------------------------------------------------------------------
       x |   0.0171674   0.0085097
       y |   0.1020408   0.0193389
---------+--------------------------------------------------------------------------
    diff |  -0.0848734   0.0211284                      -0.1262843 to -0.0434626
         |   under Ho:   0.0218448
------------------------------------------------------------------------------------
           diff = prop(x) – prop(y)                                     z = -3.8853
       Ho: diff = 0
       Ha: diff != 0                        Pr(|Z| < |z|) = 0.0001
```

Figure 8.3   Edited commands and output for the analysis of parasite clearance (data from Zongo, Dorsey, Rouamba, *et al.*, 2007)

By examining Figure 8.3 we can identify some of the results of our earlier calculations, although quoted with more decimal places. Key features here are the estimate of the treatment difference (−0.0848734), the CI (−0.1262843 to −0.0434626) and the *p*-value (0.0001). These are all close to what we have calculated. Note in particular that the output gives two standard errors, one corresponding to *SE* (0.0211284) and used for the calculation of the confidence interval, and that corresponding to SE_0 (0.0218448) and used for the *z*-test.

It is often convenient, when comparing proportions in two groups, to express these in a relative way by quoting the odds ratio, *OR*. This is defined by

$$OR = \frac{p_2(1 - p_1)}{p_1(1 - p_2)}. \tag{8.10}$$

The corresponding expressions for the standard error and confidence interval are quite complex and are given in Section 8.7 for completeness.

Example 8.7 Patients with recurrent malaria – clearance of parasites

For this example,

$$OR = \frac{p_{AQ+SP}(1 - p_{AL})}{p_{AL}(1 - p_{AQ+SP})} = \frac{0.0172(1 - 0.1020)}{0.1020(1 - 0.0172)} = 0.1540.$$

The result is then expressed as indicating a reduced risk with $AQ + SP$. The null hypothesis of equality of the proportions corresponds to $OR = 1$. Use of the expressions of Equations (8.19) and (8.20) can provide an approximate confidence interval, although we used a statistical package to obtain the 95% CI as 0.06 to 0.47 and a p-value $= 0.0001$. Both indicate a statistically significant result in favour of $AQ + SP$.

8.4.4 Ordered categorical

In certain situations binary data (such as those we have analyzed as a comparison of two proportions) may arise from an underlying categorical variable such as that summarized in Table 8.1, where response to treatment is assessed on a 6-point scale ranging from 'Worse' to 'Complete resolution'. Investigators at the analysis stage could therefore define a satisfactory response as including 'Complete resolution' or 'Striking improvement' and then summarize these rates as 16/41(36.4%) and 1/20 (5.0%). These proportions are then compared using the methods above. However, this is wasteful of the detailed information contained in the categories. In these calculations, those in the corresponding 'not assessed' groups are regarded as not having had an improvement. In practice, how such patients should be dealt with in the analysis would be specified in the trial protocol.

A more useful approach to the comparison of the treatment groups is to use the Wilcoxon test, which involves ranking the individual patients by first combining the

Table 8.1 Investigator assessed response to treatment in patients with moderate-to-severe eczema (after Meggitt, Gray and Reynolds, 2006, Table 3)

Investigator assessed	Azathrioprine	Placebo	All	Ranks	Sum of Ranks Azathrioprine	Placebo
Complete resolution	1	0	1	1	1	—
Striking improvement	15	1	16	2 to 17	142.5	9.5
Moderate improvement	9	8	17	18 to 34	234.0	208.0
Slight improvement	6	4	10	35 to 44	237.0	158.0
No change	5	5	10	45 to 54	247.5	247.5
Worse	0	1	1	55	—	55.0
Not assessed	5	1	6			
Total	41	20	61		$W_A = 862.0$	$W_P = 678.0$

Example 8.8   Patients with eczema — response to treatment

Ignoring the 6 patients of Table 8.1 who were not assessed, there remain $m = 36$ patients in one group and $n = 19$ in the other; a total of $m + n = 55$ patients are ranked. There is only one patient who had 'Complete resolution' and so has rank 1. In contrast, 16 had 'Striking improvement' so they share the ranks from 2 to 17 and are each assigned the average of these ranks $(2 + 17)/2 = 9.5$. Similarly, those 17 with 'Moderate improvement' are assigned $(18 + 34)/2 = 26$ and so on until the 1 patient who is 'Worse' has the lowest rank 55. The ranks are now apportioned among the treatment groups within each category and summed to give the entries in the final two columns of Table 8.1. Note that $W_{36} + W_{19} = (36 + 19)(36 + 19 + 1)/2 = 1540$ in this case.

Analysis command

```
ranksum Grade, by(Treat)
```

Output

```
Two-sample Wilcoxon rank-sum (Mann-Whitney) test

        Treat |      obs    rank sum    expected
 -------------+-----------------------------------
 Azathioprine |       36         862        1008
      Placebo |       19         678         532
 -------------+-----------------------------------
     combined |       55        1540        1540

 unadjusted variance      3192.00
 adjustment for ties      -210.27
                         ---------
 adjusted variance        2981.73

 Ho: Grade(Treat==Azathioprine) = Grade(Treat==Placebo)
              z =   -2.674
     Prob > |z| =   0.0075
```

Figure 8.4   Edited commands and output for the analysis of the response to treatment in patients with mild-to-moderate eczema of Table 8.1 (after Meggitt, Gray and Reynolds, 2006, Table 3)

From these, and using the Azathrioprine group, $W_0 = 36(36 + 19 + 1)/2 = 1008$ and $SE_0 = \sqrt{36 \times 19 \times (36 + 19 + 1)/12} = 3192 = 56.4978$. From Equation (8.7), $z = (862.0 - 1008)/56.4978 = -2.761$. From Table T1, the p-value $= 2(1 - 0.99711) = 0.00578$. This suggests a statistically significant advantage to A over P in these patients.

The corresponding output from a statistical package is summarized in Figure 8.4. The corresponding statistical analysis command comprises the test to be performed (**ranksum**) followed by the endpoint variable (**Grade**) and the groups to be compared (**Treat**). The output differs from our calculations in that $z = -2.674$. However, modifications to the W-test, as we have described it, should be made if there are many tied observations and hence have the same rank value. As a consequence, SE_0 is

Example 8.8 *(Continued)*

modified to become 2981.73 = 54.6052 and so is reduced in size. This adjustment leads to a larger *p*-value = 0.0075 but this has little implication for the interpretation of the results in this example. Nevertheless, this is the appropriate procedure to use and fortunately statistical packages make the necessary adjustment automatically.

two sets of data. Once again, however, a decision as to how the 'non-assessed' are to be utilized in the analysis needs to be pre-specified (for example, by all being ranked as 7 or omitted from the calculations entirely).

8.4.5 Time-to-event

As we have indicated in Chapter 4, time-to-event data are characterized by observations that may be censored. In some subjects, in whom the endpoint 'event' of interest has occurred, the actual survival time *t* is observed. However, other subjects for whom the 'event' has not yet occurred at the last point in their observation time have censored survival times, $T+$. The analysis of these data, which involves either one of *t* or $T+$ for every subject, will involve Kaplan–Meier estimates of the corresponding survival curves.

Calculating the Kaplan–Meier survival curve, even with a small dataset, is a tedious business. It has to be calculated using a large number of decimal places to avoid rounding error and is therefore prone to mistakes. The process first involves ranking the survival times of the group under consideration from smallest to largest. If, in this ordered listing, a *t* and a $T+$ take the same numerical value (i.e. are tied) then the censored observation is given the larger ranking. Alongside each rank, either 1 or a 0 is placed according to whether or not an event had occurred at that time. The *t* will essentially have a 1 attached and the $T+$ a 0.

The simplest situation is illustrated in Figure 8.5a for 15 subjects whose survival time is measured in years and all of whom have died. All survival times are known, and there are no censored observations. The Kaplan–Meier survival curve commences at $t = 0$ when 100% are alive and continues horizontally until $t = 0.088$ years, at which time one patient dies and so the survival curve drops by 1/15 and 14/15 (93.33%) remain alive. The curve then continues horizontally until $t = 0.367$ when 2 of these 14 patients die, thereby leaving (12/14) alive. At this time, 12/15 (80.00%) remain alive. This is equivalent to

$$\frac{14}{15} \times \frac{12}{14} = \frac{12}{15}$$

which is the product of those still alive after the two death times of 0.088 and 0.367 years. This process continues with the death at $t = 0.663$ and the Kaplan–Meier estimate, denoted $S(t)$, is now

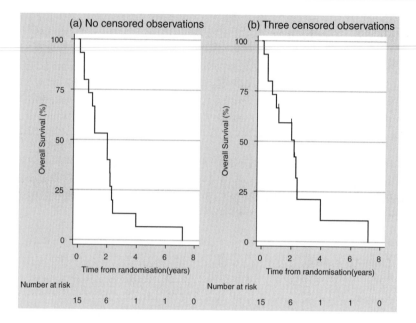

Figure 8.5   Kaplan–Meier survival curves with (a) no censored and (b) censored observations

$$S(0.663) = \frac{14}{15} \times \frac{12}{14} \times \frac{11}{12} = \frac{11}{15}$$

and so on until the final death at $t = 7.159$ when $S(7.159) = 0$. This process is summarized in the **Output** of Figure 8.6a. A step-down plot of the **Survivor Function** against **Time**, or $S(t)$ against t, gives the survival curve of Figure 8.5a.

This laborious process is not essential when there are no censored observations, as the successive survival estimates are simply 14/15, 12/15 and 11/15 (until 0/15) expressed as percentages. However following this process when censored observations are present, as in Figure 8.6b allows the Kaplan–Meier curve to be estimated as follows.

Once again, the Kaplan–Meier survival curve commences at $t = 0$ with 100% alive and continues as before until

$$S(0.942) = \frac{14}{15} \times \frac{12}{14} \times \frac{11}{12} \times \frac{10}{11} = \frac{10}{15} = 0.6667$$

and 10 patients remain. However, the next observation is censored at $T+ = 1.095$ years as no 'event' has occurred for this patient. Beyond this time, there remain only 9 patients on follow-up and at risk of having an 'event'. At $t = 1.103$ when the next event occurs this leaves 8/9 alive. Thus

$$S(1.103) = \frac{14}{15} \times \frac{12}{14} \times \frac{11}{12} \times \frac{10}{11} \times \frac{8}{9} = \frac{10}{15} \times \frac{8}{9} = 0.5926.$$

(a)

Analysis commands – No censored observations

stset OSy, fail(Dead)
sts   list

Output

```
---------------------------------------------------
             Beg.                Net      Survivor
  Time      Total    Fail       Lost      Function
---------------------------------------------------
 0.088       15       1          0         0.9333
 0.367       14       2          0         0.8000
 0.663       12       1          0         0.7333
 0.942       11       1          0         0.6667
 1.095       10       1          0         0.6000
 1.103        9       1          0         0.5333
 1.974        8       1          0         0.4667
 1.982        7       1          0         0.4000
 2.166        6       1          0         0.3333
 2.182        5       1          0         0.2667
 2.292        4       1          0         0.2000
 2.382        3       1          0         0.1333
 3.953        2       1          0         0.0667
 7.159        1       1          0         0.0000
---------------------------------------------------
```

(b)

Analysis commands – With 3 censored observations

stset OSy, fail(NewDead)
sts list

Output

```
---------------------------------------------------
             Beg.                Net      Survivor
  Time      Total    Fail       Lost      Function
---------------------------------------------------
 0.088       15       1          0         0.9333
 0.367       14       2          0         0.8000
 0.663       12       1          0         0.7333
 0.942       11       1          0         0.6667
 1.095+      10       0          1         0.6667
 1.103        9       1          0         0.5926
 1.974+       8       0          1         0.5926
 1.982        7       1          0         0.5079
 2.166        6       1          0         0.4233
 2.182+       5       0          1         0.4233
 2.382        3       1          0         0.2116
 3.953        2       1          0         0.1058
 7.159        1       1          0         0.0000
---------------------------------------------------
```

Figure 8.6 Edited commands and output for the analysis for calculating the Kaplan–Meier survival curves with (a) no censored and (b) censored observations

There is a further censored observation at $T+ = 1.974$ so that

$$S(1.982) = \frac{14}{15} \times \frac{12}{14} \times \frac{11}{12} \times \frac{10}{11} \times \frac{8}{9} \times \frac{6}{7} = 0.5079$$

and this process continues until the final event at $t = 7.159$ when $S(7.159) = 0.000$. The corresponding analysis is summarized in Figure 8.6b. We have highlighted in bold in the Survivor Function columns where the two sets of calculations begin to diverge. The step-down plot of $S(t)$ against t for the censored example is the survival curve of Figure 8.5b.

Note that in both situations, the final values of $S(7.159) = 0.000$. This corresponds to the survival time of the patient with the observed survival time $t = 7.159$, which is longer than any other but has had an 'event' at this (longest of all) time. Had this longest survivor not had the event, then the corresponding observation would be $T+ = 7.158$, and $S(7.158) = 0.1058$ retains the same value as $S(3.953)$.

In order to complete the necessary calculations, the database must contain two variables describing the time-to-event data. One variable is that which contains the individual survival times, while the second contains either 0 or 1 for each subject. Zero indicates a censored observation and 1 indicates that for the corresponding subject the event has actually occurred. In Figure 8.6, 'OSy' represents the overall survival time of these patients from randomization expressed in years, while 'Dead' obviously indicates whether or not still alive (0: alive, 1: dead). The corresponding command **stset OSy, fail(Dead)** describes the data as a time-to-event and which variable indicates the censoring, while **sts list** requests the Kaplan–Meier estimates of the corresponding survival curve.

If we have two groups to compare then each will provide a Kaplan–Meier estimate of the corresponding survival curves. Comparisons between groups can be made using the logrank test. The summary statistic used is the hazard ratio (HR) which is the ratio of the risks of an event in the two groups concerned. The test of the null hypothesis is a test of the equality of these risk rates between the groups with respect to the endpoint (event) concerned. This is expressed as H_0: $HR_0 = 1$. The logrank test is based on the same principles as the Wilcoxon test described earlier. However, the presence of censored observations again makes the calculations tedious and prone to error. Consequently we omit the details here although these can be found in, for example, Machin, Cheung and Parmar (2006a, Chapter 3).

8.4.6   Regression methods

In Section 2.10 we introduced the linear model

$$y = \beta_0 + \beta_1 \tau + \varepsilon \tag{8.11}$$

where y represents the endpoint of interest in the clinical trial, $\tau = 0$ and $\tau = 1$ the two interventions concerned and β_0 and β_1 are the regression constants to be estimated

Example 8.9   Survival of children with advanced neuroblastoma

The Kaplan–Meier estimates of the individual survival curves for children with advanced neuroblastoma, randomized to receiving either retinoic acid or placebo in a double-blind formulation, are shown in Figure 8.7.

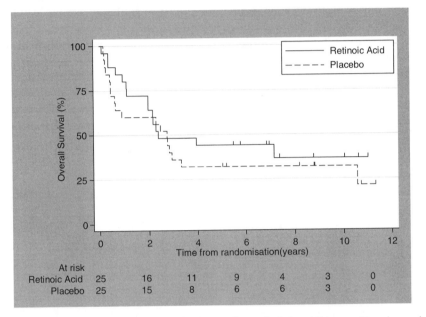

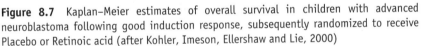

Figure 8.7   Kaplan–Meier estimates of overall survival in children with advanced neuroblastoma following good induction response, subsequently randomized to receive Placebo or Retinoic acid (after Kohler, Imeson, Ellershaw and Lie, 2000)

The corresponding computer output from a calculation of the logrank test is given in Figure 8.8 with the analysis commands indicated. In addition to **stset OSy, fail(Dead)** the logrank test command **sts test Treat** is added. Finally **sts list, by(Treat) at (1 5)** provides the Kaplan–Meier estimates for the two survival curves, printed at 1 and 5 years for each group.

The hazard ratio is estimated by the ratio of two ratios. One is the ratio of the observed number of events to those expected in the Placebo group ($56/55.22 = 1.0141$) and the other for Retinoic acid ($55/55.22 = 0.9960$). Together these give $HR = 0.9960/1.0141 = 0.98$ indicating a marginal advantage to those receiving Retinoic acid. This is very close to the null hypothesis value, $HR_0 = 1$, suggesting no significant difference between treatments. The way in which the number of expected events is calculated depends on the number of subjects within each group, the associated number of events and the total survival time within each group.

As there are only two intervention groups in this example, the familiar z-test can be obtained as the square root of **chi2(1)** in Figure 8.8. In this example,

Example 8.9   (Continued)

$z = 0.00 = 0.00$ also, as only 2 decimal places have been provided in the output. This would give a p-value $= 1$ exactly! However, the computer holds more decimal places internally and provides (**Pr>chi2 0.9669**) or a p-value $= 0.97$. In the situation when there are g (> 2) interventions being compared, the output would contain a term such as **chi2(g-1)** and the p-value would be obtained from a χ^2 (Chi-squared) distribution with $g - 1$ degrees of freedom (*df*). The output illustrated also gives the 1- and 5-year overall survival rates for the two groups (for example, the 5-year rate for Retinoic acid group is estimated to be 39.8%).

Analysis commands

```
stset OSy, fail(Dead)
sts  test  Treat
sts list, by(Treat) at (1 5)
```

Output – Number of observations and failures

```
     failure event: Dead == 1.
obs. time interval : (0, OSy]

--------------------------------------------------

    176   obs.
    111   failures

--------------------------------------------------
```

Output – Logrank test

Treat		Alive	Events observed	Events expected
Retinoic acid		33	55	55.22
Placebo		32	56	55.78
Total		65	111	111.00

chi2(1) $= 0.00$ Pr>chi2 $= 0.9669$

Output – Kaplan-Meier estimates at 1 and 5 years

Time	Total	Fail	Survivor Function	Std. Error	[95% Conf. Int.]	
Retinoic	acid					
1	69	20	0.7727	0.0447	0.6702	0.8469
5	36	4	0.3977	0.0522	0.2957	0.4978
Placebo						
1	65	24	0.7273	0.0475	0.6213	0.8081
5	34	6	0.3964	0.0523	0.2942	0.4967

Figure 8.8   Edited commands and output for the analysis using the logrank test to compare survival curves (after Kohler, Imeson, Ellershaw and Lie, 2000)

from the trial data. We also stated that ε represents the noise (or error); this is assumed to be random and have a mean value of 0 across all subjects recruited to the trial and standard deviation (SD) σ.

However, subtle changes to the form of this model may have to be made to accommodate different endpoint types. We discuss the changes necessary under the relevant sections below. We will not review the details of how the regression coefficients are estimated as this can be found in many statistical texts including Campbell, Machin and Walters (2007). We also rely on computer packages for calculation purposes as is good practice for the clinical trial team.

In this case the analysis command is **regress,** the endpoint variable concerned **SASSAD,** and the two groups are defined by **Treat.** If we compare this output with that of Figure 8.1 then there are some familiar quantities, for example, standard error **(Std.Err)** $= 2.3955$ and $t = -2.62$ (in Figure 8.1, we have 2.395528 and 2.6202, respectively). In addition, from this output the estimated regression coefficients are $b_0 = 12.9268$ and $b_1 = -6.2768$. This leads to the model:

$$y = 12.9268 - 6.2768\tau. \tag{8.12}$$

We noted in Section 2.10 that the difference between treatments is estimated by b_1, which we now compare with **diff** 6.276829 in Figure 8.1. The two methods of analysis give identical results, apart from some arithmetic rounding errors. We shall see that this approach to analysis gives greater flexibility in more complex situations.

Example 8.10   Patients with eczema – reduction in SASSAD

In order to compare the mean SASSAD reduction with Azathioprine and Placebo in patients with moderate-to-severe eczema, the regression command necessary to fit the linear model together with the resulting output is given in Figure 8.9.

Analysis command

regress SASSAD Treat

Output

```
------------------------------------------------------------------------------
  Source |     SS        df        MS                      Number of obs = 61
---------+-----------------------------------              F( 1, 59) = 6.87
   Model |    529.62      1       529.62                   Prob > F = 0.0112
Residual |   4551.33     59        77.14
---------+-----------------------------------
   Total |   5080.95     60
------------------------------------------------------------------------------

  SASSAD |   Coef.      Std. Err.      t      P>|t|       [95% CI]
---------+--------------------------------------------------------------------
   Treat |  -6.2768      2.3955      -2.62    0.011    -11.07 to -1.48
   _cons |  12.9268
------------------------------------------------------------------------------
```

Figure 8.9   Edited commands and output for the analysis from a regression package used to compare the SASSAD score for eczema between two treatment groups (after Meggitt, Gray and Reynolds, 2006, Table 3)

8.4.7   Comparing means

For this situation the model of Equation (8.11) is unchanged with the proviso that the endpoint y can be regarded as a continuous variable with an approximately Normal distribution within each of the (two) groups concerned.

8.4.8   Proportions and the odds ratio

In this situation, it is clear that the endpoint y can only take two values 0 or 1, perhaps representing Present/Absent or Yes/No. Therefore, it cannot have the Normal distribution form which has a possible range of values from $-\infty$ to $+\infty$. Equally, the proportions, p_1 and p_2, observed with the feature in each group, must lie between 0 and 1 (equivalently 0 to 100%). One solution to this is to use $y = \log [p/(1 - p)]$ on the right-hand side of Equation (8.10) instead; this is termed logit (p). Suppose $p = 0.01$, then logit $(0.01) = -4.60$; if $p = 0.5$ then logit$(1) = 0$ and if $p = 0.99$, then logit$(0.99) = + 4.60$. These values suggest a range of possible values on this scale from $-\infty$ to $+\infty$ with 0 in the middle. The linear model is then expressed

$$\text{logit}(p) = \beta_0 + \beta_1 \tau + \varepsilon. \tag{8.13}$$

The regression parameters of this model can be fitted using logistic regression.

Example 8.11   Oral lichen planus

In the randomized trial conducted by Poon, Tin, Kim, *et al.* (2006), one endpoint of concern was the clinical response at 4 weeks post-randomization to cyclosporine (C) or steroid (S). The observed response rates were $p_S = 0.5211$ and $p_C = 0.4545$, giving an odds ratio

$$OR = \frac{p_C(1 - p_S)}{p_S(1 - p_C)} = \frac{0.4545(1 - 0.5211)}{0.5211(1 - 0.4545)} = 0.7657,$$

indicating a greater response rate in favour of S. This is almost exactly reproduced in the lower section of Figure 8.10 where it is highlighted. The associated 95% CI is 0.391 to 1.499, which covers the null hypothesis value of $HR_0 = 1$ and the p-value $= 0.436$. However, preceding this section is the analysis command to fit Equation (8.13) above, yielding estimates of the regression coefficients as $b_0 = 0.0845574$ and $b_1 = -0.2668789$. From these, we have $\exp(-0.2668789) = 0.7658$, which equals the OR we had before. The analysis commands (**logit Response Treat**) and (**logistic Response Treat**) are therefore two ways of carrying out the same analysis: one expressing the results in terms of regression coefficients and the other by use of the OR.

Example 8.11 *(Continued)*

Analysis command

```
logit Response Treat
```

Output

```
Logistic regression                              Number of obs = 137
                                                   LR chi2 (1) = 0.61
                                                 Prob > chi2 = 0.4358
Log likelihood = -94.62466
------------------------------------------------------------------
Response |    Coef.    Std. Err.    z    P>|z|    [95% Conf. Interval]
---------+--------------------------------------------------------
   Treat | -0.2668789  0.3428555  -0.78  0.436  -0.9388634 to 0.4051055
   _cons |  0.0845574  0.2375685
------------------------------------------------------------------
```

Analysis command

```
logistic Response Treat
```

Output

```
------------------------------------------------------------------
Logistic regression                              Number of obs = 137
                                                   LR chi2 (1) = 0.61
                                                 Prob > chi2 = 0.4358
Log likelihood = -94.62466
------------------------------------------------------------------
Response | Odds Ratio  Std. Err.    z    P>|z|    [95% Conf. Interval]
---------+--------------------------------------------------------
   Treat | 0.7657658   0.262547   -0.78  0.436    0.3910721 to 1.499461
------------------------------------------------------------------
```

Figure 8.10 Edited commands and output from a regression package used for the analysis of data on oral lichen planus (data from Poon, Tin, Kim, *et al.*, 2006)

8.4.9 Ordered categorical

In the case of logistic regression, the endpoint has one of the two values 0 or 1. When we have ordered categorical data that can take one of J responses, it is convenient to label the response options $1, 2,\ldots, J$. We can then develop a model that is based on a generalization of logistic regression. There are a number of approaches that can be adopted, and we shall describe one of the more common methods, known as the proportional odds model.

Equation (8.13) described the logistic model as $\mathrm{logit}(p) = \beta_0 + \beta_1\tau + \varepsilon$. Since p is the probability that the outcome Y is positive (i.e. equal to 1), we could instead have written $P(Y=1)$ to mean the probability that $Y=1$. This implies logit $\{P(Y=1)\} = \beta_0 + \beta_1\tau + \varepsilon$.

The proportional odds model extends this for the J outcomes, giving:

$$\mathrm{log\,it}\{P(Y \leq j)\} = \alpha_j + \beta_1\tau + \varepsilon, \text{ for } j = 1, 2, \ldots, J-1. \tag{8.14}$$

The α_j values represent a set of constants for the $J-1$ cut-points. The model is therefore effectively analyzing each of the $J-1$ ways that the responses can be combined, ≤ 1, ≤ 2, $\leq 3, \ldots, \leq J-1$. Since β_1 does not have a subscript j, it will have the same value for all of the $J-1$ thresholds. Thus the odds-ratio β_1 is assumed to be the same no matter how we collapse the categories: hence the name 'proportional odds'. When fitting model (8.14) using a computer package, the software is effectively solving the equation for all possible $J-1$ thresholds simultaneously, in order to estimate the single best value of β_1.

Apart from the fact that there are now $J-1$ cut-points instead of the single binary one, the computer output from ordered logistic regression is very similar to that of (simple) logistic regression, and can be displayed either as coefficients or odds ratios. In fact, ordered logistic regression can be applied to the binary data of Figure 8.10, in which case identical results would be obtained. It is however more complex to use since when there are several response options it becomes important to scrutinize the validity of the assumptions. In particular, it should be determined whether the odds-ratio really does appear to be constant across all of the thresholds. If this is not the case, other models should be explored.

8.4.10   Time-to-event

Although we will not go into full details in the case of time-to-event data, the basic regression model is modified to

$$\log\ (HR) = \beta_1 \tau + \varepsilon. \tag{8.15}$$

This is termed the Cox (after DR Cox) proportional hazards regression model, more details of which can be found in Machin, Cheung and Parmar (2006). Fitting this model to the data using the command (**stcox Treat**) with the survival data of the children with neuroblastoma gives the results depicted in Figure 8.11.

The output from the command **stcox Treat** gives an $HR = 0.992151$ which is very close to that which we had calculated earlier: 0.98. The commands which corresponds more directly to the regression equation format are **stcox Treat, nohr** which leads directly to $\log\ (HR) = -0.00788\tau$ and from which, with $\tau = 1$, $\exp(-0.00788) = 0.992151$ as previously noted.

8.4.11   Extending regression models

The corresponding randomization in the trial of children with neuroblastoma was stratified by two disease stages, and this fact needs to be taken account of in the analysis. The extended command (**sts test Treat, strata(stage)**) does this. The highlighted expected number of events in Figure 8.11 is taken from the non-stratified logrank test of Figure 8.8, which can be directly compared to those obtained taking the stratification by stage into account. In this example, there is no material difference between the two analyses (unstratified or stratified), so the interpretation remains the same.

Although these results are no different from those obtained earlier, the advantage of the Cox, and any other regression model, is that it can be extended to include covariates

Analysis commands

```
stset OSy, fail(Dead)

stcox Treat
stcox Treat, nohr

sts test Treat, strata(stage)
```

Edited output

```
Cox regression -- Breslow method for ties

        failure_d:  Dead
analysis time _t:  OSy

No. of subjects = 176
No. of failures = 111

chi2(1) = 0.00, Prob > chi2 = 0.96693
-----------------------------------------------------------------
   _t | Haz. Ratio   Std. Err.    z     P>|z|        [95% Conf. Int.]
------+----------------------------------------------------------
Treat | 0.992151     0.188497   -0.04  0.967    0.683691 to 1.439779
-----------------------------------------------------------------


-----------------------------------------------------------------
   _t |    Coef.     Std. Err.    z     P>|z|        [95% Conf. Int.]
------+----------------------------------------------------------
Treat | -0.00788     0.189988   -0.04  0.967    -0.380250 to 0.36449
-----------------------------------------------------------------

Stratified log-rank test for equality of survivor functions
--------------+----------------------------------------
              |  Events      Events        From
    Treat     | observed   expected(*)   Figure 8.8
--------------+----------------------------------------
Placebo       |    56        55.89         (55.78)
Retinoic acid |    55        55.11         (55.22)
--------------+----------------------------------------
Total         |   111       111.00
--------------+----------------------------------------
(*) sum over calculations within stage
chi2(1) = 0.00, Pr>chi2 =      0.9826
```

Figure 8.11   Edited commands and output from a regression package using the Cox model for the logrank and stratified logrank test to compare survival curves (part data from Kohler, Imeson, Ellershaw and Lie, 2000)

by appropriately adapting Equation (8.12). In the case of a single covariate x, the model becomes:

$$\log{(HR)} \ = \ \beta_1\tau + \beta_2 x + \varepsilon. \tag{8.16}$$

Analysis commands

```
stcox Treat Agem, nohr
stcox Treat Agem
```

Output – giving regression coefficients

```
        failure_d:  Dead
analysis time_t:  OSy
```

Cox regression -- Breslow method for ties

No. of subjects =	176	Number of obs = 176
No. of failures =	111	
Time at risk =	748.2573582	
LR chi2(2) =	699.58	
Log likelihood = -174.50631		Prob > chi2 = 0.0000

t	Coef.	Std. Err.	z	P>|z|	[95% Conf. Int]
Treat	0.02497	0.14510	0.17	0.863	-0.2594 to 0.3094
Agem	-0.58366	0.01271	-45.91	0.000	-0.6086 to -0.5587

Output – giving HR

t	Haz. Ratio	Std. Err.	z	P>|z|	[95% Conf. Int]
Treat	1.0253	0.1415	0.17	0.863	0.7716 to 1.3626
Agem	0.5576	0.007093	-45.91	0.000	0.5441 to 0.5719

Figure 8.12   Edited commands and output from a statistical package using the Cox model to compare survival in two treatment groups taking into account patient age which is known to be strongly predictive of outcome (part data from Kohler, Imeson, Ellershaw and Lie, 2000)

For example, suppose age is *known* to be prognostic for outcome. The investigators will need to check if the treatment comparison, in this case the estimate of β_1, is modified by taking age into account. Thus in Figure 8.12 the continuous variable age in months (**Agem**) is added to the regression model using the command (**stcox Treat Agem, nohr**). This gives the regression coefficient for Treat as $b_1 = 0.02947$ rather than -0.0078 of Figure 8.11. This has changed the regression coefficient from suggesting a marginal advantage to retinoic acid to a marginal disadvantage, although the corresponding p-value $= 0.863$ indicates that there is little evidence against the null hypothesis of no difference between treatments. The corresponding hazard ratio is obtained using (**stcox Treat Agem**) and gives $HR = \exp(0.02497) = 1.025$.

Age appears to be very strongly prognostic in these patients, although taking account of age changes the estimate of the *HR* only marginally. Nevertheless, care needs to be taken to ensure this is truly the case. A more detailed scrutiny of these data is required before a firm view of how survival is influenced by age can be determined. We are using this as a statistical example – not a definitive indication. In the context of a clinical trial we are not directly interested in the influence of age, but only whether knowledge of a patient's age influences to any degree our estimate of β_1. Age therefore constitutes what is known as a 'nuisance covariate'. As we have noted, in this example, age appears to be of strong prognostic importance but does not change our estimate of β_1 materially.

The above example provides us with the rationale for using regression-based methods for the analysis of clinical trials. Seldom will a univariate comparison, whether of means, proportions or survival rates, be sufficient for the eventual analysis of any randomized trial. Consequently, most trials will require some adjustment to the simple comparison, perhaps necessitated by using a stratified design or when (as is often the case) known prognostic factors are present. In theory, the simplest model of Equation (8.11) (suitably adapted to the type of endpoint variable of concern) can be extended without end to include k variables by means of:

$$y = \beta_0 + \beta_1 \tau + \beta_2 x_2 + \beta_3 x_3 + \ldots + \beta_k x_k + \varepsilon. \tag{8.17}$$

However, the main focus still remains on estimating β_1, which measures the effect of the intervention, and good practice should confine the x variables (the covariates) to the randomization strata (if any) and at most to one or two key (and known to be) *major* influencing prognostic factors.

8.5   Other issues

8.5.1   Missing values

If information is missing on an endpoint variable, then the trial size is effectively reduced so that, at the very least, the precision of the final estimate of the difference measure between interventions will be reduced. If the number missing is considerable, then there will be some concern as to whether the comparisons between groups may be biased in some way.

In certain situations, 'missing' values may be anticipated but are not missing in the conventional sense of the relevant information being absent. In assessing the clinical response following treatment for moderate-to-severe eczema of Example 8.8 (summarized in Table 8.1), there may have been good clinical reasons why 6 patients were 'Not assessed'. However, if the possibility of these arising was anticipated at the planning stage of the trial, then suitable action if these arise should have been specified. Thus a statement in the protocol might indicate that any 'Not assessed' patients will be regarded as eczema 'Worse' (or subject 'Ignored') for trial summary purposes. Table 8.13 summarizes the results obtained if the 'missing' cases are 'ignored' or regarded as 'worse' in the example of Table 8.1.

This example illustrates a critical situation in that one analysis suggests a statistically significant advantage of Azathioprine over Placebo (p-value $= 0.008$), whereas

---

Analysis command

Missing values omitted

```
nptrend Grade, by (Treat)
```

Missing values classed as Worse

```
nptrend NewGrade, by (Treat)
```

Output

Missing values omitted

```
Treat        score        obs      sum of ranks
   0            0           36          1154
   1            1           19           386

       z = -2.67
```
Prob > **|z|** = **0.008**

Missing values classed as Worse

```
Treat        score        obs      sum of ranks
   0            0           41          1390
   1            1           20           501

       z = -1.88
```
Prob > **|z|** = **0.061**

Figure 8.13   Edited commands and output for the analysis from a regression package used to compare the SASSAD score for eczema   between two treatment groups (data from Meggitt, Gray and Reynolds,   2006, Table 3)

---

the other analysis suggest the difference is of marginal statistical significant (p-value $= 0.061$). This is one reason why Good Clinical Practice insists that the statistical analysis plan in the protocol must specify what is to be done should such circumstances arise.

8.5.2   Graphical methods

In many situations summary statistics, albeit very useful, do not necessarily convey all the salient features of the trial results. For example, although Figure 1.1 indicates an advantage to Azathioprine in patients with moderate-to-severe eczema, there is considerable variation about the respective mean values of 12.93% and 6.65%. Even in the Placebo group, the majority of patients appear to benefit from the treatment they received. Further, there are also many patients receiving Azathioprine who do not appear to benefit greatly. The graphs in the corresponding report by Meggitt, Gray and Reynolds (2006, Figure 2) provide the reader with a very useful view of what is going on. Many tips to assist with the graphical presentation of data are provided by Freeman, Walters and Campbell (2008).

8.5.3   Multiple endpoints

We have based the above discussion on the assumption that there is a single identifiable endpoint or outcome, upon which treatment comparisons are based. However, there is often more than one endpoint of interest within the same trial. For example, a trial could be assessing wound healing time, pain levels and MRSA infection rates. If one of these endpoints is regarded as more important than the others, it can be named as the primary endpoint of the trial and any statistical analysis focuses on that and that alone. A problem arises when there are several outcome measures which are all regarded as *equally* important. A commonly adopted approach is to analyze each endpoint distinctly from every other.

Unfortunately, the multiple significance tests and associated confidences intervals are all calculated using the same patients, albeit on distinct outcome variables for each. It is well recognized that this causes the p-values to become distorted. Often a smaller p-value will be considered necessary for statistical significance to compensate for this. An equivalent strategy is to multiply the p-values obtained by the number of endpoints analyzed, say k, and hence only declare those comparisons as statistically significant if the revised value is less than (say) the conventional 0.05.

However, there is no entirely satisfactory solution to this problem, so we would reiterate the importance of identifying only one, two at the most, primary endpoints and confining hypotheses testing to just these. Any analyses conducted on other endpoints should be regarded more as hypothesis generating comparisons rather than for drawing definitive conclusions concerned with treatment differences.

8.5.4   Stopping rules

We have discussed in Chapter 7 the role of a Data Monitoring Committee (DMC). Whether formally constituted, or perhaps consisting of the trial statistical and data management team, the role of the DMC is to oversee the trial as it progresses with particular emphasis on recruitment targets, appropriate trial size, safety concerns and evidence that may justify closing the trial early. One aspect of this work may be for the DMC to review planned interim analyses of the data as we discussed in Example 3.23 of Section 3.10, in which the trial protocol set out a specific requirement to review the number of local relapses after every 14 patients completing one-year on trial post diagnosis. If the observed number of relapses exceeded those specified, then 'these numbers will be an indication to resume the use of local radiation therapy'. For this trial in children with Wilms' tumour, the trial statistician was responsible for advising the TSC should such a situation occur.

In other circumstances, the interim analyses will take the form of that planned for the primary endpoint at the end of the trial and may concern a continuous, binary, ordered categorical or time-to-event variable, taking the form of one or other of the examples we have described in this chapter. No new principles are therefore concerned. However, the trial design team have to decide on the frequency of such interim analyses and also be aware that multiple looks at (ever accumulating) data on the same endpoint variable raises the same issues as those concerned with multiple endpoints. In this situation, the lack of independence of the successive analyses causes the p-values to become distorted; the

Table 8.2   Change in overall significance level and suggested nominal significance level with an increasing number of schedule interim analyses (after Pocock, 1983, pp. 148–149)

Maximum number of *interim* statistical tests of the primary endpoint	Overall significance level	Nominal significance level
0	0.05	0.05
1	0.08	0.029
2	0.11	0.022
3	0.13	0.018
4	0.14	0.016
. . .	. . .	. . .
9	0.19	0.0106

Example 8.12   Resectable hepatocellular carcinoma

As we noted in Example 7.2, Lau, Leung, Ho, *et al.* (1999) planned for a single interim analysis using a nominal significance level of 0.029 when 30 patients had entered the trial, and had a median follow-up of 2 years. They report their interim analysis as follows:

> Between April 1992 and July 1996, 30 patients (14 in the treatment group and 16 controls) entered the study and the first interim analysis was done in October 1996. There were 3 (21%) and 11 (68.8%) recurrences in the treatment and control groups respectively (p = 0.01). . . . . In view of the significant improvement in disease-free survival in the treatment group (p < 0.029, the Pocock boundary), we stopped the randomization . . . .

However during the interval, while the median follow-up was accruing to 2 years for these 30 patients and the period for analysis and examination of the interim results, a further 13 patients had entered the trial. The eventual analysis presented on all 43 patients resulted in a *p*-value = 0.037 which, while still regarded as statistically significant by the authors, is much larger than that obtained at the interim analysis.

The trial was designed to recruit 120 patients on the basis of an anticipated hazard ratio (*HR*) of $HR_{\text{Plan}} = 0.5$ in favour of lipiodol. The interim value reported was $HR_{\text{Interim}} = 0.23$ (a far larger benefit than the large benefit anticipated) and that of the final analysis based on 43 patients was $HR_{\text{Final}} = 0.37$. This latter value moves the estimate of the benefit closer to the planning value.

This example highlights the difficulties posed by any interim analysis: they are necessarily based on relatively few patients; are very sensitive to chance fluctuations; and, if declared statistically significant, provide an estimate of the treatment effect much larger than that anticipated by the design. Such analyses therefore have to be viewed with extreme caution by the DMC before making their recommendations.

greater the number of interim analyses, the greater the distortion. Consider the example of using a continuous endpoint variable for comparing two treatment groups. If the significance level planned for the final analysis of the completed trial is 5%, this level increases to 8%, 14% and 19% if 2, 5 or 10 interim looks, respectively, at the data are made, as shown in Table 8.2. Essentially these imply that the more we look at the data, the more likely are we to reject the null hypothesis even if true. This raises the distinct possibility of inappropriately claiming efficacy and stopping a trial early as a consequence. One way round this difficulty is to introduce a nominal significance level whose value depends on the number of interim analyses planned, as described by Pocock (1983). If two interim analyses are planned Table 8.2 suggests that, to declare statistical significance (at the 5% level set by the design), any p-value obtained should be less than 0.022.

8.6 Practice

As should be fully appreciated, clinical trials are a major undertaking. The precious data which have been accumulated deserve a careful and rigorous analysis based on a framework set out within the protocol. This analysis demands the full use of the statistical team and the latest in analysis techniques including graphics routines and appropriate computer software. No home-grown analysis packages should be used nor hand calculations – even of elementary comparisons. It is also important that the data are fully explored, although checking for inconsistencies and out-of-range problems should have been addressed as the trial progresses starting with the information from the first recruit. Many trials take a long time to complete, so that analysis plans set down in the protocol may not be the most appropriate when the time comes for analysis and synthesis. Although the trial team are obliged to analyze and report in the way prescribed, this should not prevent them from making full use of any new (statistical and software) developments that have arisen in the interim. Any such supplementary analysis should be reported as such and the implications on any (new) interpretations highlighted. The statistical team must be involved in all stages of the trial, from beginning to end; it is poor practice just to pass the final 'parcel' of data to an outside statistical team who are not fully integrated into the process.

8.7 Technical details

8.7.1 Standard Normal distribution

The standardized Normal distribution has a mean equal to 0 and a standard deviation (SD) equal to 1. The probability density function of such a Normally distributed random variable z is given by

$$\phi(z) = \frac{1}{\sqrt{2\pi}} \exp\left(-z^2/2\right). \tag{8.18}$$

The curve described by Equation (8.18) is shown in Figure 8.14.

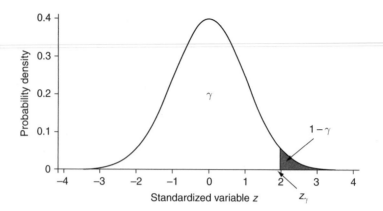

Figure 8.14   The probability density function of a standardized Normal distribution

For several purposes we shall need to calculate the area under some part of this Normal curve. To do this, use is made of the symmetrical nature of the distribution about the mean of 0 and the fact that the total area under a probability density function is unity.

Any unshaded area, such as that depicted in Figure 8.14, which has area γ (here $\gamma \geq 0.5$) has a corresponding value of z_γ along the horizontal axis that can be calculated. For areas with $\gamma < 0.5$ we can use the symmetry of the distribution to calculate, in this case, the values for the shaded area. For example if $\gamma = 0.5$, then we can see from Figure 8.14 that $z_\gamma = z_{0.5} = 0$. It is also useful to be able to find the value of γ for a given value of z_γ. For example, if $z_\gamma = 1.9600$ then $\gamma = 0.975$. In this case, the unshaded area of Figure 8.14 is then 0.975 and the shaded area is $1 - 0.975 = 0.025$.

Table T1 gives the value of z for differing values of γ. Thus for a 1-tailed or 1-sided $\alpha = 1 - \gamma = 0.025$ we have $z = 1.9600$. As a consequence of the symmetry of Figure 8.14, if $z = -1.9600$ then $\alpha = 0.025$ is also in the lower tail of the distribution. Hence $z = 1.9600$ corresponds to two-tailed or two-sided $\alpha = 0.05$.

As we have indicated following Equation (8.1), a 95% CI requires $z_{0.975} = 1.9600$. Further, from Table T1 or Table T2 for a 99% CI, $z_{0.995} = 2.5758$.

8.7.2   Recommended method for comparing proportions

Newcombe and Altman (2000, pp. 46–49) describe a recommended method for calculating a $100(1 - \alpha)\%$ confidence interval for a single proportion, with lower limit (L) to upper limit (U) defined by

$$L = (A - B)/C \quad \text{to} \quad U = (A + B)/C, \tag{8.19}$$

where $A = 2mp + z^2_{1-\alpha/2}$; $B = z_{1-\alpha/2}\sqrt{z^2_{1-\alpha/2} + 4mp(1 - p)}$; $C = 2(m + z^2_{1-\alpha/2})$, m is the number of subjects in the group and p is the observed proportion of responses.

In the case of two intervention groups of size m and n with corresponding estimated proportions of p_1 and p_2, the estimated difference is $d = p_1 - p_2$. To calculate the corresponding confidence interval, Equation (8.19) is evaluated for each group to obtain L_1, U_1 and L_2, U_2. The $100(1 - \alpha)\%$ confidence interval for the true difference in proportions δ is then

$$d - \sqrt{(p_1 - L_1)^2 + (U_2 - p_2)^2} \quad \text{to} \quad d + \sqrt{(p_2 - L_2)^2 + (U_1 - p_1)^2}. \quad (8.20)$$

Note that the difference d is not generally at the midpoint of this interval.

8.7.3 Confidence interval for an odds ratio

The estimated $100(1 - \alpha)\%$ CI for the true OR is given by

$$\exp\left[\log OR - z_{1-\alpha/2}SE(\log OR)\right] \quad \text{to} \quad \exp\left[\log OR + z_{1-\alpha/2}SE(\log OR)\right]$$
$$(8.21)$$

where

$$SE(\log OR) = \left[\frac{1}{mp_1(1 - p_1)} + \frac{1}{np_2(1 - p_2)}\right]^{1/2}. \quad (8.22)$$

CHAPTER 9

Trial Size

This chapter outlines the basic components required for trial size calculations. However, the determination of the number of patients to recruit to a trial depends on several factors. An important factor is the type of endpoint concerned, for example continuous, binary or time-to-event, and hence the form the statistical analysis will ultimately take. The approach to sample size calculation requires the concepts of the null and alternative hypotheses, significance level, power and (for the majority of situations) the anticipated difference between groups or effect size. We stress the importance of providing a realistic estimate of the latter at the design stage.

9.1   Introduction

Investigators, grant-awarding bodies and biotechnology companies all wish to know how much a trial is likely to cost them. They would also like to be reassured that their money is well spent, by assessing the likelihood that the trial will give unequivocal results. In addition, the regulatory authorities including the Committee for Proprietary Medicinal Products in the European Union, the Food and Drug Administration in the United States and many others require information on planned trial size. To this end, many pharmaceutical and related biomedical companies provide guidelines for Good Clinical Practice (GCP) in the conduct of their clinical trials, and these generally specify that a sample size calculation is necessary.

When designing a new trial, the size (and of course the design) should be chosen so that there is a reasonable expectation that the key question(s) posed will be answered. If too few patients are involved, the trial may be a waste of time because realistic medical improvements are unlikely to be distinguished from chance variation. A small trial with no chance of detecting a clinically meaningful difference between treatments is unfair to all the trial participants who are subjected to the risk and discomfort of the clinical trial. On the other hand, recruiting too many participants is a waste of resources and may be unfair if, for example, a larger than necessary number of patients receive the inferior treatment when one treatment could have been shown to be more effective with fewer patients.

Providing a sample size is not simply a matter of identifying a single number from a set of tables, but a process with several stages. At the preliminary stage, 'ball-park' figures are required that enable the investigators to judge whether or not to start the detailed planning of the trial. If a decision is made to proceed, then a subsequent stage is to refine the calculations for the formal trial protocol itself. For example, when a clinical trial is designed, a realistic assessment of the potential superiority (the anticipated benefit or effect size) of the proposed test therapy must be made before any further planning. The history of clinical trials research suggests that, in certain circumstances, rather ambitious or overoptimistic views of potential benefit have been claimed at the design stage. This has led to trials being conducted of insufficient size to reliably answer the underlying questions posed.

To estimate the number of subjects required for a trial, we have to first identify a single major outcome that is regarded as the primary endpoint for measuring efficacy.

If a trial has more than one primary endpoint, we have to evaluate the sample size for each endpoint in turn (possibly allowing for the anticipated use of a correction factor for multiple testing) and use the maximum of these estimates. The trial size calculation is therefore reduced to multiple calculations, each for a single outcome. (see Section 9.6).

Consider the regression coefficient of β_1 in the model (2.1). We showed that this corresponds to the true or population difference between two groups. Once we conduct our clinical trial, then the corresponding data estimates this quantity with b_1. However, at the planning stage of the trial, we certainly do not know β_1 since determining this is the research question. Neither do we know b_1 as the trial has not yet been conducted. Nevertheless at the planning stage, in order to calculate sample size, we need to postulate a value for b_1, which we denote by $\beta_{1\text{Plan}}$. We hope that $\beta_{1\text{Plan}}$ will be close to β_1, but we do not know this. At the end of the trial b_1 may or may not be close to $\beta_{1\text{Plan}}$ but, whether this is the case or not, we use it as an estimate of β_1. The associated confidence interval provides a measure of our uncertainty with respect to the true value.

Although for analysis purposes in Chapter 8 we focused more on confidence intervals than on testing hypotheses to obtain p-values, for the purpose of planning the size of a trial the discussion is conducted more easily in terms of testing hypotheses.

9.1.1 Caution

In what follows it is important to keep the differences between β_1, $\beta_{1\text{Plan}}$ and b_1 in mind as, sometimes, the notation we have to use in what follows does not always make this easy.

Further, using β for the power (see below) as well as for describing the regression coefficients may also cause confusion, although this usage tends to be standard practice.

9.2 Significance level and power

9.2.1 Significance level

At the planning stage of a trial we have to define a value for the significance level α so that, once the trial is completed and analyzed, a p-value smaller than this would lead to the rejection of the null hypothesis. If the p-value $\leq \alpha$, we therefore reject the null hypothesis of a zero effect size, $\delta = 0$, and conclude that there is a statistically significant difference between the interventions – in other words $\delta \neq 0$. On the other hand, if the p-value $> \alpha$ then we do not reject the null hypothesis and accept that δ could be zero. Although the value of α is arbitrary, it is often taken as 0.05 or 5%.

For example, at the end of a trial a p-value ≤ 0.05 would indicate that so extreme (or greater) an observed difference could only be expected to have arisen by *chance alone* 5% of the time or less. In consequence therefore, it is quite likely that a *real* difference between groups is present. On the other hand, the trial may result in a p-value > 0.05 and be declared 'not statistically significant'. However, such a statement may indicate that there was insufficient evidence to be able to declare that 'the observed difference between groups has *not* arisen by chance alone'. It does not imply that there is necessarily 'no (true) difference between the groups'.

Even when the null hypothesis is in fact true, there is still a risk of rejecting it. To reject the null hypothesis when it is true is to make a Type I error. Plainly, the associated probability of rejecting the null hypothesis when it is true is equal to α. The quantity α is interchangeably termed the significance level or probability of a Type I (or false-positive) error and sometimes as the test size.

9.2.2 The alternative hypothesis

Usually with statistical significance tests (see Chapter 8), by rejecting the null hypothesis we do not accept any specific alternative hypothesis. Hence it is usual, and good practice, to report the range of plausible population values of the true difference with a confidence interval. However, sample-size calculations require us to provide a specific alternative hypothesis, H_A. This specifies a particular value of the effect size δ which is not equal to zero.

9.2.3 Power

The 'power' of a significance test is the probability that such a test will produce a statistically significant result, given that a true difference between groups of a certain magnitude truly exists.

The clinical trial could yield an observed difference that would lead to a p-value $> \alpha$ even although the null hypothesis is really not true, that is, $\delta \neq 0$. In such a situation, we then accept (more correctly phrased as 'fail to reject') the null hypothesis although it is truly false. This is called a Type II (false-negative) error and the probability of this is denoted β.

The probability of a Type II error is based on the assumption that the null hypothesis is not true, that is, $\delta \neq 0$. There are clearly many possible values of δ in this instance and each would imply a different alternative hypothesis H_A and a different value for the probability β. Here specifying $\delta \neq 0$ corresponds to what is termed a two-sided alternative hypothesis, as δ can be < 0 or > 0. A one-sided alternative hypothesis would specify, for example, that $\delta > 0$.

Test statiscally significant	Difference exists (H_A true)	Difference does not exist (H_0 true)
Yes	Power $(1 - \beta)$	Type I error (α)
No	Type II error (β)	

Figure 9.1 Relationship between type I and type II errors and significance tests

The power is defined as one minus the probability of a Type II error, thus the power equals $1 - \beta$. That is, the *power* is the probability of obtaining a 'statistically significant' p-value when the null hypothesis is truly false and so δ has a value not equal to zero. The choice of power is arbitrary but is frequently taken as either 90% or 80%; the latter means there is a one-in-five chance of a false negative, that is, failure to detect a true difference of the specified magnitude (see Section 9.5).

The relationship between Type I and II errors and significance tests is described in Figure 9.1.

It is of crucial importance to consider sample size and power when interpreting statements following a completed trial and mentioning 'non-significant' results. In particular, if the power of the trial was initially very low, all we can conclude from a non-significant result is that the question of the presence or absence of differences between interventions remains unresolved. A trial with low power is only able to detect large treatment differences and, in many cases, the existence of a large difference may be clinically implausible and the hypothesis therefore unrealistic.

9.3   The fundamental equation

In a trial comparing two groups with m subjects per group and a continuous outcome variable, $\bar{x}_1$ and $\bar{x}_2$ summarize the respective means of the observations taken. Further, if the data are Normally distributed with equal and known (population) SD σ, then the standard errors are $SE(\bar{x}_1) = SE(\bar{x}_2) = \sigma/\sqrt{m}$. The estimated difference between the groups is therefore

$$\bar{d} = \bar{x}_2 - \bar{x}_1$$

and this has

$$SE(\bar{d}) = \sigma\sqrt{\frac{2}{m}}.$$

The two groups are compared using the z-test of Equation (8.2). Here we assume that $SE(\bar{d})$ is the same whether the null hypothesis H_0 of no difference between groups is true, or the alternative hypothesis H_A that there is a difference of size δ, is true.

Figure 9.2 illustrates the distribution of $\bar{d}$ under the null and alternative hypotheses. The two distributions are such that $\bar{d}$ has a Normal distribution either with mean 0 or mean δ, depending on which of the two hypotheses is true. If the observed $\bar{d}$ from a trial

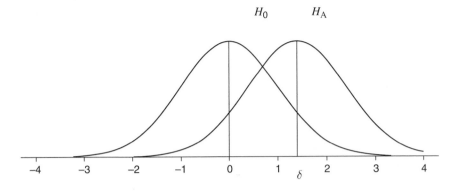

Figure 9.2   Distribution of $\bar{d}$ under the null and alternative hypotheses

exceeds a critical value, then the result is declared statistically significant. For a significance level of α (here assumed one-tailed for expository purposes only) we denote this critical value by d_α.

Under the assumption that the null hypothesis H_0 is true, $\bar{d}$ has mean 0 and the critical value for statistical significance d_α is determined by

$$\frac{d_\alpha - 0}{\sigma\sqrt{\dfrac{2}{m}}} = z_{1-\alpha} \quad \text{or} \quad d_\alpha = z_{1-\alpha}\sigma\sqrt{\frac{2}{m}}. \tag{9.1}$$

Here $z_{1-\alpha}$ is the value along the horizontal axis of the standard Normal distribution of Table T1 and correspond to an area in the upper tail of that distribution of α.

In contrast, under the assumption that the alternative hypothesis H_A is true, $\bar{d}$ now has mean δ but the same $SE(\bar{d}) = \sigma\sqrt{\frac{2}{m}}$. In this, case the probability that $\bar{d}$ exceeds d_α must be $1 - \beta$ and this implies that

$$\frac{d_\alpha - \delta}{\sigma\sqrt{\dfrac{2}{m}}} = -z_{1-\beta} \quad \text{or} \quad d_\alpha = \delta - z_{1-\beta}\sigma\sqrt{\frac{2}{m}}. \tag{9.2}$$

Here $z_{1-\beta}$ are the values along the horizontal axis of the standard Normal distribution of Table T1 and correspond to areas in the upper tail of that distribution of β.

Equating the two expressions (9.1) and (9.2) and rearranging, we obtain the sample size for each group in the trial as

$$m = 2\left[\frac{\sigma}{\delta}\right]^2 (z_{1-\alpha} + z_{1-\beta})^2 = \frac{2(z_{1-\alpha} + z_{1-\beta})^2}{\Delta^2}, \tag{9.3}$$

where $\Delta = \delta/\sigma$ is termed the standardized effect size. Equation (9.3) is termed the *Fundamental Equation* as it arises, in one form or another, in many situations for which sample sizes are calculated.

The use of Equation (9.3) for the case of a two-tailed test, rather than the one-tailed test, involves a slight approximation since $\bar{d}$ is also statistically significant if it is less than $-d_\alpha$. However, with δ positive the associated probability of observing a result smaller than $-d_\alpha$ is negligible. For the case of a two-sided test, we simply replace $z_{1-\alpha}$ in Equation (9.3) by $z_{1-\alpha/2}$. To evaluate Equation (9.3), a planning value for Δ is required and α and β have to be specified.

The fundamental equation has to be modified for the specific experimental design proposed for the trail. If the allocation ratio (the relative numbers of patients to be recruited in each group) is $1 : \lambda$, that is, different from $1 : 1$, then Equation (9.3) becomes

$$m = \left(\frac{1+\lambda}{\lambda}\right)\frac{(z_{1-\alpha/2} + z_{1-\beta})^2}{\Delta_{\text{Plan}}^2}, \lambda > 0. \tag{9.4}$$

Consequently, if the number of subjects for Group 1 is m, the number for Group 2 is $n = \lambda m$. This leads to a total trial size of $N = m + n = m(1+\lambda)$ subjects.

It must be emphasized that the standardized effect size Δ_{Plan} in these equations refers to what the investigators anticipate the true value of Δ will be. Once the trial is completed the data provide an estimate $D_{\text{TrialData}}$ of the true value $\Delta_{\text{Population}}$. This estimate may or may not correspond closely to Δ_{Plan}, although the investigators will hope that it does.

9.4   Specific situations

9.4.1   Comparing means

If the variable being measured is continuous and can be assumed to have a Normal distribution, then the number of subjects m required for Group 1 when there are λm in Group 2 is obtained from Equation (9.4), but modified to become

$$m = \left(\frac{1+\lambda}{\lambda}\right)\frac{(z_{1-\alpha/2} + z_{1-\beta})^2}{\Delta_{\text{Plan}}^2} + \frac{z_{1-\alpha/2}^2}{2(1+\lambda)}, \lambda > 0. \tag{9.5}$$

The quantity $z_{1-\alpha/2}^2/[2(1+\lambda)]$ adjusts Equation (9.4) for situations when sample sizes are likely to be small. This leads to a total trial size of $N = m + n = m(1+\lambda)$ subjects.

Example 9.1   Difference in means – change in disease activity

In Example 1.2, Meggitt, Gray and Reynolds (2006) in their trial in patients with moderate-to-severe eczema anticipated a $\delta_{\text{Plan}} = 14$-unit difference in disease activity between the Azathioprine and Placebo groups and a standard deviation

Example 9.1 *(Continued)*

of $\sigma_{Plan} = 17$ units. Together, these provide an anticipated standardized effect size $\Delta_{Plan} = \delta_{Plan}/\sigma_{Plan} = 14/17 = 0.82$, or approximately 0.8. Further their design stipulated a 2 : 1 Azathioprine : Placebo allocation ratio, $\lambda = 2$, a two-sided significance level $\alpha = 0.05$ (5%) and power $1 - \beta = 0.8$ (80%). Use of Table T2 gives $z_{1-\alpha/2} = z_{0.975} = 1.96$ and $z_{1-\beta} = z_{0.8} = 0.8416$. Substituting these in Equation (9.5) gives

$$m = \left(\frac{1+2}{2}\right)\frac{(1.96 + 0.8416)^2}{0.8^2} + \frac{1.96^2}{2(1+2)} = 19.04 \approx 20.$$

From this, $n = \lambda m = 2 \times 20 = 40$ and so a total sample size of $N = 60$ subjects is required. Had a 1 : 1 allocation ratio been used then $m = n = 25.5 \approx 26$, giving a total of 52 subjects, 8 fewer than the number required with the unequal allocation ratio $\lambda = 2$.

9.4.2 Comparing proportions

If the outcome variable of the 2-group design is binary, such as when a satisfactory response to treatment either is or is not observed, then the number of subjects required for Group 1 for anticipated difference $\delta = \pi_2 - \pi_1$ is obtained from

$$m = \frac{\left[z_{1-\alpha/2}\sqrt{(1+\lambda)\overline{\pi}(1-\overline{\pi})} + z_{1-\beta}\sqrt{\lambda\pi_1(1-\pi_1) + \pi_2(1-\pi_2)}\right]^2}{\lambda(\pi_2 - \pi_1)^2}. \qquad (9.6)$$

Here π_1 and π_2 are the proportions anticipated to respond in the respective groups, and $\overline{\pi} = (\pi_1 + \lambda\pi_2)/(1 + \lambda)$. The number to be recruited to Group 2 is $n = \lambda m$, and the total number of subjects $N = m(1 + \lambda)$.

Example 9.2 Complete response rate in multiple myeloma

The randomized trial described in Table 4.1 (Palumbo, Bringhen, Caravita *et al.*, 2006) compared Melaphalan and Prednisone (MP) with Melaphalan, Prednisone and Thalidomide (MPT) in elderly patients with multiple myeloma. A principal endpoint was complete response. At the design stage, the planning values for the response rates were set as 5% with MP and 15% with MPT. Further, their design stipulated a 1 : 1 allocation ratio, a two-sided significance level $\alpha = 0.05$ (5%) and power $1 - \beta = 0.9$ (90%).

Example 9.2   *(Continued)*

Here $\lambda = 1$, $\pi_{\text{MPT-Plan}} = 0.15$ and $\pi_{\text{MP-Plan}} = 0.05$ were the anticipated proportions with complete response in the respective groups, and hence $\bar{\pi} = (0.05 + 1 \times 0.15)/(1 + 1) = 0.1$. Use of Table T2 gives $z_{1-\alpha/2} = z_{0.975} = 1.96$ and $z_{1-\beta} = z_{0.8} = 1.2816$. Substituting these values into Equation (9.6) gives

$$m = \frac{\left[1.96\sqrt{2 \times 0.1 \times (1 - 0.1)} + 1.2816\sqrt{0.05(1 - 0.05) + 0.15(1 - 0.15)}\right]^2}{(0.15 - 0.05)^2} = 187.06 \approx 190.$$

From this $n = 190$ also, and so a total sample size of $N = 380$ subjects is required. This was the planned size used by the investigators. Had the trial been planned with a power of 80%, rather than 90%, the required sample size would have been 290.

However, because of the results obtained from an interim analysis of the accumulating data from the trial and falling enrolment, the trial steering committee stopped the trial after 331 patients had been randomized. Their report was then based on 255 patients with at least 6 months of follow-up which was the minimum required to evaluate the clinical response. The observed response rates were $p_{\text{MPT}} = 20/129 = 0.1550$ and $p_{\text{MP}} = 3/126 = 0.0238$. The first was close to the planning value, the second approximately half that which had been anticipated.

9.4.3   Ordered categorical data

With only two categories in the scale we have the binary case described above, although an alternative approach would have been to formulate this in odds ratio (OR) terms, rather than as a difference in proportions. This formulation leads to very similar sample sizes with the small differences arising due to some approximations that have to be made in that approach. However, although perhaps not as intuitive as a difference, working in terms of an OR scale leads to the extension from the binary split to the situation in which an ordered categorical variable is used for endpoint assessment. The process is quite complex so we illustrate it by means of an example.

Table 9.1 is a collapsed version of Table 8.1 from Example 8.8, in that some of the categories have been merged so that the sample size process is a little easier to describe. In this example, every patient is classified into one of the $\kappa = 4$ improvement categories at the end of the trial and the numbers falling into the respective categories in each treatment noted. The individual proportions are then calculated by dividing these by the corresponding numbers in each treatment group.

Table 9.1 Investigator assessed response to treatment in patients with moderate-to-severe eczema (adapted from Meggitt, Gray and Reynolds, 2006, Table 3)

Improve	Category	Number		Proportion		Cumulative proportion		
		Placebo (P)	Azath (A)	Placebo (P)	Azath (A)	Placebo (P)	Azath (A)	
	i			p_{Pi}	p_{Ai}	q_{Pi}	q_{Ai}	OR
None	0	6	5	0.3158	0.1389	0.3158	0.1389	—
Slight	1	4	6	0.2105	0.1667	0.5263	0.3056	2.86
Moderate	2	8	9	0.4211	0.2500	0.9474	0.5556	2.52
Marked	3	1	16	0.0526	0.4444	1.0000	1.0000	14.41
	Total	19	36	1.0000	1.0000			

The corresponding odds ratios are the chance of a subject being in a given category or higher in one group compared to the same categories in the other group. For category i, which takes values 1, 2 and 3, the odds ratio is given by

$$OR_i = \frac{q_{Pi}(1 - q_{Ai})}{q_{Ai}(1 - q_{Pi})}. \tag{9.7}$$

Using this equation in the data of Table 9.1 gives

$$OR_1 = \frac{q_{A1}(1 - q_{P1})}{q_{P1}(1 - q_{A1})} = \frac{0.3158(1 - 0.1389)}{0.1389(1 - 0.3158)} = 2.86,$$

$$OR_2 = 2.52 \text{ and } OR_3 = 14.41.$$

Although not precisely the case here, for sample size purposes, an assumption is made which specifies that these odds ratios will be the same irrespective of the category division used; for all categories defined this is equal to OR_{Plan}.

In designing a trial, the first requirement is to specify the proportion of subjects anticipated in each category of the scale, for one of the groups. For $\kappa = 4$ categories, these anticipated or planning proportions for one group are set as $\pi_{P1}, \pi_{P2}, \pi_{P3}$ and π_{P4} respectively, where $\pi_{P1} + \pi_{P2} + \pi_{P3} + \pi_{P4} = 1$. Consequently, we define planning $Q_{P1} = \pi_{P1}, Q_{P2} = \pi_{P1} + \pi_{P2}, Q_{P3} = \pi_{P1} + \pi_{P2} + \pi_{P3}$ and $Q_{P4} = \pi_{P1} + \pi_{P2} + \pi_{P3} + \pi_{P4} = 1$.

From these, and using the specified OR_{Plan}, the planning values for the comparator group are then calculated as

$$Q_{Ai} = \frac{Q_{Pi}}{[(1 - Q_{Pi})OR_{Plan} + Q_{Pi}]}.$$

Once these are obtained, the planning values $\pi_{A1}, \pi_{A2}, \pi_{A3}$ and π_{A4} can be determined. Finally $\bar{\pi}_i = (\pi_{Ai} + \pi_{Pi})/2$, the average proportion of subjects anticipated in each category i, is required.

In the case of κ categories (not just equal to 4 as in this illustration), the required sample size for a $1:1$ randomization for one intervention group is

$$m_\kappa = \frac{6(z_{1-\alpha/2} + z_{1-\beta})^2}{\Gamma \times (\log OR_{Plan})^2}, \tag{9.8}$$

where $\Gamma = (1 - \sum_{i=1}^{\kappa} \bar{\pi}_i^3)$ and the total trial size is $N_\kappa = 2m_\kappa$.

If the number of categories is large, it is clearly difficult to postulate the proportion of subjects who would fall into a given category. However, if the number of categories *exceeds* five, then Γ in Equation (9.8) is approximately unity. This then simplifies the calculations a great deal, as they now only depend on OR_{Plan}, the significance level α and power $1 - \beta$.

The assumption of constant OR implies that it is justified to use the Mann–Whitney U-test at the analysis stage in this situation. It also means that we can use the anticipated OR from *any* pair of adjacent categories for planning purposes.

Example 9.3   Patients with moderate-to-severe eczema

Suppose a confirmatory trial of that conducted by Meggitt, Gray and Reynolds (2006) is planned on the basis of the information from the Placebo group provided in Table 9.1. The corresponding odds ratios are all greater than what would be regarded as a clinically useful improvement. As a consequence, the investigators set $OR_{Plan} = 2$, but used the observed proportions in each improvement category with Placebo as the basis for their planning. Use of Table 9.1 and $OR_{Plan} = 2$ then lead to Table 9.2.

From Table 9.2, $\Gamma = 1 - (0.2553^3 + 0.1900^3 + 0.4822^3 + 0.0726^3) = 0.8640$, then with two-sided $\alpha = 0.05$, $z_{0.975} = 1.96$, power $1 - \beta = 0.8$, $z_{0.8} = 0.8416$ and from Equation (9.8):

$$m_4 = \frac{6(1.96 + 0.8416)^2}{0.8640 \times (\log 2)^2} = 113.45 \approx 120 \text{ per group.}$$

Hence, on a $1:1$ allocation, $N = 2m_4 = 240$ patients would be required.

Table 9.2   Planning values for the confirmatory trial of that conducted by Meggitt, Gray and Reynolds (2006)

Improvement	Category i	Placebo (P) π_{Pi}	Q_P	Azathrioprine (A) Q_A	π_A	$\bar{\pi}_i$
None	0	0.32	0.32	0.1905	0.1905	0.2553
Slight	1	0.21	0.53	0.3605	0.1700	0.1900
Moderate	2	0.42	0.95	0.9048	0.5443	0.4822
Marked	3	0.05	1.00	1.0000	0.0952	0.0726
	Total	1.00	—	—	1.0000	

As it has become clear, sample size calculation in this situation is not a straightforward process. The book by Machin, Campbell, Tan and Tan (2009) has specialist software included to enable this to be done.

9.4.4 Time-to-event

As indicated in Chapter 8, comparisons between groups when summarizing time-to-event data can be made using the logrank test; the summary statistic used is the hazard ratio (HR). The test of the null hypothesis of equality of event rates between the groups with respect to the event (endpoint) concerned provides the basis for the sample size calculations. This is expressed as H_0: $HR = 1$.

Pre-trial information on the endpoint, either as the anticipated median 'survival' for each group or as the anticipated proportions 'alive' at some fixed time point, will usually form the basis of the anticipated difference between groups for planning purposes. The corresponding effect size is HR_{Plan}. If proportions alive at a chosen time point are anticipated to be π_1 and π_2 then

$$HR_{Plan} = \frac{\log \pi_2}{\log \pi_1}. \tag{9.9}$$

On the other hand, if a planning value of the median survival time M_1 of one of the groups is given, this implies that at that median time half are alive and half not, so that $\pi_1 = 0.5$. Further if M_2 is given, then $HR_{Plan} = M_1/M_2$, and use of Equation (9.9) allows a planning value of $\pi_2 = \exp(\log 0.5/HR_{Plan}) = \exp(-0.6932/HR_{Plan})$ to be obtained.

Once HR_{Plan} is obtained, then the number of events required to be observed in Group 1 is

$$e_1 = \frac{1}{\lambda} \left(\frac{1 + \lambda HR_{Plan}}{1 - HR_{Plan}} \right)^2 (z_{1-\alpha/2} + z_{1-\beta})^2. \tag{9.10}$$

For the second group, $e_2 = \lambda e_1$ events are required or a total of $E = e_1 + e_2$ for the trial as a whole.

The corresponding number of subjects needed in order to observe these events for Group 1 is

$$m = \frac{1}{\lambda} \left(\frac{1 + \lambda HR_{Plan}}{1 - HR_{Plan}} \right)^2 \frac{(z_{1-\alpha/2} + z_{1-\beta})^2}{[(1 - \pi_1) + \lambda(1 - \pi_2)]}. \tag{9.11}$$

For Group 2, $n = \lambda m$, leading to $N = m + n = m(1 + \lambda)$ subjects in total.

Example 9.4   Differences in survival – gastric cancer

Cuschieri, Weeden, Fielding, *et al.* (1999) compared two forms of surgical resection for patients with gastric cancer. The primary outcome (event of interest) was time to death. The authors state:

> Sample size calculations were based on a pre-trial survey of 26 gastric surgeons, which indicated that the baseline 5-year survival rate of D_1 surgery was expected to be 20%, and an improvement in survival to 34% (14% change) with D_2 resection would be a realistic expectation. Thus 400 patients (200 in each arm) were to be randomized, providing 90% power to detect such a difference with $P < 0.05$.

Here $\pi_1 = 0.2$, $\pi_2 = 0.34$ and so from Equation (9.9), $HR_{Plan} = \log 0.34/\log 0.2 = (-1.078)/(-1.609) = 0.6667$. The authors set $1 - \beta = 0.9$ and imply a two-sided significance level $\alpha = 0.05$ and a randomization in equal numbers to each group, hence $\lambda = 1$. Table T1 implies $z_{1-0.025} = z_{0.975} = 1.9600$ and $z_{1-0.9} = z_{0.1} = 1.2816$, then substituting all the corresponding values in Equation (9.11) gives.

$$m = \left(\frac{1 + 0.6667}{1 - 0.6667} \right)^2 \frac{(1.9600 + 1.2816)^2}{[(1 - 0.2) + (1 - 0.34)]}$$

$$= 25 \times \frac{10.5080}{1.46} \approx 180 \text{ per surgical group.}$$

9.5   Practical considerations

9.5.1   Trial objectives

It is customary to start the process of estimating sample size by specifying the size of the difference required to be detected, and then to estimate the number of participants required to allow the trial to detect this difference if it really exists. Given that this is a plausible and a scientific or medically important change then, at the planning stage, the

Design Option	
Effect size, δ	The anticipated (planning) size of the difference between the two groups
Type I error, α	Equivalently the significance level of the statistical test to be used in the analysis
Type II error, β	Equivalently the power, $1 - \beta$
Withdrawal rate, W	Anticipated withdrawal or lost to follow up rate
Allocation ratio, λ	The relative numbers of subjects to be included in each of the 2 intervention groups

Figure 9.3   Components necessary to estimate the size of a comparative trial

investigators should be reasonably certain to detect such a difference after completing the trial. 'Detecting a difference' is usually taken to mean 'obtain a statistically significant difference with p-value ≤ 0.05'. Similarly the phrase 'to be reasonably certain' is usually interpreted to mean something like 'have a chance of at least 90% of obtaining such a p-value' if there really is a difference of the magnitude anticipated. The major components of this process are summarized in Figure 9.3.

9.5.2 The anticipated effect size

A key element in the design is the 'effect size' that it is reasonable to plan to observe – should it exist. The way in which possible effect sizes are determined will depend on the specific situation under consideration. Sometimes there may be very detailed prior knowledge which then enables an investigator to anticipate what effect size between groups is likely to be observed, and the role of the trial is to confirm that expectation. In general, estimates of the anticipated effect size may be obtained from the available literature, formal meta-analyses of related trials or may be elicited from expert opinion.

In practice, a range of plausible effect size options are usually considered before the final planning effect size is agreed. For example, an investigator might specify a scientific or clinically useful difference that it is hoped could be detected, and would then estimate the required sample size on this basis. These calculations might then indicate that an extremely large number of subjects is required. As a consequence, the investigator may next define a revised aim of detecting a rather larger difference than that originally specified. The calculations are repeated, and perhaps the sample size becomes realistic in that new context.

One problem associated with planning comparative clinical trials is that investigators are often optimistic about the magnitude of the improvement of a new treatment over the standard. This optimism is understandable, since it can take considerable effort to initiate a trial and, in many cases, the trial would only be launched if the investigator is enthusiastic enough about the new treatment and is sufficiently convinced about its potential efficacy. However, experience suggests that as trial succeeds trial there is often a growing realism that, even at best, earlier expectations were optimistic. There is ample historical evidence to suggest that trials that set out to detect large treatment differences nearly always result in 'no significant difference' being detected. In such cases there may have been a true and worthwhile treatment benefit that has been missed, since the level of detectable differences set by the design was unrealistically high and hence the sample size too small to establish the true (but less optimistic) size of benefit.

For circumstances where there is little prior information available, Cohen (1988) has proposed a standardized effect size Δ_{Cohen}. In the case when the difference between two groups is expressed by the difference between their means $\delta = (\mu_2 - \mu_1)$ and σ is the SD of the endpoint variable which is assumed to be a continuous measure, then

$$\Delta_{\text{Cohen}} = (\mu_2 - \mu_1)/\sigma = \delta/\sigma. \qquad (9.12)$$

A value of $\Delta_{\text{Cohen}} \leq 0.2$ is considered a 'small' standardized effect, $\Delta_{\text{Cohen}} \approx 0.5$ as 'moderate' and $\Delta_{\text{Cohen}} \geq 0.8$ as 'large'. Experience has suggested that, in many areas of clinical research, these can be taken as a good pragmatic guide for planning purposes.

Example 9.5   Anticipated effect size

As we noted in Example 9.1, Meggitt, Gray and Reynolds (2006) stipulated $\delta_{Plan} = 14$ units with standard deviation $\sigma_{Plan} = 17$ units as their design criteria for assessing the difference in disease activity between Azathioprine and Placebo. The corresponding anticipated standardized effect size is $\Delta_{Plan} = \delta_{Plan}/\sigma_{Plan} = 14/17 = 0.82$. This would be regarded as a large effect using the Cohen criteria and so would suggest (at the design stage) that the possibility of a more modest outcome should be reviewed before finally deciding on patient numbers.

When comparing two proportions, the standardized effect size becomes

$$\Delta_{Cohen} = \frac{\pi_{2Plan} - \pi_{1Plan}}{\sqrt{\bar{\pi}_{Plan}(1 - \bar{\pi}_{Plan})}},$$

where $\bar{\pi}_{Plan} = (\pi_{1Plan} + \pi_{2Plan})/2$. In the design of the trial of Example 9.2 conducted by Palumbo, Bringhen, Caravita et al. (2006) in elderly patients with multiple myeloma, they set $\pi_{MPT-Plan} = 0.15$, $\pi_{MP-Plan} = 0.05$ and so $\bar{\pi}_{Plan} = (0.15 + 0.05)/2 = 0.1$ giving

$$\Delta_{Plan} = \frac{0.15 - 0.05}{\sqrt{0.1(1 - 0.1)}} = 0.33.$$

This represents a modest-to-small effect size using the Cohen criteria and therefore seems to provide a realistic scenario for planning purposes.

9.5.3   Significance level and power

The choices of the significance level and power for use in the sample size calculations are essentially arbitrary. However, accepted practice has built up over the years so the conventional value for α is 0.05 (5%), or less often 0.01 (1%). In contrast, although $1 - \beta = 0.8$ (80%) for the power is recognized as a minimum requirement, many investigators fail to realize that 80% power means that they have a very high risk of a false negative. Assuming the new intervention really is superior, this means there is a serious risk of a wasted effort in conducting their trial. There has been a move to increase this to 0.9 (90%), although the greater the power the greater the required sample size. The main reason for this is to ensure that clinical trials are able to provide convincing evidence of relative efficacy of the interventions being compared. Meggitt, Gray and Reynolds (2006) used a power of 80% for their trial while Palumbo, Bringhen, Caravita et al. (2006) used a power of 90%. Both sets of investigators chose a two-sided significance level of 5%.

9.5.4 Allocation ratio

From a statistical perspective, an allocation ratio of 1 : 1 is usually the most efficient in that it produces a minimum sample size for given effect size, α and β. However, there may be situations where other ratios may be indicated. For example, Meggitt, Gray and Reynolds (2006) used a 2 : 1 randomization in favour of azathioprine over placebo in patients with moderate-to-severe eczema. They used this ratio 'to encourage recruitment . . . and to increase the likelihood of identifying infrequent adverse events'. Part of their rationale was therefore concerned with obtaining information on a secondary endpoint; in this case the occurrence of possible adverse events.

Another situation in which unequal allocation may be useful is, for example, when there is a restricted supply of the new or test intervention whereas the standard is more readily available. For example, Erbel, Mario, Bartunek, *et al.* (2007) in Example 1.12 were investigating a new bioabsorbable stent for coronary scaffolding. We might foresee the supplies of the 'experimental' stent being limited, while those used in current practice are readily available. In such cases, the number of patients for which the test stent can be given is fixed (perhaps at a relatively small number), but recruiting more than this number to receive the control stent could increase the statistical efficiency of the design. However, this is a case of 'limited resources' and might equally be discussed in the following section.

9.5.5 Limited resources

A common situation is one where the number of subjects (often patients) that can be included in a trial is governed by non-scientific forces such as time, money or human resources. With a predetermined (maximal) sample size, the researcher may then wish to know what probability he or she has of detecting a certain effect size with a trial confined to this size. If the resulting power is small, say < 70%, then the investigator may decide that the trial should not go ahead. A similar situation arises if the type of subject under consideration is uncommon, as would be the case with a clinical trial in rare disease groups. In either case the sample size is constrained and, instead of estimating the sample size, the researcher is interested in calculating the size of effects which could be established for a reasonable power, say, 80%.

Example 9.6 Homeopathic arnica

One trial which identified limited resources as defining sample size was that of Stevinson, Devaraj, Fountain-Barber, *et al.* (2003), described in Example 1.9. The trial was concerned with pain relief using homeopathic arnica, and the authors state:

> Because of the preliminary nature of the trial and the number of patients expected to be available, a minimum sample size of 60 was considered feasible.

9.5.6   Subject withdrawals

One aspect of a clinical trial which can affect the number of patients recruited is the proportion of patients who are lost to follow-up before the endpoint variable concerned can be determined. For example, in patients with eczema (Table 8.1) the endpoint was clinical response 12 weeks following commencement of treatment. The planning team should try and foresee the potential loss of required patients and ensure the trial procedures minimize this possibility. They should also have a strategy for dealing with it if and when it occurs. As we discussed in Section 8.6, one option is to exclude the patient from any evaluation; another is to regard such patients as failures. Neither option is satisfactory, although our preference is for the latter. Whatever the team decides, it should be stated in the protocol analysis plan rather than made as an ad hoc strategy if such losses occur. These losses or withdrawals are a likely problem for trials in which patients are monitored over a long period of follow-up time. If the endpoint is a time-to-event variable, then any such 'lost' patients also have censored observations. This is also the case for whom the event of interest has not occurred at the end of the trial or, more, precisely at the time-point when the analysis is to be conducted.

Whatever the circumstances, as a precaution against withdrawals the planned number of patients is often adjusted upwards to

$$N_W = N/(1 - W) \qquad\qquad (9.13)$$

where W is the anticipated withdrawal proportion. The estimated size of W can often be obtained from reports of trials conducted by others. If there is no such experience to hand, than a pragmatic value may be to take $W = 0.1$.

Example 9.7   Adjusting for withdrawals

Palumbo, Bringhen, Caravita *et al.* (2006) calculated that a sample size of $N = 380$ was necessary to demonstrate an anticipated increased response rate from 5% with MP to 15% with MPT. Among the subsequent 331 elderly patients with multiple myeloma randomized, 5 withdrew their consent to participate and a further 10 were lost to follow-up. This corresponds to an actual loss of 15/331 (4.5%). Had they applied our suggested $W = 0.1$ to their intended (as opposed to actual) recruitment, then their planned trial size would have been increased from 380 to 418 or 420 patients. With the experience of one completed trial, the investigating team of a possible future follow-on trial in the same type of patients may more realistically set $W = 0.05$.

9.6   Further topics

9.6.1   Several primary outcomes

We have based the above discussion on the assumption that there is a single identifiable endpoint or outcome, upon which comparisons are based. There is often more than one endpoint of interest, such as the relative survival time and response rates, as well as quality of life scores of subjects in the two groups. If one of these endpoints is regarded as more important than the others, it can be named as the primary endpoint and sample-size estimates are based on that alone. A problem arises when there are several outcome measures that are regarded as equally important. A commonly adopted approach is to repeat the sample-size estimates for each outcome measure in turn, and then select the largest of these as the sample size required to answer all the questions of interest.

However, it is well recognized that if many endpoints are included in one trial and the groups are tested for statistical significance for all of these, then the p-values so obtained are distorted. To compensate for this, smaller observed p-values may be required to declare 'true' statistical significance at level α. In such cases, the sample-size calculations will be similarly affected so that, to retain the level at α for all the tests conducted, a value depending on the number of endpoints k is sometimes substituted in, for example, Equations (9.14) and (9.15). A common value taken is simply α/k, which is commonly known as the Bonferroni correction. Even when $k = 2$, this substantially increases the size of the planned trial.

Example 9.8 Two major endpoints – disease activity

In the randomized trial described by Meggit, Gray and Reynolds (2006) there was one primary endpoint specified: disease activity using SASSAD. However, several secondary endpoints, including reduction in percentage body area involved, were reported. We repeat the sample size calculations previously made in Example 9.1, but with (two-sided) α replaced by $\alpha/2$ since $k = 2$ in this case. From Table T1, using the value 0.025, this gives $z_{1-\alpha/4} = z_{0.9875} = 2.2414$. The $z_{1-\beta} = z_{0.8} = 0.8416$ remains the same, and so from Equation (9.5) with $\lambda = 1$ we have

$$m = \left(\frac{1+2}{2}\right)\frac{(2.2414 + 0.8416)^2}{0.8^2} + \frac{2.2414^2}{2(1+2)} = 23.11 \approx 25.$$

This gives the planned trial size with two endpoints as $N = m(1 + \lambda) \approx 75$ patients in this case. This would increase the trial size by 25% compared to the earlier calculations.

9.6.2 Revising trial size

As we have indicated, in order to calculate the sample size of a trial we must first have suitable background information together with some idea regarding what is a realistic difference to seek. Sometimes such information is available as prior knowledge from the literature or other sources, but at other times a pilot trial may need to be conducted.

Traditionally, a pilot trial is a distinct preliminary investigation, conducted before embarking on the main trial. However, the use of an internal pilot trial has been explored. The idea here is to plan the clinical trial on the basis of best available information, but to regard the first patients entered as the 'internal' pilot. When data from these patients have been collected, the sample size can be re-estimated with the revised knowledge so generated.

Two vital features accompany this approach: firstly, the final sample size should only ever be adjusted upwards, never down; and secondly, we should only use the internal pilot in order to improve the components of the sample size calculation which are independent of the observed difference between groups. This second point is crucial. It implies that when estimating the difference in the means of two groups, it is valid to re-estimate the planning SD, σ_{Plan} but not the planning effect size, δ_{Plan}. Both these points should be carefully observed to avoid distortion of the subsequent significance test and a possible misleading interpretation of the final trial results.

Example 9.9   Internal pilot to modify trial size – gastric emptying time

Lobo, Bostock, Neal, *et al.* (2002) estimated their required sample size by assuming a reduction in gastric emptying time of 30 minutes, significance level $\alpha = 0.05$ and power $1-\beta = 0.9$ to obtain $N = 40$. However, after recruiting 10 patients to their trial, they observed a gastric emptying time reduction of 74 minutes. As a consequence of this observed but interim value being greater than that used at the planning stage, the sample size was recalculated and *reduced* from the initial 40 patients to 20. Such a step breaks all the rules attached to the use of internal pilot trials. Although misguided, they did at least report exactly what they did.

The advantage of an internal pilot is that it provides an insurance against misjudgement regarding the baseline planning assumptions. It is, nevertheless, important that the intention to conduct an internal pilot trial is recorded at the outset and the full details are given in the trial protocol.

9.7   Other methods and software

Since sample size determination is such a critical part of the design process, we recommend that all calculations are carefully checked before the final decisions are made. This is particularly important for large and/or resource intensive studies. In-house checking by colleagues is also important.

Sources of sample size calculation details are provided by:

Biostat (2001) *Power & Precision: Release 2.1*, Englewood, NJ.

Dupont, W.D. and Plummer, W.D. (1997) PS: power and sample size, *Controlled Clinical Trials*, **18**, 274.

Lenth, R.V. (2006) Java Applets for Power and Sample Size, www.stat.uiowa.edu/~rlenth/Power

Machin, D., Campbell, M.J., Tan, S.B. and Tan, S.H. (2009) *Sample Sizes Tables for Clinical Studies*, 3rd edn, Wiley-Blackwell, Oxford.

This describes sample size calculation methods for a wide choice of designs for clinical research including clinical trials.

A CD-Rom for sample size calculations is provided with each copy.

National Council for Social Studies (2005) *Power Analysis and Sample Size Software (PASS): Version 2005*, Kaysville, UT.

SAS Institute (2004) *Getting started with the SAS power and sample size application: Version 9.1*, SAS Institute, Cary, NC.

StataCorp (2007) *Stata Statistical Software: Release 10*, College Station, TX.

Statistical Solutions (2006) *nQuery Adviser: Version 6.0*, Saugus, MA.

9.8 Guideline

ICH E9 Expert Working Group (1999). Statistical principles for clinical trials: ICH Harmonised tripartite guideline. *Statistics in Medicine*, **18**, 1907–1942.

Considerations with respect to determining an appropriate sample size at the planning stage of a trial are discussed in Section 3.5, while issues when addressing the possibility of sample size adjustment during the course of a trial are in Section 4.3.

CHAPTER 10

Reporting

Once the trial is completed then dissemination of the trial results is an important part of the whole process. This is most often done by publication in the clinical research literature, presentation at conferences and also by less formal processes such as press releases. In this chapter, we consider the important procedures to follow when presenting the results from a clinical trial. Clinical journals publish guidelines for reporting, and we caution authors to respect these in order to give their trial the greatest chances of being accepted for publication – ideally in the most appropriate journal within the speciality concerned.

10.1 Introduction

10.1.1 Preliminaries

We emphasized in Section 7.6 that the preparation for publishing the trial results should begin at the very earliest stages, perhaps even before the first patient is recruited. There is no need to wait until the last patient is recruited and the final interventions completed. We stressed there that it is important to identify the journal (or other publication outlet) and be very mindful of the corresponding 'Instructions to Authors'. Often the more mundane aspects of the submission process are overlooked, such as who is responsible for preparing the top copy of the manuscript, obtaining conflict of interest statements from each author, summarizing and acknowledging the funding sources, checking how the article is to be submitted (many are web-based) and finally identifying who will receive the editorial correspondence.

10.1.2 When to publish

The first rule after completing a clinical trial is to report the results – whether they are positive, negative or equivocal. Despite this mandate to publish, not least so that any benefits that may have been demonstrated can be passed to future patients as quickly as possible, some care has to be taken in deciding the appropriate time for this. If all

Randomized Clinical Trials: Design, Practice and Reporting   David Machin and Peter M Fayers
© 2010 John Wiley & Sons, Ltd

patients have been recruited and complete efficacy details obtained from every patient as specified in the protocol, publication can be immediate. In contrast, if the trial involves long-term follow-up of patients, perhaps eventually recording their survival time from randomization, then it may be a long time before all patients have died. As we have indicated, survival trials depend on the number of events observed and not just the numbers of subjects recruited. An appropriate time to publish is once the number of events specified in the protocol has been accrued. The time when this will occur should be estimated during the trial design and affects the calculation of sample size requirements. It should be refined as the trial progresses, as it will be affected by the recruitment rates and the actual event rate. As this date approaches, steps can be taken for preparing the publication to minimize delays.

There will be circumstances where, for example, the new treatment in a trial may be much more efficacious than had been anticipated at the design stage. The temptation is then to publish interim findings. Seldom however, if ever, will it be justified to publish interim results while the trial is still open, since it will certainly disturb the equipoise necessary for the randomization and will affect the 'fully informed' consent process. The decision to publish interim results should not be made without prior consultation with an independent data monitoring committee (DMC) who should be the only ones, at that stage, who are fully conversant with all the data and any interim analyses. Smith, Procter, Gelber, *et al.* (2007) of Example 1.8 justify early publication of some aspects of their trial results as follows:

> The independent data monitoring committee continues to review data about deaths, compliance, and safety every 6 months. On the basis of a review in March, 2006, they recommended that the overall survival results for observation alone versus treatment with trastuzumab for 1 year with a median follow-up of 2 years should be made public. Results from the group of patients treated with trastuzumab for 2 years remain blinded because the comparison with the group treated for 1 year continues to mature.

Similarly, even if large differences appear to be emerging before trial completion, any decision to stop the trial early should only be made following advice from a DMC. Once a randomized trial is stopped early, for whatever reason, it may not be possible to start again and the consequences of an inconclusive result arising are of real concern.

10.2   Publication guidelines

Although there is a range of clinical trial designs and they are used in a very wide variety of situations, they all have to be analyzed, interpreted and the conclusions reported. The research is not complete without this final step. For those designing clinical trials, it is clearly important to be aware of the demands that will be made at the reporting stage. A careful investigating team will therefore take due note of these requirements, modify the design as necessary and ensure that, as the trial progresses, the necessary information is accumulated.

Several guidelines and associated checklists have been published to assist authors in preparing their work for publication. These guidelines outline the essential features of clinical trial reports. In particular, they clarify how aspects pertinent to their design should be described. However, an investigating team may have a target journal in mind even in the early stages of planning a trial and, consequently, should also take note of any specific journal requirements concerned with aspects of their potential trial. Before embarking on the trial, it is therefore prudent to cross-check the intended design against these requirements. Anything overlooked at the initial design stage can then be taken into account with a design modification *before* embarking on the trial. In contrast, it may be too late to discover such an omission at the time of analysis and reporting.

Guidelines for reporting also give hints on what seemingly extraneous detail needs to be collected and documented. These may include the details of the consent procedures, outcomes in subjects who do not fully comply with the protocol as stipulated or precise details of with whom the trial is formally registered.

For those trials that do not fit into specific guidelines, it is nevertheless useful to cross-check aspects of design with selected items from available guidelines. In these circumstances, it may also be useful for investigators to compile their own checklists that can be updated by their own experience as the trial proceeds. As a first trial is often only one step in a development process, such a personal checklist will be a useful guide for any subsequent trial in the series.

For certain types of trials, including those used in the development stages of a new drug, there may be mandatory guidelines imposed by the regulatory authorities. These may set minimum standards or very specific requirements. Any investigating team ignoring such advice would need to provide cogent reasons for doing so. Such departures may be entirely appropriate as new information and new situations are always arising. Should these occur, then cross-checking with the regulatory bodies at the design stage is clearly prudent. For non-regulatory situations, teams may be free to have a more flexible approach. However, although flexibility is desirable, care should be taken to ensure this does not lead to lower standards.

Considerable effort is required in order to conduct a clinical trial of any type and size and this effort justifies reporting of the subsequent trial results with careful detail. However, there is a wide variation in the quality of the standard of reporting of clinical trials. Some reports even omit key details such as the numbers randomized to each intervention group. Nevertheless, major strides in improving the quality of the reporting of randomized trials have been made. Pivotal to this has been the Consolidation of the Standards of Reporting Trials (CONSORT) statement described by Begg, Cho, Eastwood, *et al.* (1996) and amplified by Moher, Schultz and Altman *et al.* (2001). CONSORT has been extended by Boutron, Moher, Altman, *et al.* (2008) to address non-pharmacologic treatment trials; Zwarenstein, Treweek, Gagniere, *et al.* (2008) for reporting pragmatic trials; and widened to cluster randomized trials by Campbell, Elbourne and Altman, *et al.* (2004). CONSORT describes the essential items that should be reported in a trial publication in order to give assurance that the trial has been conducted to a high standard. This internationally agreed recommendation has been adopted by many of the leading medical journals, although there are still some who do not appear to insist that their authors comply with the requirements. Some of the key items from CONSORT are listed in Figure 10.1.

One particular feature of the CONSORT statement is that the outcomes of all participants randomized to a clinical trial are to be reported, in particular how many

Participants	Eligibility criteria for participants and the setting and locations where the data were collected
Interventions	Precise details of the interventions intended, and how and when they were actually administered
Objectives	Specific objectives and hypotheses
Outcomes	Clearly defined primary and secondary outcome measures
Sample size	How sample size was determined
Randomisation	Details of method used to generate the random allocation sequence – including details of strata and block size.
	Method used to implement the random allocation – numbered containers, central telephone, or web-based
Blinding	Description of the extent of the blinding in the trial – investigator, participant.
Statistical methods	Statistical methods used for the primary outcome(s)
Participant flow	Flow of participants through each stage of the trial
Recruitment	Dates defining the periods of recruitment and follow-up
Follow-up	As many patients as possible to be followed up. Drop-outs should be reported by treatment group

Figure 10.1   Selected key items to be included in a clinical trial report (adapted and abbreviated from that recommended for a randomized trial by Moher, Schultz and Altman, 2001)

were excluded from any of the analyses and the reasons why. For example, it must be stated how many participants were randomized but then refused the allocation and perhaps insisted on the competitor intervention.

Complementing the CONSORT statement which emphasizes the need to describe the participant flow through the trial process, guidelines for statistical referees of clinical papers have been published in several journals. These include those of the British Medical Journal as described by Altman, Gore, Gardner and Pocock (2000), now updated and available in BMJ (2006), together with the checklist for the statistical review of papers devised by Gardner, Machin, Campbell and Altman (2000). To give one example of a requirement, the checklist specifies that confidence intervals (on the treatment effect size) are to be given for the main results, supplementing the p-value from the associated hypothesis test.

These guidelines and checklists are clearly useful for those designing trials, who will eventually become the authors and then be exposed to the peer review system of the journal concerned. It simplifies the submission process to have prior knowledge of exactly what statistical and other referees will be looking for.

10.2.1   Evidence-based medicine

The purpose of publication should be to influence clinicians who treat future patients. By following established guidelines and adopting a high standard of reporting of clinical trials, the reader is better able to appreciate the clinical messages that arise from the trial that has been published. This in turn allows the reader to determine the relevance of the results to his or her clinical or research practice. Looking further ahead, this clarity facilitates the task of those who conduct systematic reviews. It enables them more readily to identify the key features of the trial to be included in their overview, ultimately leading to more reliable synthesis and a firmer basis for evidence-based medical practice. Further, if the data from the trial (rather than just the summary information within the trial publication) can be made available to such an overview, clearly this may further enhance the process. This care need not always be entirely altruistic, as it is possible that the investigator for the current trial may become an investigator (or even the lead investigator) in a future systematic overview of the trials in their specific area of interest.

10.2.2 Plain language

It should be emphasized how important it is that that authors use care with their choice of wording, particularly when trying to capture the essence of a trial's findings with respect to the primary endpoint. This is especially important for the abstract and conclusion section of the associated publication, when there is often a word limit set by the journal concerned. As a consequence of these difficulties, Pocock and Ware (2009) have made some very useful suggestions as to how these results may be phrased (Figure 10.2). In this figure, treatment differences and their 95% CI, p-value, strength of evidence and appropriate comment for use in conclusions are displayed. For non-inferiority scenarios, the non-inferiority margin δ (referred to as η in Chapter 11.3) is shown and p_{NI} is obtained from the consequent test of non-inferiority.

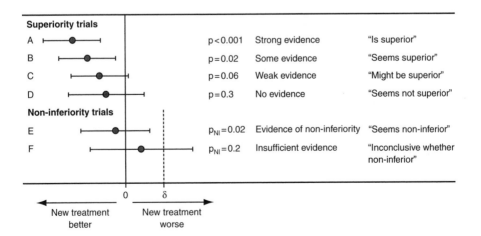

Figure 10.2 Scenarios for primary endpoint of a randomized trial comparing new and standard treatment groups (after Pocock and Ware, 2009)

10.3   Responsibilities

10.3.1   Authorship

> *Ensure the reporting is to the highest of standards*

The successful conduct of a randomized controlled trial involves a multidisciplinary team of a size and make-up depending on the scale and complexity of the trial being undertaken. Although there may be a single instigator of the research idea who can perhaps be identified as the principle investigator, it is clear that due recognition of the whole team is needed at the trial publication stage. In many cases, the journals demand that the roles of named authors to a publication should be made clear and that only those making a substantial contribution to the trial should be cited on the title page. Such a policy makes it very difficult for those conducting, for example, trials with extensive multicentre involvement. Some journals allow extensive lists of names to be detailed, thus the paper by Kahn, Fleischhacker, Boter, *et al.* (2008), which we have quoted as Example 2.4, includes 19 named authors. Some groups, such as the Singapore Lichen Planus Study Group (2004), publish under a collective authorship. They then list in an appendix to the paper the members of the writing committee, the coordinating centre team, members of the data monitoring committee, those from the individual clinical centres contributing patients (together with their number) and any other groups of individuals as appropriate.

10.3.2   Registration

As recommended by Dickersin and Rennie (2003), it is increasingly a requirement by national authorities and funding agencies that clinical trials are registered *before* the first patient is randomized. Those conducting trials need to be aware of these obligations. The same is true for some clinical journals which require a statement to this end in any submitted article; this should be checked before the trial is launched. This statement can be brief as in the following four articles (two published in the *Lancet*, one in the *BMJ* and one in *Diabetologia*).

Hancock, Maher, Latimer, *et al.* (2007, p. 1638) declare:

> This trial was registered with the Australian Clinical Trials Registry, ACTRN0 12605000036616.

Zheng, Kang, Huang, *et al.* (2008, p. 2013) state:

> This trial is registered with the Japan Clinical Trials Registry (http://umin.ac.jp/ctr/index/ htm) number UMIN-CRT C000000233.

Hay, Costelloe, Redmond, *et al.* (2008, p. 1) simply state:

> **Trial registration** Current Controlled Trials ISRCTN26362730.

Jenni, Oetliker, Allemann, *et al.* (2008, p. 1457) similarly state:

> *Trial registration*: ClinicalTrials.Gov NCT00325559.

10.3.3   Funding sources

There is always a concern that if a trial is sponsored by a particular agency then this agency may have a vested interest in the outcome. The worst-case scenario would be if that agency manipulated the reporting of the trial results, perhaps by selectively reporting only favourable outcomes as they perceive it or by suppressing the publication of unfavourable findings. As a consequence, most journals insist on declarations of any conflict of interest – financial or otherwise.

The trial conducted by Smith, Procter, Gelber, *et al.* (2007, p. 31) of Example 1.8 openly acknowledges the support of a pharmaceutical company by stating in their *Lancet* article:

> The trial was sponsored and funded by Roche. The collection, analysis, and interpretation of the data were done entirely independently, under the auspices of the Breast International Group. The corresponding author led the writing of the paper with input from the HERA executive committee, which includes a Roche representative who was not allowed to influence the paper in any way other than as approved by the executive committee. All authors had access to all the data. The trials' steering committee had final responsibility to submit the manuscript for publication.

In this statement the authors address the potential conflict with the funding body and make it very clear who has final responsibility. Other articles may not contain such explicit detail, since what is required will depend on the house rules of the particular journal concerned and the specifics of the relationship with the funding body. Thus Lo, Luo, Fan and Wei (2001, p. 463) in *Caries Research* simply state:

> This study was supported by a grant from Dentsply DeTrey and a grant from the University of Hong Kong.

On the other hand, in describing a trial of patients with nasopharyngeal cancer published in the *Journal of Clinical Oncology*, Wee, Tan, Tai, *et al.* (2005, p. 6732) are more explicit:

> Role of the funding source
>
> The National Medical Research Council of Singapore sponsored the study. The sponsor had no role in the study design, data collection, data analysis, data interpretation, writing of the report, or decision to summit the report for publication.

Any potential conflict of interest is often incorporated into statements concerning the funding source as there is often some overlap. However, whatever the format, the position has to be made evident. Thus Erbel, Di Mario, Bartunek, *et al.* (2007, p. 1875) of Example 1.12 name those who may have a conflict of interest in their *Lancet* article:

> Conflict of interest statement
>
> The study was sponsored by Biotronik, Germany. RE, JB, JK, MH, RW, and TFL acted as consultants for Biotronik, Berlin, Germany. The other authors declare that they have no conflict of interest.

10.4   Background

> *Objective of the trial sufficiently described?*

It is difficult to be specific about what should be contained in the Background or Introduction section on the rationale for why the trial being reported was undertaken. This will be very trial specific and hence may vary considerably in content, extent and complexity. Nevertheless, one crucial component of the background is to summarize succinctly the purpose and objectives of the trial being described. It is not always the case that the objectives of a trial are clearly stated.

The objectives of the trial of Example 2.1 in patients with oral lichen planus (OLP) are described by Poon, Goh, Kim, *et al.* (2006, p. 47) as follows.

> This randomized controlled trial compared the efficacy of topical steroid (triamcinolone acet-onide 0.1% in oral base; Kenalog; Bristol-Myers Squibb, New York, NY) and topical cyclosporine (Sandimmun Neoral solution containing 100 mg cyclosporine/mL; Novartis Intl AG, Basel, Switzerland) in patients with histologically confirmed OLP, with respect to response rate (by clinical scoring) and alleviation of pain and burning sensation (by patient-self assessment at weeks 4 and 8.

It is not always easy to encapsulate all the details in a single sentence or short paragraph but the authors in this example mention: the disease, randomized trial, the two interventions and three endpoints. In contrast, Levie, Gjorup, Skinhøj and Stoffel (2002, p. 610) of Example 1.11 include in the final sentence of their introduction a clear rationale for the trial of the novel hepatitis B vaccine.

> The rationale behind testing a 2-dose regimen was that fewer injections should improve com-pliance and be more convenient for those being immunized.

10.5   Methods

10.5.1   Participants

> *Satisfactory statement of diagnostic criteria for entry to the trial?*
> *Satisfactory statement of the source of participants?*

Hancock, Maher, Latimer, *et al.* (2007, p. 1638), in a trial in patients with acute low back pain, describe in the following the source of the participants (presenting to GPs in Sydney) and give a detailed summary of inclusion and exclusion criteria:

> All patients with low back pain (with or without leg pain) of less than 6 weeks duration presenting to any of 40 participating GPs in Sydney, Australia, were invited to participate. The inclusion criterion was a complaint of pain in the area between the 12th rib and buttock crease causing moderate pain and moderate disability (measured by adaption of items 7 and 8 of SF-36). Exclusion criteria were: present episode of pain not preceded by a pain-free period of at least 1 month, in which care was not provided; known or suspected serious spinal pathology; nerve root

compromise (with at least two of these signs: myotomal weakness, dermatomal sensory loss or hyporeflexia of the lower limb reflexes); presently taking NSAIDs or undergoing spinal manipulation; any spinal surgery within the preceding 6 months; and contraindication to paracetemol, diclofenac, or spinal manipulative therapy.

In contrast to this rather complex inclusion and exclusion criteria, although this degree of complexity is by no means unusual, those given by Stevinson, Devaraj, Fountain-Barber (2003, p. 60) of Example 1.9 are relatively straightforward:

> All patients between the ages of 18 and 70 years undergoing elective hand surgery for carpel tunnel syndrome by one surgeon (VSD) at the Royal Devon & Exeter Hospital or a private plastic surgery clinic were eligible for the trial. Patients were excluded if they were currently taking homeopathy remedies, reported previous hypersensitivity to homeopathy, were taking aspirin, or were unable to complete the study diary or attend follow-up appointments. Patients were not included in the trial a second time if they subsequently underwent surgery on the other hand.

In specifying these relatively straightforward criteria, the investigators were clearly mindful of the possibility of patient losses from the trial and hence stipulated requirements with respect to the ability to complete the study diary and to attend follow up clinics.

10.5.2 Procedures

> *Interventions well defined?*
> *Potential degree of blindness used?*

The three interventions in Example 2.6 of a trial for the treatment of fever in children of Hay, Costelloe, Redmond, *et al.* (2008, p. 2) were straightforward to describe as all parents received (double-blind) two medicine bottles, either (i) one containing active paracetemol and the other active ibrufen, (ii) one containing active paracetemol and the other placebo ibrufen or (iii) one containing placebo paracetemol and the other active ibrufen to give to their children. Thus the description of the interventions was precisely the same for whichever of the three options the child was randomized to receive.

> Intervention
>
> Parents were given standardized verbal and written advice on the appropriate use of loose clothing and encouraging children to take cool fluids. The intervention was the provision of, and advice to give, the study drugs for up to 48 hours: paracetemol every 4–6 hours (maximum of four doses in 24 hours) and ibuprofen every 6–8 hours (maximum of three doses in 24 hours).
>
> In this interesting example, the parents and children would know there were two different types of bottle that had to be used as the frequency of administration of the drug depended on the bottle contents.

10.5.3   Assessments

> *Satisfactory statement of criteria for outcome measures?*
> *Outcome measures appropriate?*

Although it may be relatively straightforward for a reader to judge if the endpoint criteria are well described, it is not necessarily so easy to judge if this primary (and any other outcome measure) is indeed the most appropriate, although some justification for the choice may well be included in the Background. In any event, one would expect that the specialist referees appointed by the journal concerned would view this aspect of the trial report critically. Nevertheless, it is the responsibility of the authors to indicate the importance and relevance of the endpoints chosen.

Drucker, Buse, Taylor, *et al.* (2008, p. 1240) list, for their trial of exenatide once weekly versus twice daily for the treatment of type 2 diabetes, the following endpoints:

> The primary endpoint in this study was the change in HbAκ at 30 weeks. Secondary endpoints included examining safety and tolerability, and analysis of fasting and postprandial plasma glucose concentrations, bodyweight, fasting glucagon, fasting lipids, blood pressure, exenatide pharmacokinetics, and paracetamol absorption. We also recorded the proportion of patients achieving target HbAκ concentrations of 7.0% or less, 6.5% or less, and 6.0% or less, overall and by baseline HbAκ strata; HbAκ by antibody titre; and body weight in the presence and absence of nausea.

In the above example, the primary endpoint is clear (except that 'change' requires a comparison which is not stipulated and their choice of '30 weeks' needs justifying). However, the plethora of secondary outcomes is too many and too confusing for sensible reporting and interpretation of the trial findings.

In the trial of Example 2.3, Chow, Tai, Tan, *et al.* (2002, p. 1222) define the primary endpoint for patients with inoperable hepatocellular carcinoma as:

> The primary endpoint was overall survival. Survival time was computed from the date of randomization to the date of death or the date of last contact.

The authors give a clear statement of just what the primary outcome is and then define precisely how it is determined for each patient.

10.5.4   Consent

> *Consent procedures appropriate and adequately described?*

In contrast to the trial protocol itself, which will require careful detail, in most instances the consent process can be described in very general terms such as that given in Example 1.9 by Stevinson, Devaraj, Fountain-Barber (2003, p. 62), who state:

> Ethical Approval
>
> The study protocol was approved by the Exeter Research Ethics Committee. Approval was also obtained from the Royal Devon and Exeter Healthcare NHS Trust. All participants gave written informed consent.

However, there may be particular concerns in some situations. Kahn, Fleischhacker, Boter, *et al.* (2008, p. 1086) in their trial of Example 2.4 in patients with schizophrenia and schizophreniform disorder take due account of the particular types of patients involved in the consent process. They state:

> All participants – or their legal representatives – provided written informed consent. The trial complied with the Declaration of Helsinki, and was approved by the ethics committees of the participating centres. The Julius Centre for Health Sciences and Primary Care monitored the trial according to Good Clinical Practice and International Conference on Harmonisation guidelines.

An even more complex consent process was necessary for the trial conducted by Tyrer, Oliver-Africano, Ahmed, *et al.* (2008, p. 58), who wished to randomize patients with intellectual disability who had aggressive challenging behaviour to receive, in a double-blind manner, placebo, haloperidol or risperidone. They summarize the consent process:

> Written informed consent was obtained on the basis of information that was understandable to the individuals concerned, which sometimes included considerable explanation and representation of the trial in simple picture format, so that the notion of the study could be appreciated. For patients who were not able to give informed consent, we approached relevant carers, including relatives and care staff at supported homes or related residential settings to give assent to the trial. Consent was given in writing and witnessed.

This declaration demonstrates due concern for the particular patients in question and underlines the difficulty in the truly informed consent process in some situations. However, such patients should not be denied the possibility of entering trials, particularly when the objective is targeted specifically at improving the care of such individuals.

In other situations, rather less stringent requirements have been permitted such as for the trial of Larsson and Carlsson (2002, p. 136). They evaluated the role of metronidazole in reducing vaginal cuff infection rates after abdominal hysterectomy among women with bacterial vaginosis, and state:

> Women gave verbal informed consent to participate in the study.

However, verbal consent alone is rare, even for the most minor of ailments and therapies; it provides no evidence at all that the clinical teams really did follow the rules for informed consent. Indeed, many ethical review bodies and many journals insist that evidence of informed consent is always formally recorded for each patient.

10.5.5 Monitoring

Although it is not essential for all trials to have an independent DMC, if one was established then brief details of the remit should be reported. Comi, Pulizzi, Rovaris, *et al.* (2008, pp. 2086–2087) who conducted a trial in patients with relapsing-remitting multiple sclerosis established an external data safety monitoring board. They describe the process:

> The Steering Committee supervised the conduct of the study. An independent external data safety monitoring board met six times via teleconference and three times in face-to-face meetings during

the trial period, to review the study conduct and the unblinded safety and efficacy results. An interim analysis was done at the discretion of the data safety monitoring board who had the authority to recommend discontinuation of the trial.

The members of data safety monitoring board were also listed in the trial report and, although one interim analysis was undertaken, the trial continued until the planned recruitment target was achieved.

10.5.6 Randomization

> *Method of randomization described?*
> *Acceptably short delay from allocation to start of intervention?*

Central to the conduct of a randomized controlled trial is the randomization process itself, and this is one major focus for the statistical guidelines of BMJ (2006) and a key consideration when judging the quality of a clinical trial. This process should have been carefully established following the procedures outlined in Chapter 5. However, some trials are likely to have unique features and so necessary adjustments may have to be made. Major points to consider are who carried out the randomization (e.g. randomization by telephoning the central trials office), the number of interventions under test, identification of suitable stratifying variables that are prognostic for outcome, whether the trial was single- or multicentre and the appropriate levels of masking. Investigators will have to detail their choice of allocation strategy, whether based on (simple) randomization principles, randomized blocks of a specific size, or by a method such as minimization. There should also be a clear statement of any delay between the time of randomization and the start of the interventions.

In the double-blind randomized trial conducted by Chow, Tai, Tan, *et al.* (2002, p. 1222) of three doses of tamoxifen in patients with non-operable hepatocellular carcinoma, the authors state:

> Randomization was performed in balanced blocks of 5, stratified by center and corresponding to P, TMX60, and TMX120 in the respective ratios of 2:1:2.

In this trial, in which 329 patients were recruited, the stratification by recruiting centres in Hong Kong, Myanmar, Singapore and elsewhere was done to ensure that the proportions of patients receiving the different doses remained approximately constant, at all points in time during the recruitment period, in all centres.

Szefler, Mitchell, Sorkness, *et al.* (2008, p. 1066) describe a randomized trial in which adolescents and young adults with persistent asthma were randomized on a 1 : 1 basis to either standard treatment or standard treatment modified on the basis of exhaled nitric oxide (NO). The authors state:

> ..., we used centralised block randomization, with a block size of ten, to assign patients to receive either guideline-based care or guideline-based care supplemented by NO monitoring. The randomization sequence was generated from a random number table and was stratified by site by use of SAS statistical software (version 9.1.3). A computer program generated a treatment option for

each patient according to the study allocation, so that investigators and patients were not aware of individual treatment assignments.

By the latter phrase we presume the authors mean 'before the allocation takes place', as this was not a double-blind trial.

In contrast to a simple yet balanced randomization procedure, Meggitt, Gray and Reynolds (2006, p. 840) in their single-centre trial of Example 1.2 used a minimization approach to randomize 63 patients, outlined as follows:

Azathioprine or placebo was allocated in a ratio of 2:1 ..... Treatment allocation was done with minimisation (Minim computer program, version 1.5) by an independent clinician after informed consent had been obtained. With this method, group allocation does not rely solely on chance (randomisation), but ensures that baseline differences in the distribution of possible outcome determinants are kept to a minimum. Minimisation variables were: (i) TMPT range, normal (>7.5 nmol/h per mL red blood cells [RBC]) versus intermediate (2.5–7.5); (ii) referring centre, (iii) body surface area involved of more than 50% versus 50% or less (used as surrogates for severe vs moderate disease activity); and (iv) severe skin infection needing oral antibiotics in the mouth before starting the trial.

The four minimization variables imply $2^4 = 8$ prognostic categories as well as treatment itself. It is difficult to imagine this complex process would work satisfactorily with, for example, only 21 assigned to placebo, as this would imply less than three patients per minimization cell. The likelihood is that some cells would in fact be empty. Essentially, the authors use too many stratifying variables for a trial of only 63 patients, and grouping continuous variables into categories may not be advisable either.

Computer-based randomization is often initiated by means of a telephone or fax call to a central randomization office which then queries the computer system with the relevant details. The allocated intervention is then output in some format and relayed to the investigating team concerned. However, the investigators participating in the trial of Example 2.4 by Kahn, Fleischhacker, Boter, et al. (2008, p. 1086) had access to a web-based system which is described in the trial report as:

Patients were randomly assigned by a dedicated web-based online system – which was developed in-house by the Data Management Department of the Julius Center for Health Sciences and Primary care (version 1.2) – to daily doses of: haloperidol 1–4 mg, amisulpride 200-800 mg, olanzapine 5–20 mg, quetiapine 200–750 mg, or ziprasidone 40–160 mg.

The authors then went on to state:

Since some study drugs were not registered at all participating centres, we used a minimisation procedure to prevent unequal group sizes at the end of the trial – ie, treatment assignment of new patients depended on the distribution of participants over the treatment groups. Randomisation to ziprasidone was blocked between December, 2003, and October, 2004, because the minimisation procedure used during randomization assigned ziprasidone to too many patients, in the few countries where ziprasidone was available.

The above detail describes several interesting features of this 50-centre, 14-country, 498-patient randomized trial. The first is that not all the five drugs under test were available at all sites, so that a key aspect of patient eligibility may have been compromised to some extent as *all* patients should be suitable for *all* interventions on offer prior to randomization. For example, if one of the drugs (say drug X) is thought to have a particular and likely side-effect but the others not, then susceptible patients should not be entered on trial. However, if X is not available for part of the recruitment period then these 'susceptible' patients might be randomized during this interval. Such a possibility raises issues of interpretation once the analysis is complete, particularly since, as is evident here, one of the drugs was assigned to twenty fewer patients than the other options. Secondly, the five drugs cannot be randomized in balanced blocks within centres. We would imagine that the consent process may also be difficult in such circumstances. Finally, this illustrates that any software developed for the randomization requires vigorous testing and continual monitoring as trial recruitment progresses. Nevertheless, what happened is clearly stated and so the readers of the article can judge for themselves the importance or otherwise of these features in influencing their own interpretation of the trial results.

In some patient allocation processes the investigator may access an on-line system. The trial of Smolen, Beaulieu, Rubbert-Roth, *et al.* (2008, p. 988) utilized 'an interactive voice response system' for randomization. This method of randomization brings the added advantage of being accessible 24 hours per day and every day, which facilitates multicentre multinational cooperation and enables 'out-of-hours' patients to be entered on the trial without delay.

10.5.7   Statistical considerations

10.5.7.1   Justification of trial size

> *Pre-trial calculation of sample size reported?*
> *Duration of post intervention follow up stated?*

The size of the trial needs to be fully justified. The most important aspect of this is that the anticipated effect size should reflect a difference between the interventions which is clinically or scientifically meaningful. If, as recommended above, the description of the Background to the trial already indicates the anticipated consequences of the intervention, only a short summary is required here. As two-sided significance tests of 5% are usual, any departures from this standard need to be justified. Although a minimum power of at least 80% is to be expected, trials of a greater power are desirable. There should be sufficient information provided, as well as an explicit reference to the sample size formula used, for the potential statistical reviewer and any reader of the article to verify the calculations made.

In a trial concerned with a ventilator-weaning protocol for mechanically ventilated patients in intensive care, Girard, Kress, Fuchs, *et al.* (2008) justified their chosen trial size to compare control, comprising usual care including spontaneous breathing trials (SBT), against an intervention comprising spontaneous awakening trials (SAT) plus SBT as follows:

> On the basis of a pilot database, we expected a mean of 12.9 (SD 10.4) ventilator-free days in the control group. Thus, we calculated that a sample size of 334 patients would be needed to detect a

25% increase in ventilator-free days to 16.1 days within the intervention group with 80% power and a two-sided significance level of 0.05.

This corresponds to a standardized effect size of the continuous measure of ventilator-free days of $\Delta = (16.1 - 12.9)/10.4 = 0.31$ which, according to Cohen's criterion, would suggest a moderate-to-small effect size. The authors indicate that their calculations use the sample size program of Dupont and Plummer (1997) which essentially evaluates Equation (9.5) in this situation. Although mathematically correct, it is somewhat misleading to quote the calculations to three significant figures as there is usually much uncertainty surrounding the anticipated effect size. Thus 334 would be better rounded to a more realistic 340 or perhaps 350 in this case.

Poon, Goh, Kim, *et al.* (2006, p. 49) use the binary variable response rate as their primary endpoint and, on this basis, explained their trial size in the following terms:

> It was anticipated that the response rate with steroids at 4 weeks would be approximately 60% and that this may be raised to as much as 80% with cyclosporine. With a 2-sided test size of 5% and power of 80%, the number of patients planned for the trial was 200 (Machin, Campbell, Fayers and Pinol, 1997*).

*Now updated as Machin, Campbell, Tan and Tan (2009).

The authors indicate the two-sided test size 5%, power 80%, effect size 20% and give a source reference to a whole book (rather than to the specific formula used for the calculation). In fact, the authors used Equation (9.6) for comparing two proportions but then factored in a possible patient loss of 10%. This factoring should have been made more explicit in their description.

In this example, the duration of post-intervention follow-up to determine the end-point of 4 weeks is included within the sample size statement. The observed response rates turned out to be 52% and 48%, much lower than the planning values and in the reverse magnitude to that anticipated. In addition, the trial was closed prematurely after 137 patients due to slow recruitment but without reference to the relative efficacy of the treatments concerned.

In contrast, the overall survival time of patients with nasopharyngeal cancer was the main focus of the trial by Wee, Tan, Tai, *et al.* (2005, p. 6731) and they justify patient numbers by:

> On the basis of a two-sided test size of 5% and a power of 90%, it was anticipated that a minimum of 200 patients would need to be recruited to detect the difference in absolute survival at 2 years of 25% that was observed by Al-Sarraf et al. This assumes that the survival rate was 55% for RT alone and 80% for CRT.

With these assumptions, the use of Equation (9.11) for this time-to-event endpoint leads to a trial size of 162 patients but, without stating it, the investigators then factored in a potential loss of patients of 15% bringing the numbers to 186, further rounded up to 200 in recognizing two things: (i) the fact that confirmatory trials often report less favourable outcomes than the original trial and should be larger, and (ii) that sufficient numbers should be recruited to provide convincing evidence of the benefit and its probable magnitude. The investigators should have made these considerations more explicit in their description.

Motzer, Escudier, Oudard, *et al.* (2008, p. 450) very carefully define progression-free survival (PFS) for their trial in patients with advanced renal cell carcinoma as:

> Progression-free survival, . . ., defined as the time from randomization to the first documentation of disease progression or death (from any cause).

However, one difficulty which sometimes arises with reports of time-to-event trials is that the precise definition of exactly what is regarded as an 'event' is not always explicitly included. In contrast to the PFS of the above example, other authors do not always count non-cancer deaths as indications of progression yet still use the term PFS. In situations where there are multiple possibilities for patient failure, the occurrence of any of which is regarded as *the* event of interest, special care has to be taken by the authors to make this clear.

Despite the above examples of formal justification of sample size, vague qualitative justifications do appear in the literature from time to time. One example is Zheng, Kang, Huang, *et al.* (2008, p. 2015) when investigating the effect of carbocisteine in patients with chronic obstructive pulmonary disease, who state:

> Accurate calculation of sample size had been an issue of great attention when planning the trial, but we were unable to do so because of scarcity of reference data from previously published studies. Consequently, the sample size was determined on the experiences of Chinese respiratory doctors and by the steering committee. The estimated sample size was deemed to be powered for this study.

In our view this statement is insufficient. Even the subjective views must have led to some quantification since the trial subsequently randomized 709 patients with chronic obstructive pulmonary disease, 354 to carbocisteine and 355 to placebo. One way of quantifying the anticipated effect would have been for the design team to conduct a survey of potential investigators and ask them for a personal estimate of (say) the 1-year exacerbation rates with no treatment (the placebo group) and also to ask how much this might improve if carbocisteine were used – answers might range from a negative, zero or positive impact. The distribution of their responses could then be summarized and, for example, the minimum, median and maximum anticipated effect size used to provide a range of planning options for the eventual sample size. A summary of the ensuing discussion and the rationale for the final choice can then be reported in the trial publication itself.

A similar situation arises in the trial conducted by Tyrer, Oliver-Africano, Ahmed, *et al.* (2008, pp. 58–59) who also experienced difficulty in determining an appropriate sample size. However, they adopt a rather more systematic approach to the problem.

> We had initial difficulty in establishing a sample size, since the MOAS scale has not been used often in studies of intellectual disability. However, from our previous study of MOAS scores in this population (Oliver, Crawford, Rao, et al., 2007), we obtained means and standard

deviations, and also developed a good idea of a clinically meaningful difference in scores. We calculated that with 96 patients allocated in total to the two active drugs (total number of patients needed in study = 144), we had 80% power at the 5% level to detect a difference in MOAS score of 4, with a standard deviation of 8 and an unpaired t test with an allocation ratio of 2 : 1.

The investigators therefore set $\delta_{Plan} = 4$ and $\sigma_{Plan} = 8$ to define a clinically mean-ingful standardized effect size of $\Delta_{Plan} = \delta_{Plan}/\sigma_{Plan} = 4/8 = 0.5$ which corresponds to a moderate effect following the Cohen (1988) suggestions. For this trial, this repre-sented the anticipated difference between one arm (placebo) and the average of the second and third arms (risperidone and haloperidol). The three arms were to be randomized on a 1 : 1 : 1 basis. The sample size calculations using Equation (9.5) with an allocation $\lambda = 2$ give $m = 48$ for the placebo arm and 96 for the two arms combined. These were then to be allocated equally amongst these two. In fact, randomizing 50 per group would seem more realistic. However, no direct reference to the method of calculation of sample size is given.

We return to this example when addressing sample size and analysis issues related to this type of three-group design in Chapter 13.3.

10.5.7.2 Interim analysis for data monitoring

If a DMC is established to monitor a trial then some statistical guidelines to assist in the monitoring process should have been specified in the protocol, which need to be summarized. We have given one such summary in Example 7.2, which was included in the report by Lau, Leung, Ho, et al. (1999, p. 798), describing their trial in patients with resectable hepatocellular carcinoma. In that example, a formal stopping rule was described and this triggered the early termination of the trial to patient entry.

In the equivalence or conservative trial (see Chapter 11.4) comparing intravenous immune globulin and plasma exchange in Guillain–Barré syndrome of van der Meché and Schmitz (1992), part of the stopping rule is described as follows:

Stopping rule for a conservative trial

> ... a stopping rule based on a test of significance was applied in the protocol: the trial should be terminated if one of the two treatments proved superior after the accrual of 100 patients (P < 0.030, after correction for two analyses). . . . .

However, the monitoring appears to have been made by the investigators themselves rather than by establishing an independent DMC to advise them. In contrast to Lau, Leung, Ho, et al. (1999) and van der Meché and Schmitz (1992), both of which describe their stopping rules, many trials that invoke such rules omit precise details of how these are determined in the corresponding publication. It is important, whether or not these rules are indeed stopping rules (or merely advisory indications) for the DMC, that they should be carefully described and clearly justified.

10.5.7.3   *Intended final analysis*

> *All statistical procedures adequately described or referenced?*
> *Statistical analyses appropriate?*
> *Prognostic factors adequately considered?*

There are a multitude of different methods available for analysis, the choice of which will depend on the type of endpoint(s) being summarized and the design itself. In general, the more straightforward the analysis and consequently its description, the easier it is to communicate the trial findings. Details of the analytical methods will have been summarized in the trial protocol. What is required here is a résumé of that description plus any modifications or additions that may have become relevant with the passage of time.

Poon, Goh, Kim, *et al.* (2006) describe their method of analysis as:

> Analyses were made on an intention-to-treat basis. Comparisons of clinical response rates, VAS and grid measures of the marker lesion were made using logistic and linear regressions adjusted for baseline symptoms as appropriate (Frison and Pocock, 1992). 95% confidence intervals (CI) for treatment differences were calculated using CIA (Bryant, 2000) statistical software.
>
> The longitudinal data, using all the individual measures available, were summarized graphically and, to give an indication of trends over time, fractional polynomials permitting an estimate of treatment differences were fitted using Stata (StataCorp, 2001). These models take into account the correlated nature of the repeated measures on each patient.

In this example, the authors specify the software used to calculate the confidence intervals for treatment difference. They also indicate that baseline variables thought prognostic for outcome were taken into account if they affected the estimated treatment differences.

Part of the very detailed statistical methods section of Girard, Kress, Fuchs, *et al.* (2008, p. 129) states:

> . . . . Kaplan-Meier analysis, and the log-rank test were also used to assess the effect of the treatment protocols on 1-year survival; patients were censored at the time of last contact alive or at 1 year from enrolment, whichever was first. The unadjusted hazard ratio (HR) of death was obtained with Cox proportional hazards assumption by examining scaled Schoenfeld's partial residuals (Schoenfeld, 1982) for the independent variable included in the model: no violation of the assumptions was detected.

Although the statistical methods summarized here are very explicit, the one reference given is rather old, very technical in nature and unlikely to be understood by many readers. A more up-to-date and accessible description of the method should have been provided. It is unfortunate if statistical methods are presented as a technical 'black-box' which gives little insight into the processes concerned rather than by reference to, for example, Bradburn, Clark, Love and Altman (2003). This article is one part of a tutorial series explaining aspects of time-to-event analysis designed specifically for a clinical audience.

10.6   Findings

> *High proportion of participants followed up?*
> *High proportion of participants complete intervention?*
> *Were participants who dropped out from the intervention and control groups described adequately?*
> *Intervention and control groups comparable in relevant measures?*

The information necessary to comply with each component of the above panel may be placed in various parts of the Results section. Important details will be provided in the flow diagram suggested by the CONSORT statement and what will often be the first figure of the Results section, describing the basic features of the participants in the randomized intervention groups.

10.6.1   CONSORT

Figure 10.3 gives an example of the CONSORT style patient flow though the two-group trial of Example 1.2 conducted by Meggitt, Gray and Reynolds (2006, Figure 1) in

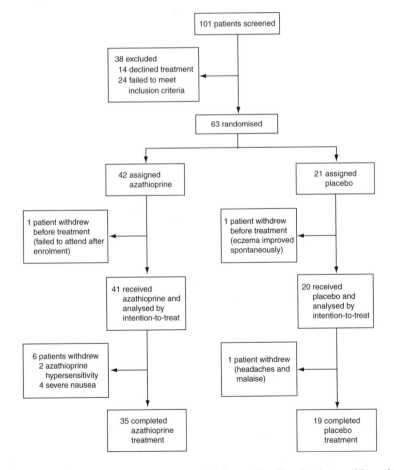

Figure 10.3   Trial profile following the CONSORT guidelines (after Meggitt, Gray and Reynolds, 2006, Figure 1)

patients with moderate-to-severe eczema. The schema clearly shows that, of those screened, 63 are randomized in the 2 : 1 ratio as planned. There were only two patients who withdrew before treatment commenced, one of which was perhaps caused by a delay from randomization to the commencement of treatment. Details of those who withdrew from protocol treatment are also given, two showing hypersensitivity to azathiprine, four experiencing severe nausea and one having headaches and malaise. As one might anticipate, there were no withdrawals of this type in those receiving placebo. This will not always be the case, however, as placebos are as effective in producing side-effects as they are in inducing therapeutic responses.

A rather more complex CONSORT diagram is depicted in Figure 10.4 summarizing key features of the trial of Szefler, Mitchell, Sorkness, *et al.* (2008, Figure 1). In this trial, there are numerous reasons why many of the 709 patients screened are excluded

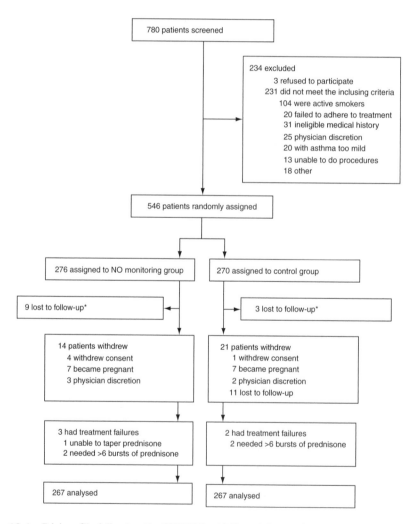

Figure 10.4   Trial profile following the CONSORT guidelines (after Szefler, Mitchell, Sorkness, *et al.*, 2008, Figure 1)

from the randomization. This illustrates that, at least as far as this example is concerned, a great deal of unnecessary work is devoted to examining patients who will not be considered for randomization. In other circumstances, this may be a sufficiently added burden to prevent the planned trial from ever being conducted. Another interesting feature is the 'physician discretion' option which was the reason given for 25 (presumably otherwise eligible for the trial) not being randomized and five withdrawals post randomization. Of course the attending physician has, and quite rightly so, the ultimate responsibility for the care of the patient. However, when such discretion is exercised the underlying rationale for it should be recorded – certainly for any made post randomization. It is also worthy of note that 14 women (7 in each group) who became pregnant were also withdrawn and it is a possible cause for concern that 11 were lost to follow-up in the control group but none in those receiving NO. Such unbalanced losses may cause bias in the final treatment comparison although, in this case, the loss only represents 4% (11/270) and is unlikely to have a major impact. Despite these potential difficulties, the CONSORT diagram provides the reader of the article with the necessary information to make a judgement on whether or not this attrition of patients will have any impact on the clinical interpretation of the findings presented.

10.6.2   Participant characteristics

> *Intervention and control groups comparable in relevant measures?*

Although the eligibility criteria are specified in the protocol, it is clearly important to describe in the trial report the types of patients actually included and randomized. The (baseline) characteristics summarized usually include some basic demographic data, information on the condition under investigation and variables that are known or suspected to be prognostic for outcome. This has been done with patients with eczema in Table 10.1 which summarizes baseline demographic and clinical characteristics of the participants in the trial of Meggitt, Gray and Reynolds (2006, Table 1). This tabulation extends beyond the demographics of age and gender to details concerning markers such as genetic polymorphism in thiopurine methyltransferase (TMPT) and immunoglobin E (IgE), concomitant disease, hayfever and asthma, previous treatment for eczema and baseline assessments of several endpoint measures, disease activity (SASSAD), body area involved and itch score. The authors also indicate that more complete information is available in an accompanying web-based table which has been published online with the corresponding article.

Although not a critical point, it is important to remember that the purpose of such a table is not for *estimating*, for example, the mean age of the participants within the placebo group, but merely for *describing* them. Thus the range of ages, rather than the standard deviation (SD) is a more appropriate summary measure here. This equally applies to the other continuous variables within the table such as TMPT activity and patient-assessed itch score.

Although a randomized trial, it is clear from Table 10.1 that the characteristics of those in the placebo and azathioprine groups are not exactly identical although there

Table 10.1   Demographic and clinical characteristics together with baseline assessments of disease of patients with moderate-to-severe eczema (selected from Meggitt, Gray and Reynolds, 2006, Table 1)

	Treatment	Placebo	Azathioprine
Demographic	Number of patients	20	41
	Age (years)	36 (12)	30 (11)
	Men (%)	16 (80%)	19 (46%)
Potentially prognostic	TPMT activity (nmol/h/mL RBC)	10.4 (2.1)	10.3 (2.2)
	TPMT heterozygous range	2 (10%)	5 (2%)
	Previous systemic therapy or phototherapy for eczema	16 (80%)	30 (73%)
	Hayfever	14 (70%)	29 (71%)
	Asthma	13 (65%)	27 (66%)
	Raised serum IgE	15/15 (100%)	34/35 (97%)
Baseline assessment of endpoints	Disease activity (SASSAD)	32.7 (8.9)	32.3 (13.2)
	Body area involved	58.3 (17.9)	51.0 (21.0)
	Patient-assessed itch score	5.7 (1.8)	5.4 (2.1)
	Patient-assessed loss-of-sleep score	4.9 (2.6)	4.4 (2.5)
	Quality of life score (DLQI)	9.4 (6.1)	9.7 (5.0)

Data are mean (*SD*) or number (%).

are no major disparities. However, what happens if we do statistical tests to see if disparities actually occur? In this case, Fayers and King (2008) point out:

> ... we already know what the answer must be. Because the treatments are allocated by randomization, any differences in the baseline characteristics must be purely due to chance. Even when randomization is done properly, we expect approximately 5% of the characteristics tested to have P-values that are less than 0.05, and we expect 1% of characteristics to be significant with P < 0.01. In other words, if there were 20 baseline characteristics being explored, on average we would expect, purely by chance, that one characteristic would be significant with P < 0.05.

Significance tests of baseline imbalances are only useful as a means of testing whether there may have been a violation of the randomization procedure. Despite these remarks, D'Haens, Baert, van Assche, *et al.* (2008, Table 1) in their trial in patients with newly diagnosed Crohn's disease inappropriately conducted 12 statistical tests of baseline characteristics illustrated in Table 10.2, although none turned out to be statistically significant at the 5% level. In contrast Meggitt, Gray and Reynolds (2006, p. 842) correctly noted:

> By chance, there was a sex imbalance between groups at baseline (table 1, webtable 2) . . . .

It is important to remember that many of the variables in the first table of a report are purely descriptive in nature. However, any that are identified as *major prognostic features* for outcome *at the design stage* of the trial should be used to determine if the estimate of treatment effect changes substantially when the analysis is adjusted for these

Table 10.2 Baseline characteristics illustrating the inappropriate use of a statistical significance tests for comparing groups which have been randomized (after D'Haens, Baert, van Assche, *et al.*, 2008, Table 1)

	Early combined immunosuppression (n = 65)	Conventional management (n = 64)	p value
Sex (female)	43 (66.2%)	37 (57.8%)	0.33^a
Race (white)	64 (98.5%)	61 (95.3%)	0.37^b
Age (years)	30.0 (11.8)	28.7 (10.9)	0.50^c
Weeks from diagnosis to treatment	2.0 (1.0–5.0)	2.5 (1.0–11.0)	0.65^b
Height (m)	1.71 (0.09)	1.71 (0.10)	0.93^c
Weight (kg)	63.1 (13.4)	62.5 (12.1)	0.82^c
Smoking			0.18^a
Current	28 (43.1%)	23 (35.9%)	
Former	8 (12.3%)	16 (25.0%)	
Never	29 (44.6%)	25 (39.1%)	
Mesalazine use	3 (4.6%)	2 (3.1%)	1.00^b
Disease location			0.90^a
Small bowel	14 (21.5%)	15 (23.4%)	
Ileocolitis	31 (47.7%)	28 (43.8%)	
Colitis	20 (30.8%)	21 (32.8%)	
CDAI score^d	330 (92)	306 (80)	0.12^b
IBDQ^e	122 (33)	136 (28)	0.11^b
C-reactive protein concentration (mg/L)	19 (5–75)	25 (8–59)	0.22^b

Data are number (%), mean (SD) or median (IQR) unless otherwise specified.
^{a} χ^2 test for dichotomous variables.
^{b} Student's *t* test for continuous variables.
^{c} Fisher's exact test.
^{d} Crohn's Disease Activity Index scores range from 0–600; higher scores indicate greater disease activity.
^{e} Inflammatory Bowel Disease Questionnaire scores range from 32–224; higher scores indicate better health-related quality of life.

using regression techniques. Any baseline characteristics that are of major prognostic value should be used as covariates or as stratification factors, especially if there appears to be an imbalance in these characteristics (irrespective of whether or not that imbalance is statistically significant)

10.6.3 Endpoints

> *Presentation of statistical material satisfactory?*
> *Confidence intervals given for the main results?*
> *Conclusions drawn from the statistical analysis justified?*

It is important to emphasize that the main focus of any report on the outcome of a randomized clinical trial must be on the relative efficacy of the alternative interventions under test with respect to the primary endpoint(s) specified in the protocol. Thus, the intention of the eventual analysis is to enable a statement such as that of Girard, Kress,

Table 10.3   Drug efficacy at 12 weeks in patients with moderate-to-severe eczema treated by either placebo or azathioprine (part data from Meggitt, Gray and Reynolds, 2006, Table 2)

Treatment	Placebo	Azathioprine	Difference (95% CI)
Number of patients	20	41	
Reduction in disease activity (SASSAD)	6.6	12.0	5.4 (1.4 to 9.3)
Reduction in % body area involved	14.6	25.8	11.2 (1.6 to 20.7)
Reduction in itch score	1.0	2.4	1.4 (0.1 to 2.7)
Reduction in loss-of-sleep score	1.2	2.5	1.3 (−0.1 to 2.6)
Improvement in quality of life (DLQI)	2.4	5.9	3.5 (0.3 to 6.7)
Reduction in soluble CD30	−12.6	3.3	16.0 (−0.3 to 32.3)
Median reduction in combined moderate/potent topical steroid use (g per month)	12.5	22.5	4.8 (−14.0 to 39.0)

Fuchs, *et al.* (2008, p. 126) to be made. In the structured abstract of their paper, they summarize:

> Interpretation: Our results suggest that a wake up and breathe control protocol that pairs daily spontaneous awakening trials (ie interruption of sedatives) with daily spontaneous breathing trials results in better outcome for mechanically ventilated patients in intensive care than current standard approaches and should become routine practice.

The results obtained from seven different endpoint variables are summarized in Table 10.3 (Meggitt, Gray and Reynolds, 2006; Table 2) This table does not, for example, report the simple difference between mean reduction in disease activity (SASSAD), but those obtained after adjustment for the four variables in the minimization algorithm used for the dynamic method of treatment allocation (see Section 5.3). However, this detail is lost as an obscure footnote to their table. Differences between groups after such adjustments are not necessarily easy for the reader to interpret. It is therefore usual to first give the unadjusted values and then point out whether or not these differences, once adjusted, substantially alter the interpretation of the trial results. In Table 10.3 the simple differences all appear to equal the unadjusted difference, except for reduction in soluble CD30 (15.9, which is trivially different than 16.0) and median reduction in combined moderate/potent topical steroid use (10.0, which is very different from 4.8).

Section 4.4 provides a more satisfactory analysis available for this design, using regression techniques to include the baseline (pre-treatment) assessment of SASSAD as a covariate and the values at 12 weeks as the dependent variable y.

Nevertheless, Table 10.3 clearly sets out the values of the estimated treatment difference for each endpoint variable concerned, and quotes the corresponding 95% confidence intervals. A further useful addition would be the corresponding p-values for each comparison.

10.6.4   Adverse events

Adverse effects of interventions reported?

Table 10.4 Incidence of adverse events in patients with dyslipidaemia (part data from Krishna, Anderson, Bergman, *et al.*, 2007, Table 2)

		Anacetrapib (mg)			
	Placebo 0	10	40	150	300
Number of patients	10	10	10	10	10
Nausea	1	—	1	—	1
Headache	3	3	3	3	1
Diarrhoea	—	—	—	1	1
Pain in extremity	1	—	—	—	—
Abdominal pain	1	—	—	—	—
Dizziness	1	2	—	—	1

In some situations one or more of the interventions may raise concerns about safety issues, which then have to be balanced against its other merits. For example, in the trial described in Example 3.7, relating to the use of alternative mattresses to reduce pressure sores, there was a concern that one mattress type (with the greater physical depth) might be associated with more patients falling from the bed. The corresponding protocol will therefore have identified the 'adverse events' that should be documented and these should be reported in the trial-associated publications.

In the trial of Example 1.3 involving 40 patients with dyslipidaemia, Krishna, Anderson, Bergman, *et al.* (2007) recorded 28 different types of adverse events. Some of these are listed in Table 10.4 by the five doses of anacetrapib received, which varied from 0 mg (Placebo) to 300 mg. In their article, the Placebo results were placed as the final column of their table, but are placed here in the column to the left of that for 10 mg, to facilitate a visual inspection of trends over increasing dose. In fact, no patterns seem to be present but this is quite a small trial and clear patterns may not be expected. However, headache, the *most* common adverse event affecting 13/50 (26%) of patients, is *least* common in those receiving the highest dose of 300 mg.

The authors conclude, without any statistical comparisons, that:

> Anacetrapib was generally well tolerated . . . in patients with dyslipidaemia. There were no serious adverse events and no discontinuations due to clinical or laboratory adverse experiences. . . . All adverse experiences were transient and resolved without treatment.

In contrast, when reporting the adverse events given in Table 10.5, Meggitt, Gray and Reynolds (2006, Table 4) make a statistical comparison but not between the two randomized treatment groups. Neither are the details of this analysis described in the Statistical Methods section, but only added as a footnote to their table. They compare TMPT activity among the groups experiencing different levels of nausea. It is unclear whether those from both the azathiprine and placebo groups are included or whether standard deviation or standard error is within the brackets [.], no confidence interval is quoted and the form of analysis by grouping nausea into two categories (None and Mild versus Moderate and Severe) is less than optimal in

Table 10.5 Adverse events and laboratory abnormalities reported in patients with moderate-to-severe atopic eczema (after Meggitt, Gray and Reynolds, 2006, Table 4)

		Treatment group	
		Azathiprine (%)	Placebo (%)
	Number of patients	41	20
Adverse events			
Nausea[a]	None	20 (49%)	15 (75%)
	Mild	10 (24%)	5 (5%)
	Moderate (dose-limiting)	7 (17%)	—
	Severe	4 (10%)	—
Headaches		5 (12%)	3 (15%)
Abdominal pain		4 (10%)	2 (10%)
Lightheadedness		3 (7%)	1 (5%)
Malaise		1 (2%)	2 (10%)
Folliculitis		3 (7%)	2 (10%)
Respiratory tract	Lower	2 (5%)	—
Infection	Upper	2 (5%)	1 (5%)
Abnormalities in laboratory measures			
> 1 episode neutropenia ($1-2 \times 10^9$/L)		2 (5%)	—
> 1 episode mild lymphopenia ($1-1.5 \times 10^9$/L)		18 (43%)	6 (30%)
> 1 episode moderate lymphopenia ($1-1.5 \times 10^9$/L)		10 (24%)	4 (20%)
Alanine transaminase increase >15% above upper normal limit		4 (10%)	2 (10%)
Alanine transaminase increase >50% above upper normal limit		2 (5%)	1 (5%)

[a] TMPT activity was not significantly different ($p = 0.5$) between participants with no nausea or mild nausea, and moderate or severe nausea (10.3[2.3] vs. 10.7 [2.1] nmol/h/mL RBC).

any event. Considerable caution is required as to how one should interpret such apparently ad hoc analyses.

10.6.5 Graphics

One method of presentation of trial results that should not be overlooked is pictorial. If results can be displayed graphically and also show the actual and individual trial data that have been collected, they can be particularly informative. In the dot-plot of Figure 1.1, based on the results of the trial by Meggitt, Gray and Reynolds (2006, Figure 1A), it is easy to see that there has been a reduction in disease activity (scores greater than 0) as assessed by SASSAD for the vast majority of the patients following treatment for their eczema. Further, those receiving azathioprine tend to show greater improvement than their counterparts receiving placebo. However, it is also very clear that there is considerable overlap between the reductions achieved in the two groups. Despite the usefulness of Figure 1.1, an even more informative presentation would have been to present a dot-plot – one for each treatment group – of the actual rather than the percentage change in SASSAD scores at baseline and at 12 weeks, and to join the corresponding individual patient values. Such plots might indicate, for example, consistently lower values of SASSAD in all patients over the period but a steeper drop among those receiving azathioprine.

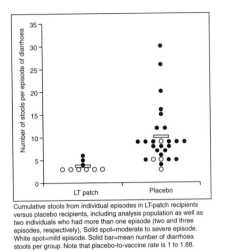

Cumulative stools from individual episodes in LT-patch recipients versus placebo recipients, including analysis population as well as two individuals who had more than one episode (two and three episodes, respectively), Solid spot=moderate to severe episode. White spot=mild episode. Solid bar=mean number of diarrhoea stools per group. Note that placebo-to-vaccine rate is 1 to 1.88.

Figure 10.5 Dot-plots of severity of diarrhoeal episodes and numbers of stools by treatment group (after Frech, DuPont, Bourgeois, *et al.*, 2008, Figure 2)

The very informative plot of Figure 10.5 is provided in the report by Frech, DuPont, Bourgeois, *et al.* (2008) and gives a clear indication of how a patch containing heat-labile toxin reduces problems associated with travellers' diarrhoea. For those patients with diarrhoeal episodes, it illustrates the variation in the number of stools per episode with the corresponding mean by treatment group, as well as the severity of the individual episodes.

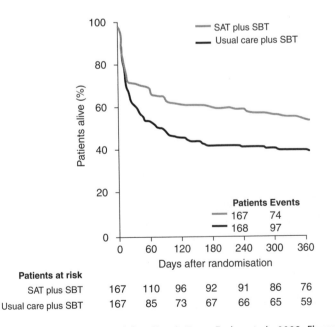

Figure 10.6 Survival at 1-year (after Girard, Kress, Fuchs, *et al.*, 2008, Figure 4)

Graphical representations are commonplace when reporting trials with a time-to-event endpoint and are particularly useful and informative. These graphs usually show the Kaplan–Meier estimates of the corresponding survival curves. An example is Figure 10.6, taken from the trial of Girard, Kress, Fuchs, *et al.* (2008). The figure clearly shows an improved survival in these mechanically ventilated patients of the 'SAT plus SBT' regime over those receiving 'Usual care plus SBT'. It gives the number of patients randomized to each intervention group and indicates how the number at risk declines within each intervention group as the year following randomization progresses. A useful addition to the graphics may have been a text box indicating the value of the HR of 0.68, the 95% confidence interval (0.50 to 0.92) and the corresponding *p*-value (0.01).

10.7   When things go wrong

Even in the most carefully planned and conducted clinical trials things can go wrong. Some of these may be mistakes made by the design team in the original concept, but others may arise through unforeseen circumstances. Whatever their importance, the wisest thing for the writing team to do is to admit them, explain how they have arisen and discuss how they might have influenced the conclusions drawn. The worst thing which can be done (and this is essentially dishonest in any event) is to try to camouflage such occurrences, perhaps hoping the referees will not spot them if they cannot be entirely concealed.

In Section 10.4, we gave one example where things went wrong. In that case the (computerized) minimization randomization process in the trial of Kahn, Fleischhacker, Boter, *et al.* (2008) malfunctioned resulting in a lack of balance in the numbers randomized to the five intervention groups. Nevertheless, their paper has been accepted for publication by a reputable journal. The referees and editors must have judged that the technical problem did not compromise the reliability of the trial conclusions.

A potentially more serious problem arose in the randomized double-blind trial of the use of tamoxifen in patients with advanced (inoperable) hepatocellular carcinoma conducted by Chow, Tai, Tan, *et al.* (2002). The possible problem with the placebo and tamoxifen tablets was only discovered when the analysis was complete; the results had indicated a reverse trend compared to that anticipated by the design. The results therefore appeared to show that high-dose tamoxifen carried an adverse survival outcome compared to placebo, with an intermediate dose giving intermediate survival outcome. This raised the possibility that the labelling for the double-blind code had become switched in some way. In fact this was not the case but it was found, after crushing and examining unused but still packaged tablets from the different centres involved, that somewhere in the production-to-packaging process some batches of placebo and active had been switched. The investigation led by a senior medical statistician concluded that despite this contamination, the results if anything would underestimate the adverse effect of high-dose tamoxifen. All this was explained in the submitted paper and the article accepted for publication in a high-impact journal.

10.8   Conclusions

We have stressed on several occasions that an important strategy for the trial team is to anticipate what the chosen journal might expect in general terms with respect to many sections of the article which is to be submitted. The major requirement is to summarize the key results and consider the consequences for clinical care and/or research. It is likely to be easy to describe the results of the trial if it addresses what many would agree is an important question, and if the outcome provides a clear and unequivocal answer to this. Summarizing the results may be more of a challenge when there still remains considerably uncertainty surrounding the conclusions, and this can happen even when a trial is well planned and executed but the results are contrary to expectations. Although the trial protocol will have reviewed the current state of knowledge at the time of planning the trial, this must be updated here with any developments that have been made during the period of the trial. In particular, the results should be compared with those from any related clinical trials that may have been published in this interim. It is also important to consider any shortcomings, for example perhaps a larger proportion of patients were lost to follow-up than had been anticipated; however, care should be taken to ensure that such limitations are reviewed in a balanced manner and are not overemphasized to the detriment of the trial's importance.

In many circumstances the trial being reported will raise further questions, perhaps requiring subsequent trials. An indication of what these might be would be a valuable addition.

10.9   Guidelines

10.9.1   General

General guidelines for the structure of reports following the completion of a clinical trial are available. These essentially describe the very detailed requirements necessary to support, if appropriate, the documentation needed for regulatory approval of the test product for subsequent clinical use. Nevertheless, even for a trial not seeking such approval, they provide a useful checklist of key features that need to be included in any published clinical trial report.

ICH E3 (1995) *Structure and Content of Clinical Study Reports.* CPMP/ICH/137/95, EMEA, Canary Wharf, London, www.emea.eu.int

10.9.2   CONSORT

The original CONSORT statement was intentionally generic and did not consider in detail specific types of trials. However, extensions to the CONSORT statement have been developed for non-inferiority and equivalence, cluster randomized designs, reporting of abstracts, data on harm, trials of herbal interventions, nonpharmacological interventions and pragmatic trials. Up to date guidelines can be found on the CONSORT web site www.consort-statement.org.

Begg, C., Cho, M., Eastwood, S., Horton R., Moher D., Olkin I., Pitkin R., Rennie D., Schultz K.F., Simel D., and Stroup D.F., (1996) Improving the quality of reporting randomized controlled trials: the CONSORT statement, *Journal of the American Medical Association*, **276**, 637–639.

Boutron, I., Moher, D., Altman, D.G., Schultz K.F., and Ravaud P., (2008) Extending the CONSORT statement to randomized trials of nonpharmacologic treatment: explanation and elaboration, *Annals of Internal Medicine*, **148**, 295–309.

Gagnier, J.J., Boon, H., Rochon, P., Moher D., Barnes J., and Bombardier C., (2006) Reporting randomized, controlled trials of herbal interventions: an elaborated CONSORT statement, *Annals of Internal Medicine*, **144**, 364–367.

Hopewell, S., Clarke, M., Moher, D., Wager E., Middleton P., and Altman D.G., (2008) CONSORT for reporting randomised trials in journal and conferences abstracts, *Lancet*, **371**, 281–283.

Ioannidis, J.P., Evans, S.J., Gotzsche, P.C., O'Neill R.T., Altman D.G., Schultz K., *et al.* (2004) Better reporting of harms in randomized trials: an extension of the CONSORT statement, *Annals of Internal Medicine*, **141**, 781–788.

Piaggio, G., Elbourne, D.R., Altman, D.G., Pocock, S.J., and Evans, S.J.W. (2001) Reporting of noninferiority and equivalence randomized trials: an extension of the CONSORT statement. *Journal of the American Medical Association*, **295**, 1152–1160.

Zwarenstein, M., Treweek, S., Gagniere, J.J., Altman D.G., Tunis S., Haynes B., Oxman A.D., and Moher D., (2008) Improving the reporting of pragmatic trials: an extension of the CONSORT statement, *BMJ*, **337**, 1223–1226.

10.9.3 Editorial

Many journals provide online versions of guidelines for authors. For example, the Journal of Clinical Oncology, at www.jco.ascopubs.org/, contains sections on: conflicts of interest; authorship contributions; clinical trial registration; and statistical guidelines.

BMJ (2006) Editors' checklist, www.bmj.com/advice/checklists.shtml

10.9.4 Statistical

Altman, D.G., Gore, S.M., Gardner, M.J. and Pocock, S.J. (2000) Statistical guidelines for contributors to medical journals, in *Statistics with Confidence*, 2nd edn (eds D.G. Altman, D. Machin, T.N. Bryant and M.J. Gardner), British Medical Journal, London, 171–190.

CHAPTER 11

Adaptations of the Basic Design

In this chapter, additional possibilities for the basic parallel two-group randomized trial are considered. One is concerned with designs which allow repeated (outcome) measures within the same individual trial participant to be taken into account. We also describe cluster trials, in which the randomization to the intervention is not made on an individual participant basis. Contrasts are made between trials designed to detect superiority, with those to demonstrate non-inferiority or equivalence. Methods of analysis and for estimating the numbers of participants to be recruited to such trials are given. We also comment on some practical issues arising and implications for reporting.

11.1 Introduction

So far in this book we have based our discussions around the parallel two-group design in which individual subjects are randomized. This is the most common design in use and it illustrates the main features of clinical trials methodology. One adaptation of the basic design is to keep the original structure, but to use as an outcome a feature that can be repeatedly measured on the individuals over an interval starting immediately post-randomization. Immediately prior to randomization, there are also situations in which this measure (the baseline measurement) is taken and even situations where such measures might also be taken on earlier occasions. Designs including such repeated measures data are termed longitudinal.

Another adaptation of the basic design is to allocate the interventions at random to collections or clusters of participants rather than to individuals. The basic design structure of a parallel two-group design may be retained again, but issues of informed consent, trial size and analysis are somewhat unique.

With the exception of Example 1.7, we have focused on clinical trials designed to establish a difference in efficacy between the alternatives. Often these compare a standard treatment or intervention and a new or alternative approach anticipated to be more effective. In general, these are termed superiority trials. In other circumstances an alternative therapy (perhaps one that is cheaper, less toxic or easier to administer) may be suggested to replace the standard, provided its efficacy is no worse than the

Randomized Clinical Trials: Design, Practice and Reporting   David Machin and Peter M Fayers
© 2010 John Wiley & Sons, Ltd

standard. Such trial types are termed non-inferiority trials and, although the basic design may appear to be the same as for a superiority trial, there are issues that affect the size of the trial as well as their conduct, analysis and interpretation.

11.2   Repeated measures

11.2.1   Autocorrelation

The problem with longitudinal data obtained from an individual is that successive measurements (of the same variable) are likely to be correlated. Alternatively phrased, the successive observations are unlikely to be independent. A key consideration in planning a trial involving repeated measures is the nature and strength of this correlation. Correlation coefficients are a measure of the degree of association between two variables. To measure the association between successive continuous measures in time, say at t_1 and t_2, we use the auto- or serial-correlation, estimated by:

$$\rho_T(1,2) = \frac{\sum (y_1 - \bar{y}_1)(y_2 - \bar{y}_2)}{\sqrt{\sum (y_1 - \bar{y}_1)^2 \sum (y_2 - \bar{y}_2)^2}}. \tag{11.1}$$

Here y_1 and y_2 represent the values of two successive assessments of the same measure made on the same subject (or on specimens taken from the subject). The expression is symmetric in terms of y_1 and y_2 and hence $\rho_T(1, 2) = \rho_T(2, 1)$ (T is included here to emphasize the time element).

11.2.2   Design

If the outcome variable in a clinical trial of a new hypertensive agent is the systolic blood pressure (SBP), this can be ascertained not just at a fixed time post-randomization (say at 12 weeks) but at any stage of the active treatment period, before the intervention commences and also after the intervention is complete. In certain circumstances, these repeated measures can ensure a more efficient comparison between the interventions on test and thereby may result in a reduction of the numbers of participants needed to be recruited.

11.2.3   Analysis

Suppose in a two-group comparative trial we make v observations of the same measure on each patient before randomization to treatment, and then make a further w observations after. The object of the therapy, once initiated, is to cause a change in these values (perhaps to lower them).

Example 11.1   Azathioprine for the treatment of atopic eczema

As described in Example 1.2, Meggitt, Gray and Reynolds (2006) randomized patients with moderate-to severe eczema to receive either azathioprine or placebo in a double-blind formulation, to ascertain the relative reduction in disease activity as assessed by the SASSAD score between the treatment groups. In fact, SASSAD was measured on several occasions including 2 weeks before, at baseline (time zero) immediately before randomization and at post randomization at 4, 8 and 12 weeks.

In the context of a parallel group trial, the repeated measures design extends the regression model of Equation (2.1) to include a term describing changes with time, t. In the simplest case, the model for the post-randomization situation takes the form:

$$y = \beta_0 + \beta_{\text{Treat}}\tau + \beta_{\text{Time}}t + \xi, \tag{11.2}$$

where y represents the continuous endpoint of interest in the clinical trial. Once again, $\tau = 0$ and $\tau = 1$ represent the two interventions concerned. We now have three regression constants, β_0, β_{Treat} and β_{Time}, to be estimated from the trial data. This model assumes that any changes in y with time will be linear.

In Equation (2.1) we stated that ε represents the noise (or error) and this is assumed to be random and have a mean value of 0 across all subjects recruited to the trial and standard deviation (SD) σ. However, in Equation (11.2) we have replaced ε by ξ, because now this 'error' term not only includes variation *between* different participants recruited to the trial but also variation in the repeated measures taken within the same participant. The degree and type of autocorrelation therefore has to be specified when fitting this regression model with an appropriate computer package.

One type of autocorrelation assumes that observations made at any time t_1 (say) on a particular individual have the same auto-correlation ρ_T with observations made at any other time, t_2. This type of correlation structure is termed 'compound symmetry' and values of between 0.6 and 0.75 are commonly found for this.

The main focus of the statistical analysis is as before: to compare the treatment groups, that is, is to estimate β_{Treat} and the corresponding confidence interval and to test the null hypothesis $\beta_{\text{Treat}} = 0$.

A repeated measure design can also include a pre-randomization or baseline observation y_{Baseline}. This is often denoted y_0, indicating that it is taken at time $t = 0$. The model can account for y_{Baseline} by expanding the right-hand side of Equation (11.2) to become

$$y = \beta_0 + \beta_{\text{Treat}}\tau + \beta_{\text{Treat}}t + \beta_{\text{Baseline}}y_{\text{Baseline}} + \xi. \tag{11.3}$$

Essentially, this model now implies that the value of a (post randomization) observation y depends on the treatment received, the time when the observation was made and also the initial value of that observation before treatment commenced. Added to these in the model is the random variation component, ξ.

In order to fit such regression models, specialist statistical packages are required which enable, for example, different autocorrelation structures to be specified. To fully describe the options available is however beyond the scope of this text. Nevertheless a simple but efficient method of analysis is to compute the mean of an individual's *post*-randomization values of the outcome, $\bar{y}_{\text{Post}}$, and use this value as the observation for analysis. These can then be summarized for each intervention group by the mean of these means, and interventions then compared perhaps using an unpaired Student's *t*-test. This effectively modifies Equation (11.2) to

$$\bar{y}_{\text{Post}} = \beta_0 + \beta_{\text{Treat}} T$$

and avoids having to specify the particular autocorrelation structure of the individual endpoint values. This approach to analysis also forms the basis for the sample size estimates that we describe in the next section.

Further, if *pre*-randomization values are also available, then the means from those observations can be used in a regression analysis of the post-randomization means. In this case, Equation (11.3) becomes

$$\bar{y}_{\text{Post}} = \beta_0 + \beta_{\text{Treat}} T + \beta_{\text{Baseline}} \bar{y}_{\text{Pre}}.$$

It should be emphasized that when the design includes baseline covariates, this should *not* lead to the 'change scores' (i.e. $y_{\text{Treat}} - y_{\text{Baseline}}$) used as the variable for each patient in the analysis. Instead, such results should always be analyzed with y_{Baseline} as a covariate in a regression model, as shown in Equation (11.3).

11.2.4   Trial size

To estimate trial size, we make the assumption that the autocorrelation structure is that of compound symmetry with a fixed value of ρ_T. In the case when two interventions are to be compared and the observations come from a Normal distribution then, with the anticipated standardized effect size specified as Δ, the sample size in each group for a two-sided test α and power $1 - \beta$ is

$$m_{\text{Repeated}} = R \left[\frac{2(z_{1-\alpha/2} + z_{1-\beta})^2}{\Delta^2} + \frac{z_{1-\alpha/2}^2}{4} \right], \qquad (11.4)$$

where

$$R = \left[\frac{1 + (w-1)\rho_T}{w} - \frac{v\rho_T^2}{[1 + (v-1)\rho_T]} \right]. \qquad (11.5)$$

Apart from the multiplying factor R, Equation (11.4) is the same as Equation (9.5) when the allocation ratio $\lambda = 1$.

For the case of no pre-randomization or baseline observations, $v = 0$ and Equation (11.5) becomes

$$R = \left[\frac{1 + (w - 1)\rho_T}{w} \right].$$

(11.6)

Further, if there is only a single post-randomization measure $w = 1$, then $R = 1$.

We shall see that R is very similar in form to Equation (11.8) for the design effect (DE) arising from a cluster design trial, except that w here is replaced there by k to distinguish the two situations. In addition here there is a divisor, again w, arises here because we are using the mean of the w observations as the unit of analysis for each patient.

Example 11.2 Placebo or sapropterin dihydrochloride in patients with phenylketonuria

Levy, Milanowski, Chakrapani, *et al.* (2007) compared sapropterin dihydrochloride with (double-blind) placebo in patients with phenylketonuria to assess its role in reducing blood phenylaline concentration, and therefore its potential for preventing mental retardation in these patients. Their design consisted of three pre-treatment initiation and four post-randomization measures, taken at weeks $-2, -1, 0$ (baseline), 1, 2, 4 and 6 weeks. For sample size purposes they used a comparison between groups of the respective mean changes in blood phenylaline from baseline to 6 weeks. The mean change for one group is obtained by calculating for each patient the difference between the two values, that is $C = y_6 - y_0$, then calculating the mean $\overline{C}$ of all these values from the m patients in the group. For sample size determination purposes, the investigating team would therefore need to specify anticipated values of $\overline{C}$ for each group and their common standard deviation. Alternatively, they might simply specify a Cohen standardized effect size, Δ_{Cohen}.

In fact, the authors set $1 - \beta = 0.95$, two-sided $\alpha = 0.05$ and randomization in equal numbers to each group, and obtain a total of $N = 80$ patients or 40 per group. By use of Equation (9.5), this implies that they set a planning value of the effect size as $\Delta_{\text{Plan}} = 0.82$, although this detail is not made explicit in their report. Further, they do not appear to have taken the repeated measures nature of their design into the sample size determination.

An alternative approach to sample size calculation would be to assume the measure of outcome for each patient will be the mean level of their blood phenylaline levels over the four post-randomization values. Thus $\overline{y}_{\text{Post}} = (y_1 + y_2 + y_4 + y_6)/4$ is the unit of observation for each patient. Such mean values would be averaged over all m patients within one group, to obtain a

Example 11.2 *(Continued)*

mean of means. The results of their trial, summarized in Figure 11.1, indicate that the post-randomization observations of mean blood phenylaline appear relatively constant from week 1 within each group, with a difference between them of about 300 μmol/L. For our illustration, we take this value as the anticipated difference between the two groups (δ_{Plan}). The widths of the corresponding 95% confidence intervals are in the region of 240 μmol/L, based on approximately 40 individuals per group which implies a standard deviation of approximately 400 μmol/L. We take this as σ_{Plan}.

If we were considering a confirmatory trial, the planning effect size might be taken as $\Delta_{Plan} = \delta_{Plan}/\sigma_{Plan} = 300/400 = 0.75$. This is somewhat smaller than that apparently used by the trial team itself. Had this standardized effect size rather than 0.82 been used, then Equation (9.5) would have suggested increasing the planned trial size from 80 to 96.

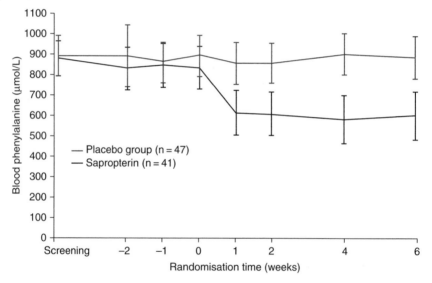

Figure 11.1   Mean blood phenylalanine concentration over time. Bars indicate 95% confidence intervals (after Levy, Milanowski, Chakrapani, *et al.*, 2007)

However, if we now consider in our sample size estimation that this is a repeated measures design with $v = 3$ and $w = 4$, we still need to provide a value for the auto-correlation between successive observations to complete the sample size calculations of Equations (11.4) and (11.5). In some situations, previous experience may suggest a planning value for this but, more often, such information may not be available. In the latter case, the planning team might explore how the final sample size will change depending on the value set for ρ_{TPlan}. Thus Table 11.1 provides trial sizes for a range of auto-correlation values with two-sided $\alpha = 0.05$, $1 - \beta = 0.95$ (as used by Levy, Milanowski, Chakrapani, *et al.*, 2007) but now with $\Delta_{Plan} = 0.75$.

Example 11.2   *(Continued)*

Table 11.1   Possible sample sizes for a hypothetical confirmatory, repeated measures trial design of that conducted by Levy, Milanowski, Chakrapani, *et al.* (2007)

Repeated measures design	$v = 3, w = 4$					
Standardized effect size	$\Delta_{Plan} = 0.75$					
Test size and power	Two-sided $\alpha = 0.05$, $1 - \beta = 0.95$					
Possible planning values of the auto-correlation coefficient, ρ_T	0.001	0.05	0.1	0.2	0.3	0.4
Total sample size, $N = 2m$	26	28	30	32	30	25
Total number of observations required, $O = N \times (v + w)$	182	196	210	224	210	175

This shows that even with very little autocorrelation, $\rho_T = 0.001$ implying successive measures on the same patient are almost independent. This repeated measures design requires only 26 patients or 13 per group. This is far fewer than the $N = 96$ if we use the 6-week value alone as the endpoint measure. This is because, for $\sigma_{Plan} = 400$, any observation at week 6, say y_6, has this standard deviation. On the other hand, the mean of the four observations $\bar{y}_{Post} = (y_1 + y_2 + y_4 + y_6)/4$ has a smaller standard deviation of $400/\sqrt{4} = 200$. This then gives a revised planning effect size of $\Delta_{PlanRepeated} = 300/200 = 1.5$. This is twice the size of $\Delta_{Plan} = 0.75$ that was originally formulated. The size of trial required is therefore much reduced.

Without recourse to the original trial data we cannot estimate a planning value for ρ_T. A pragmatic approach is therefore required for the worst-case scenario situation. Table 11.1 suggests that the largest trial size corresponds to the situation $\rho_T = 0.2$, which implies a size of 16 patients per group or $N = 32$ patients. This is still a far smaller number for the trial than that used by the investigators. This implies that making full use of the repeated measures data in the analysis of the Levy, Milanowski, Chakrapani, *et al.* (2007) trial may have reduced the need for such a large sample size.

If the number of pre-randomization assessments v in the repeated measures design is reduced to 2, 1 or 0, then the corresponding total number of patients required increases to $N = 34$, 36 and 40, respectively.

In summary, the number of patients required can be reduced at the expense of increasing the numbers of observations made on each patient. This strategy implies that the total number of observations required is greater than would have been the case if only a single assessment on each individual recruited had been made. This increase clearly has resource implications in terms of the number of examinations that have to be made. Further, it increases the complexity of the follow-up scheduling and thereby increases the possibility of patient non-compliance in this respect.

Example 11.2   *(Continued)*

We should caution that we are planning this hypothetical confirmatory trial with the hindsight of the previous trial outcome. Our armchair planning is now based on a much sounder basis than the information from the pilot studies alluded to by Levy, Milanowski, Chakrapani, *et al.* (2007) when considering their options for design.

11.3   Cluster-randomized trials

11.3.1   Design

In certain situations, the method of delivery of the intervention prevents it from being given on an individual participant basis; instead, it can only be delivered to collections of individuals. For example, if a public health campaign conducted through the local media is to be tested, it may be possible to randomize locations (termed clusters) to either receive or not the planned campaign. It would not be possible to randomize individuals. Fayers, Jordhøy and Kaasa (2002) therefore commented that cluster trials are particularly relevant when evaluating interventions at the level of clinic, hospital, district or region level.

In a two-group cluster-randomized trial, several (usually half) of the clusters will receive one intervention and the remainder the other. A whole cluster, consisting of a number of individuals who then become the trial participants, is therefore assigned as en-bloc. Nevertheless, just as for the individual specific random allocation design, the outcome is measured on every individual.

In general, cluster trials will compare $g = 2$ or more interventions. They will involve c clusters, a fraction of which (often $1/g$) will receive one of the interventions, and each cluster comprises k subjects. Design options include the choice of c and k, both of which may include non-statistical considerations in their choice. Perhaps c and k are determined by the number of clusters willing to participate and the practical limitations with respect to the number of participants recruited per cluster.

Example 11.3   Cluster design – enhanced diabetes care

Bellary, O'Hare, Raymond, *et al.* (2008) used a cluster randomized controlled trial in which 21 inner-city medical practices in the United Kingdom were assigned by simple randomization to intervention or control groups, with the object of improving diabetes prevention and care among a high-risk group. The intervention was assigned to nine medical practices, encompassing 868 patients of south

---

Example 11.3 *(Continued)*

Asian ethnic origin in total, and consisted of enhanced care including additional time with the practice nurse and support from a link worker and diabetes specialist nurse. The remaining 12 practices, comprising 618 patients, were assigned to standard care. The numbers of individuals within each of the 21 clusters is not given. Primary outcomes were changes in blood pressure, total cholesterol and glycaemic control (haemoglobin A_k) after 2 years. The results suggested that 'small but sustained improvements in blood pressure can be achieved' by use of enhanced care.

A further situation where cluster designs are useful is where there is a possibility of *contamination* in the delivery of the intervention itself. For example, in the trial of Bellary, O'Hare, Raymond, *et al.* (2008), it would not be easy to randomize half the individuals to 'enhanced care' and the other half to 'standard care' within the same medical practice. Conceptually this could be done but it would then be very difficult for the practice team involved in the 'enhanced care' group to disappear or change their mode of operation while 'standard' care is being delivered to an individual. This difficulty raises the possibility of contamination in the way 'standard care' is delivered and/or received in a similar way to that of the carry-across problem of the split-mouth design (Section 12.2). Any resulting contamination will almost certainly diminish the observed magnitude of any differences resulting from using the two approaches. A cluster design, where the specialist team is either in place in the cluster or it is not, therefore ensures that the trial results will be free from this form of contamination.

11.3.2 Consent

In a cluster-randomized trial, it is the healthcare professionals involved who consent to take part in the trial. Following randomization of the intervention to the clusters, the patients within each cluster are later informed that randomization has occurred and that they are part of a trial. This is more of a one-off process in that consent will be obtained before the trial is opened and will not directly concern (the possibly many) participants recruited within each cluster. Edwards, Braunholtz, Lilford and Stevens (1999) highlight some of the associated ethical difficulties and requirements.

11.3.3 Intraclass correlation

Despite the lack of individualized randomization and the receipt of a more group-based intervention, the assessment of the relative effect of the interventions is made at the level of the individual participant receiving the respective interventions. As a consequence, the observations of the patients within a single cluster are positively correlated as they are not completely independent of each other. Patients treated by one healthcare professional team will tend to be more similar among themselves, with respect to the outcome measure concerned, than those treated by a different healthcare team. If we know which team is involved with a particular patient, we can therefore predict the outcome for that patient by reference to experience with similar patients treated by the same team. The strength of this dependence among observations is measured by the intra-cluster correlation (ICC) or $\rho_{Cluster}$, defined as

$$\rho_{Cluster} = \frac{\sigma_{Between}^2}{\sigma_{Within}^2 + \sigma_{Between}^2}, \tag{11.7}$$

where $\sigma_{Between}$ is the between clusters standard deviation and σ_{Within} the within clusters standard deviation. In general, the more heterogeneity there is between the clusters, the greater the value of $\sigma_{Between}$ which inflates the value of $\rho_{Cluster}$. Campbell, Fayers and Grimshaw (2005) discuss the size of ICCs in a variety of settings.

Example 11.4 Magnitude of some intraclass correlation coefficients

The values of several ICCs in a medical practice setting are quoted in the methods section of the report of the cluster randomized trial of Bellary, O'Hare, Raymond, *et al.* (2008), summarized in Table 11.2.

Table 11.2 The value of some intra-class correlations (ICC) quoted by Bellary, O'Hare, Raymond, *et al.* (2008)

Variable	ICC ($\rho_{Cluster}$)
Systolic blood pressure	0.004
Total cholesterol	0.05
Haemoglobin A_k	0.05

11.3.4 Randomization

In individual-patient randomized trials, the patients will most likely present one-at-a-time and be randomized accordingly. In contrast, for cluster-randomized trials, all the clusters are usually identified before the trial is started. Any stratification and randomization (within strata) can therefore be carried out, and the clusters then informed of their allocation before beginning patient entry. Consequently, as is the case with the consent process, the clusters are all randomized to the interventions concerned before any recruitment begins. In general, the number of clusters is often quite limited but nevertheless it is the clusters themselves that are randomized rather than the individuals within each cluster.

The purpose of randomization is to try to balance characteristics associated with the *cluster* although, as their number is usually small, the scope for randomization to achieve balance between them is limited. However, as the number of clusters increases, we would expect cluster characteristics to balance (on average) across the intervention groups. Patient characteristics should therefore also balance across intervention groups.

Even in a trial with a very small number of clusters where there is little possibility of balancing patient characteristics, it is still worthwhile randomizing so that we can claim complete objectivity in the intervention allocation process. In addition, if the clusters are of variable size, then even in the situation where they are few in number it is worthwhile stratifying the randomization to the interventions by cluster size. In trials that require newly diagnosed patients, it may not be possible to specify the cluster size exactly at the planning stage. In this case, a proxy measure of cluster size, such as the size of the clinic from which the patients are drawn, can be used instead for stratification purposes.

In carrying out randomization, there may be two steps to take in a cluster design. One may be the random selection of clusters from a larger body of potential clusters to include in the trial. Once selected, the chosen clusters are assigned randomly (within strata if appropriate) to the alternative interventions.

Example 11.5   Random sample – selecting the clusters

In some circumstances there may be more clusters available than are necessary for the purposes of the trial. For example, when randomizing medical practices in rural areas of which there are 100, considerations of the total trial size might stipulate that 30 clusters would be sufficient. The team would then have to select practices for the trial, best done at random. They therefore choose $c = 30$ at random from $N_{Clusters} = 100$. In principle, this can be done by first numbering the practices in any order from 01 to 100 (using 00 to represent practice 100). Using the first two digits in (say) the first column of Table T5, we find the first 30 numbers in the range 00 to 99 are successively 75, 80, 94, 67, . . ., 87, 63. However, 03, 43, 50, 67, 90 and 94 are repeated in this list and so the next six random number pairs are taken. These are 73, 69, 64, 31, 35 and 57, but 57 has been used previously so we choose the next which is 50. This too has to be ignored and so the next, which is 48, is taken. Now that the numbered list of 30 is complete, the corresponding medical practices are then identified from the list and these are the clusters. This process is more easily achieved with a suitable computer program. Good practice now requires that this selection should be reproducible (if it should become necessary) and the process documented.

Once the clusters are identified, then the interventions are allocated to these clusters using the methods of Chapter 5. As we have stated, in this situation randomization is a one-off allocation as the actual patients within each cluster are not individually randomized.

Example 11.6   Number of clusters

In Example 1.6 we described the trial concerned with the use of hip protectors in elderly people resident in nursing homes, conducted by Meyer, Warnke, Bender and Mülhauser (2003). Their trial included a large number of clusters. Twenty-five

---

Example 11.6   *(Continued)*

nursing homes (comprising a total of 459 residents) were assigned to the intervention group and 24 homes, with 483 residents, were assigned to the control.

   In contrast, the trial of Bellary, O'Hare, Raymond, *et al.* (2008) of Example 11.6
involved less than half this number of clusters. Twenty-one inner-city medical
practices were included, with an unbalanced randomization of the clusters which
assigned 9 practices to the intervention (comprising 868 patients) and 12 practices
to control (comprising 618 patients). This is 250 patients fewer than for the
intervention group. In this case, the total number of patients of 1486 from
fewer clusters exceeded that of the nursing home trial with 942 residents. A better
design might have been first to stratify the practices into two groups of small and
large practices, then allocate these to interventions or control on a 1 : 1 basis as
closely as possible. This would certainly balance the numbers of patients within
the intervention and control groups more evenly, and perhaps balance more
closely practice characteristics and hence patient characteristics.

11.3.5   Trial size

The sample size calculation process begins by assuming the trial is to be an *individually
randomized* trial for a given effect size, significance level and power. Thus, depending
on the type of endpoint (continuous, binary, categorical or time-to-event), the number
of subjects required per intervention group $m_{\text{Individual}}$ is obtained from Equations (9.5),
(9.6), (9.8) or (9.11).

   Once obtained, $m_{\text{Individual}}$ is then inflated to give the sample size appropriate for the
cluster design. The inflation required is termed the design effect (*DE*). This is given by

$$DE = 1 + (k - 1)\rho_{\text{Cluster}}, \tag{11.8}$$

where k is the anticipated number of subjects per cluster. As we have previously pointed
out, *DE* is similar to Equation (11.6) of the repeated measures design.

   From this, the total number of patients required in each intervention group comprising c clusters of size k subjects is

$$m_{\text{Cluster}} = m_{\text{Individual}} \times DE. \tag{11.9}$$

For a trial involving g (≥ 2) interventions, when the total number of clusters c is already
determined, Campbell (2000) shows that the number of subjects required per cluster is
given by

$$k = \frac{m_{\text{Individual}}(1 - \rho_{\text{Cluster}})}{(c/g) - m_{\text{Individual}}\rho_{\text{Cluster}}}. \tag{11.10}$$

The number of participants per cluster increases rapidly as $m_{Individual}/\rho_{Cluster}$ approaches c/g, since the denominator of Equation (11.10) becomes smaller and smaller. However, Donner and Klar (2000) noted that it is seldom worth having more than about $k = 60$ individuals per cluster.

Example 11.7   Trial size – systolic blood pressure levels

Bellary, O'Hare, Raymond, *et al.* (2008) give the intra-primary care practice correlation for SBP as 0.035. An investigator wishes to repeat this trial, using the same design criteria but involving a more intensive intervention package, in $c = 30$ medical practices with SBP the main focus of the intervention. Although the previous trial had anticipated an effect size of 7 mmHg (SD 21.25) it was felt, bearing in mind the previous results, that a more realistic but still worthwhile effect size would be $\delta_{Plan} = 5$ mmHg, which is equivalent to a standardized effect size of $\Delta_{Plan} = 5/21.25 = 0.24$. This represents a *small* effect using the Cohen (1988) criterion.

Assuming a two-sided test size $\alpha = 0.05$, power $1 - \beta = 0.8$ and a $1 : 1$ allocation, Equation (9.5) gives $m_{Individual} = 274$ per group. Then with $g = 2$ interventions ('new intervention' or 'no-intervention') to be allocated equally among the medical practices, implies $c/g = 30/2 = 15$ practices per group are required. Further, with $\rho_{Cluster} = 0.035$, Equation (11.10) gives

$$k = \frac{274(1 - 0.035)}{[15 - (0.035 \times 274)]} = 48.87$$

or approximately 50 patients per practice. The total number of subjects involved with this cluster-randomized design will therefore be $N_{Cluster} = c \times k = 30 \times 50 = 1500$.

In contrast, were individuals to be randomized then this would require $m_{Individual}/15 = 274/15 = 18.27$, or approximately 20 patients per practice or $N_{Individual} = 30 \times 20 = 600$ in total. A much smaller trial would therefore be needed. Nevertheless, whichever design is chosen, conducting the trial would be a considerable undertaking.

In reality, it might be that $k = 50$ is the planned *average* number of subjects per cluster. If there is likely to be considerable variation around this figure, then the sample size may need to be adjusted upwards to account for this heterogeneity. In such a case, a cautious approach may be used by the planning team to increase the numbers by (say) 10% to give an average of 55 subjects per practice.

11.3.6   Analysis

Although the measures taken in a cluster-randomized trial are on the individuals, a straightforward comparison of those receiving the intervention against those who do not is no longer possible, except in the situation where there are exactly equal numbers of clusters assigned to each intervention and the number of subjects within each cluster are also all equal.

In the model for a cluster design comparing two interventions, Equation (2.1) has to be modified to take note of the different clusters involved. The model for a subject in cluster i is:

$$y_i = \beta_0 + \beta_{\text{Treat}}\tau + \gamma_i + \varepsilon. \qquad (11.11)$$

Here the coefficients β_0 and β_{Treat} have the same interpretation as in Equation (2.1) and $\tau = 0$ for one intervention and $\tau = 1$ for the other. In addition, γ_i is the effect for cluster i and is assumed random with a between-clusters standard deviation of σ_{Between}. The error term ε is assumed to be random with mean 0, but with a within-clusters standard deviation of σ_{Within}.

In the model-fitting process, the last terms, $\gamma_i + \varepsilon$, can be thought of as representing the residual or error variance. The structure of this variance, in relation to the actual number of clusters used within each intervention, has to be specified. Each subject is therefore categorized by which cluster they are in, the intervention received, and their individual endpoint measure. We illustrate the method of analysis using an artificial example.

Example 11.8   Cluster design comparing two interventions among five clusters

Suppose there are two interventions, randomized to five clusters which are individual General medical Practitioners (GP). Two receive the test intervention and three receive the standard. Further, the number of patients within each practice eventually recruited to the trial differs markedly from practice to practice. The endpoint measure of concern is SBP, and the results from each cluster are summarized in Table 11.3.

Table 11.3   Illustrative example of the analysis of a cluster trial

Intervention	$g = 2$	Standard				Test	
	GP	A	B	C		D	E
Number of subjects	k	8	15	27		36	14
SBP (mmHG)	Mean	139.22	141.62	139.52		128.96	129.83
	SD	16.29	21.59	19.37		20.84	27.82
	Mean				140.101		129.204
	Difference				10.897		

The corresponding regression model is that of Equation (11.1) which, in previous applications, would have been fitted by specifying **regress SBP Intervention** but this ignores the clusters. However, in this case, the fact that there are clusters affects the error structure for the fitting process, so the term **vce(cluster GP)** has to be specified. This identifies the variable **GP** as the cluster and **vce**, an abbreviation of variance,

Example 11.8 *(Continued)*

indicates that the analysis needs to consider which cluster each participant belongs to. The corresponding output for the data of Table 11.3 is given in Figure 11.2. As can be seen from the output, when compared to the Standard, the Test intervention has reduced the SBP by 10.9 mmHg (95% CI 9.0 to 12.8, *p*-value = 0.001).

Commands

```
]table GP Intervention, contents(mean SBP) row
regress SBP Intervention, vce(cluster GP)
```

Edited outputs

```
]------------------------------
       |    Intervention
  GP   | Control    Test
-------+----------------------
   A   |  139.217
   B   |  141.621
   C   |  139.519
   D   |             128.962
   E   |             129.826    Difference
-------+------------------------------------
 Total |  140.101    129.204    10.897
-------+------------------------------
Linear regression                         Number of obs = 100
                     F(1, 4) = 242.65        Prob > F = 0.0001
                                          Root MSE = 21.059

                 (Std. Err. adjusted for 5 clusters in GP)
---------------------------------------------------------------------
             |              Robust
           Y | Coef.     Std. Err.    t      P>|t|    [95% Conf. Interval]
-------------+-------------------------------------------------------
Intervention |  10.8972   0.6996     15.58   0.001    8.9549 to 12.8395
        _cons| 129.2041   0.2768
-------------+-------------------------------------------------------
```

Figure 11.2 Edited commands and output for the analysis of the cluster trial of Table 11.3

Ignoring the clusters in the analysis would still have resulted in the same estimated difference of 10.9 mmHG, but a much wider 95% CI from 2.5 to 19.5 and *p*-value = 0.011.

11.3.7 Reporting

Campbell, Elbourne and Altman (2004) have extended the CONSORT statement for reporting the results of individually randomized trial designs to those in which randomization is to clusters rather than individuals. Many points pertinent to the design as well as analysis and reporting of this type of trial are included.

11.3.8   Practical issues

For practical reasons, a cluster-randomized trial will often have a preset duration and so the numbers of subjects per cluster cannot be fixed in advance. Consequently, there can be considerable differences in the number of subjects recruited per cluster. This leads to problems at the analysis stage. If the condition under study is relatively rare, and some clusters small, there is a real possibility that in some clusters no patients will be recruited. This possibility needs to be considered at the design stage, since it can adversely affect the ability of the trial to detect differences between the interventions involved.

As noted, cluster trials may require considerably more participants (the subjects within the clusters) than would be the case for an individually based randomization design.

Fayers, Jordhøy and Kaasa (2002) warn that cluster trials carry serious design and analysis implications. In particular, an adequate number of clusters is essential as is the correct approach to analysis. Jordhøy, Fayers, Ahlner-Elmqvist and Kaasa (2002) also warn that concealment is frequently impossible in cluster randomized trials; at the time of recruiting patients to the trial the intervention or treatment allocation is already known. This can lead to severe selection bias which can invalidate the results from a cluster trial. It is essential to minimize these risks by, for example, using an independent person to screen and recruit patients into the trial.

A full discussion of cluster trials is given by Donner and Klar (2000) and Ukoumunne, Gulliford, Chinn, *et al.* (1999), while Peters, Richards, Bankhead, *et al.* (2003) make a comparison of methods for analyzing such trials. Using an example of four interventions in a factorial design structure, they compare methods to increase breast screening uptake in women.

11.4   Non-inferiority trials

11.4.1   Introduction

Implicit in a comparison between two groups in a randomized trial is the presumption that, if the null hypothesis is rejected, then there is a difference between the groups being compared. If this involves a comparison of treatments, then we therefore hope to conclude that one treatment is superior to the other irrespective of the magnitude of the difference observed. In certain situations, however, a new therapy may bring certain advantages over the reference of the current standard. There is possibly a reduced side-effects profile or easier administration or cost, but it may not be anticipated to be better with respect to the primary efficacy variable. In such a situation, we may only wish to be sure that one treatment is 'not worse than' or is 'at least as good as' another treatment: if it is better, that is fine (even though superiority would not be required to recommend it for current use). All we need to obtain is convincing evidence that the new treatment is not worse than the reference. For example, if the two treatments to be compared are for an acute but not serious condition, then the cheaper but not so efficacious alternative may be an acceptable replacement for the reference.

11.4.2   Limit of non-inferiority

In this situation, the effect size is replaced by a measure of non-inferiority of the Test intervention when compared to the reference or Standard. If the observed difference between groups is less than this in magnitude, this would imply that the Test intervention is *not inferior* to the Standard.

Under such conditions, the Test intervention may be required to be at least 'non-inferior' to the reference in relation to efficacy if it is to replace it in future clinical use. This implies that 'non-inferiority' is a pre-specified maximum reduction between two groups which, if observed to be less after the clinical trial is conducted, would render the test as non-inferior to the reference.

A key concern at the planning stage of such a trial is to define an appropriate level of 'therapeutic non-inferiority', η. The value of η is usually small and represents a difference that is considered clinically unimportant. Non-inferiority therefore means that the new intervention is, at most, only less effective than the Standard by η, and may well be better than the Standard. However, if the new intervention is instead worse than the Standard by more than η, the implication is that it could be noticeably worse and so cannot be recommended as a replacement for the Standard.

Instead of using hypothesis tests and p-values, the simplest way to analyze the results from a non-inferiority trial is by using confidence intervals. Having conducted a *superiority* trial to compare groups with respect to a particular outcome, we could calculate a two-sided $100(1 - \alpha)\%$ confidence interval for the true difference δ between two groups. This confidence interval covers the true difference with a given probability, $1 - \alpha$. However, for a non-inferiority trial, the one-sided $100(1 - \alpha)\%$ confidence interval for δ is more appropriate. This is:

$$[\text{Difference} - z_{1-\alpha}\text{SE(Difference)}]\text{to UL}, \tag{11.12}$$

where $z_{1-\alpha}$ replaces $z_{1-\alpha/2}$ of a two-sided confidence interval and the upper confidence limit UL depends on the context but not on the data. For a comparison of two proportions in a non-inferiority setting, $UL = +1$. When comparing means, $UL = \infty$. These correspond to the largest possible difference that can occur between two outcomes. The requirement for non-inferiority is that the lower limit of Equation (11.12) falls wholly above the pre-specified non-inferiority limit of $-\eta$. For example, if the response rate of a 'reference' but toxic drug is 0.5 (50%), this may be replaced by the less toxic 'test' provided the response rate is not less than 0.45 (45%). In this case, the limit of non-inferiority $\eta = 0.45 - 0.5 = -0.05$.

The concept of non-inferiority is illustrated in Figure 11.3 by considering the range of options possible for the one-sided confidence interval for a comparison of two proportions. In this figure, both situations A and B represent non-inferiority so that the Test could replace the Standard. Situation C represents inferiority, in which case the Test could not replace the Standard.

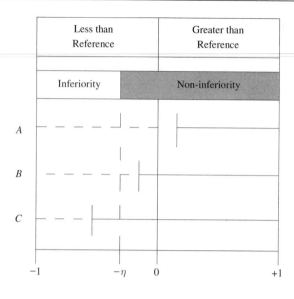

True difference : $\delta = \pi_{Test} - \pi_{Reference}$

Figure 11.3 Schematic diagram to illustrate the concept of non-inferiority by using a series of possible comparative trial outcomes, as summarized by their reported one-sided confidence intervals non-inferiority status (Trial A – *confirmed; Trial B –confirmed; Trial C – not accepted*)

Example 11.9   Non-inferiority – treatment of uncomplicated falciparum malaria

In the trial conducted by Zongo, Dorsey, Rouamba, *et al.* (2007) described in Example 1.7, the authors set a difference in risk of recurrent parasitaemia as no greater than 3% with artemether-lumefantrine (AL) as compared to amodiaguine plus sulfadoxine-pyrimethamine (AQ+SP). They observed a recurrence rate of symptomatic malaria with AQ+SP of 11/233 (4.72%), while for AL it was 37/245 (15.10%) i.e. a difference of −10.38%; with standard error

$$SE(Difference) = \sqrt{\frac{0.1510(1 - 0.1510)}{245} + \frac{0.0472(1 - 0.0472)}{233}} = 0.0268.$$

For a one-sided 90% *CI* Table T2 gives $z_{1-0.10} = z_{0.90} = 1.2816$, so that the corresponding confidence interval is −0.1038 − 1.2816 × 0.0268 to +∞ or −13.81% to +∞. The difference observed of −10.38% is clearly well below the limit of non-inferiority, set at −3%, so that replacing AQ+SP by AL would not be recommended.

11.4.3 Analysis

As we have indicated above in Equation (11.9), the one-sided confidence interval provides the appropriate method of data summary. The 'non-inferiority' measure may be the difference between two means, two proportions or expressed by the hazard ratio depending on the context.

11.4.4 Trial size

For a one-sided confidence interval approach with one-sided α and power (one-sided) β, the sample size per group required to demonstrate the non-inferiority of two means in a $1:1$ randomized design based of anticipated means $\mu_{Standard}$ and μ_{Test} with common standard deviation σ and level of non-inferiority set as η is given by

$$m_{\text{Non-Inferiority}} = \frac{2\sigma^2(z_{1-\alpha} + z_{1-\beta})^2}{\left[|\mu_{Standard} - \mu_{Test}| - \eta\right]^2}. \tag{11.13}$$

Similarly, the total sample size required for a trial to test for non-inferiority of proportions from two groups of equal size and anticipated to have the response proportions $\pi_{Standard}$ and π_{Test} is

$$m_{\text{Non-Inferiority}} = \frac{2\overline{\pi}(1 - \overline{\pi})(z_{1-\alpha} + z_{1-\beta})^2}{\left[|\pi_{Standard} - \pi_{Test}| - \eta\right]^2}, \tag{11.14}$$

where $\overline{\pi} = (\pi_{Standard} + \pi_{Test})/2$.

Example 11.10   Home or institutional care in the elderly

Regidor, Barrio, de la Feunte, *et al.* (1999) anticipated that, following a period in hospital, elderly patients are likely to have a mean and standard deviation of social functioning (SF) of about 65 and 25 respectively, if assessed by the SF-36 health questionnaire. Suppose that such patients, with no potential family support, can either be discharged to their *own* home with additional home-help provided or to institutional care. Home care is considered the best option, as there is concern that health-related quality of life may be compromised in those referred for institutional care.

If the clinical team regard institutional care to be non-inferior to home care provided SF-36 is not more than $\eta = 5$ points below those who are discharged home, what size of non-inferiority trial is needed?

On the assumption that $\mu_{Standard} = \mu_{Test}$, $\sigma_{Plan} = 25$ and the non-inferiority value is set at $\eta = 5$, we can use Equation (11.13) to determine sample size. Further assuming $\alpha = 0.1$, $\beta = 0.2$, Table T2 gives $z_{1-\alpha} = z_{0.9} = 1.2816$ and $z_{1-\beta} = z_{0.8} = 0.8416$. Together these imply

$$m_{\text{Non-inferiority}} = \frac{2 \times 25^2(1.2816 + 0.8416)^2}{5^2} = 225.4,$$

Example 11.10 *(Continued)*

giving a total of approximately $N_{\text{Non-inferiority}} = 2 \times 225 = 450$. To allow for drop-outs, perhaps we would recruit approximately 500. In the trial, elderly patients would then be randomized half to be discharged home with additional support and half to institutional care.

Example 11.11   Treatment of HIV infection

Eron, Yeni, Gathe, *et al.* (2006) describe a non-inferiority trial which compared fosamprenavir-ritonavir with lopinavir-ritonavir, each in combination with abacavir-lamivudine for the initial treatment of HIV infection. They assumed a 70% success rate with fosamprenavir-ritonavir and one of 72% with lopinavir-ritonavir. They used a one-sided 0.025 level of significance, a 90% power and set the limit of non-inferiority for fosamprenavir-ritonavir as $\eta = 12\%$ below the rate with lopinavir-ritonavir. Use of Table T2 gives $z_{0.975} = 1.96$ and $z_{0.9} = 1.2816$ while $\bar{\pi} = (0.72 + 0.70)/2 = 0.71$. Setting these values in Equation (11.12), we have

$$m_{\text{Non-Inferiority}} = \frac{2 \times 0.71(1 - 0.71)(1.96 + 1.2816)^2}{[|0.72 - 0.70| - 0.12]^2} = 432.7 \approx 450 \text{ patients,}$$

implying a total trial size of close to 900 patients. In the event, Eron, Yeni, Gathe, *et al.* (2006) randomized 887 individuals.

11.4.5   Equivalence

A special case of non-inferiority is that of equivalence. In such cases, the Test treatment is required to be neither less nor more efficacious than the Standard. Such equivalence may be very important if an alternative for the same pharmaceutical compound is being formulated. In this case, once equivalence is established the compounds are then termed bioequivalent. In such cases, the Test is designed to be the same as the Standard, at least to within specified limits. In estimating the size of equivalence trials, the Type II error β is replaced by $\beta/2$ in Equations (11.13) and (11.14).

Jones, Jarvis, Lewis and Ebbutt (1996) state that, when assessing equivalence, two types of error can occur. We can decide that the treatments are equivalent when they are not (type I error with probability α) or that the treatments are not equivalent when they are (type II error with probability β). The corresponding power of the trial, $1 - \beta$, is the probability of correctly declaring equivalence when $\delta = 0$. The null hypothesis H_0 is the combination of: $\delta \leq -\eta$ and $\delta \geq \eta$ (non-equivalence), whereas the alternative hypothesis H_A is: $-\eta < \delta < \eta$ (equivalence).

11.4.6 Reporting

Detailed requirements for reporting the results of non-inferiority (and equivalence) trials can be found in Piaggio, Elbourne and Altman (2001) who extend the CONSORT statement appropriately. They meticulously illustrate how all the key aspects of a trial should be addressed and provide useful examples and commentary. Their report also highlights features of the reporting process which relate specific design features, such as a choice of the non-inferiority limit and sample size, so this paper also serves well as a checklist for planning purposes.

11.4.7 Practical issues

As we discussed in Chapter 2, the application of the intention-to-treat (ITT) principle to a superiority trial is a conservative procedure. ITT will therefore tend to dilute the difference between the randomized interventions (since they become more similar whenever a participant refuses the randomized option and then receives the alternative, for example) and thereby reduces the chance of demonstrating efficacy should it exist. However, Piaggio and Pinol (2001) point out that, for non-inferiority and equivalence trials, the dilution caused by ITT will not act conservatively. In these cases any dilution will tend to favour, as appropriate, the non-inferiority or equivalence hypothesis. Although analysis and interpretation can be quite straightforward, the design and management of equivalence trials is often much more complex.

In general, careless or inaccurate measurement, poor follow-up of patients, poor compliance with study procedures and medication all tend to bias results towards no difference between treatment groups. This underlines why an ITT analysis is not likely to be appropriate since we are trying to offer evidence of non-inferiority. Poor study design and logistical procedures may therefore actually help to hide differences between the intervention groups. In general, therefore, the conduct of such trials demands high compliance of the patients with respect to the treatment protocol. Indeed, Jones, Jarvis, Lewis and Ebbutt (1996) suggest that a per protocol as well as an ITT analysis should be conducted in any non-inferiority or equivalence trial. Too many patients failing to adhere to their allocated treatment, for whatever reason, will clearly dilute the respective treatments to such an extent that each becomes like the other and hence falsely 'equivalent'. We can very easily demonstrate non-inferiority by conducting the trial rather badly, so the converse should be the case and extra care should be taken to prevent any 'dilution of the effect'.

11.5 Guidelines

Guidelines and other useful documents relevant to the content of this chapter are collated here.

Campbell, M.K., Elbourne, D.R. and Altman, D.G. (2004) CONSORT statement extension to cluster randomised trials. *BMJ*, **328**, 702–708.

Medical Research Council (2002) *Cluster Randomised Trials: Methodological and Ethical Considerations*. MRC clinical trials series, Medical Research Council, London.

Piaggio, G., Carolli, G., Villar, J., *et al.* (2001) Methodological considerations on the design and analysis of an equivalence stratified cluster randomization trial. *Statistics in Medicine*, **20**, 401–416.

Piaggio, G., Elbourne, D.R., Altman, D.G., *et al.* for the CONSORT Group (2001) Reporting of noninferiority and equivalence randomized trials: an extension of the CONSORT statement. *Journal of the American Medical Association*, **295**, 1152–1160.

CHAPTER 12

Paired Designs

This chapter introduces designs in which, in the case of two interventions, each participant in the trial receives both. In the cross-over trial, the two interventions are given one after the other over two periods of time in one of two possible sequences. These sequences are then randomized so that half the participants are allocated one sequence and half the other. In the split-mouth design, of particular relevance to dental studies, one side of the mouth receives one of the interventions and the other side of the mouth the other intervention. The interventions are randomized to the sides. These designs enable a within-subject comparison of the alternative interventions and hence have the potential to estimate differences between treatments more efficiently, although there are limitations to their use which we outline. Appropriate methods for determination of sample size and analysis are included. We also describe trials associated with paired organs such as eyes and kidneys and discuss how special care is needed at the trial size determination and analysis stages.

12.1 Cross-over trials

12.1.1 Design

In certain situations it is possible to test the alternative interventions within the same subjects. This brings immediate statistical advantages, since an estimate of the relative efficacy is then based on a *within*-patient comparison — one measurement taken while receiving one intervention and one while receiving the other. Such a trial has what is termed a cross-over design. This design contrasts with two trial participants, each receiving only one of the interventions concerned, where the difference between their observed outcome measures will have components of both *within*- and *between-individual* variability. Within-subject variability tends to be smaller than between-subject variability. Further, if it can be removed by comparing interventions within each individual, this should then lead to a more sensitive comparison. This in turn implies that the trial may be conducted on fewer participants than the two parallel (independent) group design discussed so far. Although this design brings statistical advantages, there are constraints on its application.

Randomized Clinical Trials: Design, Practice and Reporting   David Machin and Peter M Fayers
© 2010 John Wiley & Sons, Ltd

12.1.1.1 Two periods – two treatments

In the case of a cross-over trial comparing two drugs A and B, one of the drugs, say A, is given to a group of patients and then sometime later in a second period, the same patients are all challenged with the alternative drug B. Conversely, other patients receive B in the first period and then subsequently receive A in the second. Although each patient receives both of the treatments, some receive these in the order AB and some in the reverse order BA. Once again randomization is important. In this two-treatment two-period cross-over trial, the participants are therefore randomized to one of the sequences AB and BA. In these circumstances, double-blind trials are particularly recommended.

Example 12.1 Cross-over trial – anacetrapib and blood pressure

As indicated in Example 1.3, Krishna, Anderson, Bergman, *et al.* (2007) describe a randomized placebo (P) controlled, two-period cross-over trial of anacetrapib (A) in healthy volunteers and their trial design is summarized in Figure 12.1. During the course of the trial, 24 hour-ambulatory blood was monitored on day 10 of each treatment period. The trial participants and investigators were blinded to the order in which the trial medication was administered.

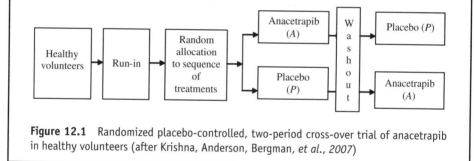

Figure 12.1 Randomized placebo-controlled, two-period cross-over trial of anacetrapib in healthy volunteers (after Krishna, Anderson, Bergman, *et al., 2007*)

12.1.1.2 Washout to reduce carry-over

It is now evident that those patients randomized to receive the sequence AB receive B (in Period II) after they have previously received A in period I. Any residual or carry-over effect of A could therefore influence the effect of B. If it does, we are actually really comparing A with B-after-A, rather than A with B. On a similar basis, with the other sequence we will be comparing B with A-after-B. This is a situation we wish to avoid, and consequently a 'wash-out' period following Period I is usually introduced before the intervention of Period II. The wash-out is intended to avoid the potential contamination of the treatment given in the first period upon the outcome in the second. The length of the wash-out period will depend on, for example, how long the drug remains active within the individual. If it has a transient effect on the endpoint of concern, and thereafter is soon eliminated from the body, then it may be presumed that the wash-out period can be relatively short and that there is little chance of a carry-over effect. In contrast, if the drugs are more likely to be excreted over a longer time, then an extended wash-out period will be required.

12.1.1.3 Run-in

In some cases, as in Figure 12.1, a 'run-in' period may also be a feature of a cross-over design. In this example, the purpose of the run-in was to screen volunteers for their eligibility by ensuring that they had a maximum blood pressure of less than 140/90 mmHg and a diastolic blood pressure that did not differ by more than 10 mmHg measured on days −4 and −1 prior to randomization to the treatment sequence.

12.1.2 Difficulties

The complexity of the cross-over design, with a possible run-in, Period I, wash-out, and Period II, impacts on the type of subject that can be studied in this way. The wash-out has to ensure not only that the drug has been completely excreted but any residual effect on the subject is entirely eliminated. This implies, for example, that every patient recruited will return, prior to commencing Period II treatment, to the disease state they were in before the Period I drug had been given. The disease or condition therefore needs to be relatively stable over time within the patient concerned, so that when treatment is withdrawn (at the end of Period I) the patients' condition will return to the pre-treatment state.

An extreme example of when the cross-over trial should not be used is when there is a potential for cure with the Period I treatment. In such cases, challenging any cured patient with the Period II intervention would be entirely inappropriate. In the investigation of ambulatory blood pressure changes of placebo or anacetrapib in the trial conducted by Krishna, Anderson, Bergman, et al. (2007), there was a reasonable expectation that the healthy volunteers would return to their pre-Period I blood pressure after a suitable washout period and no carry-over was therefore anticipated. The authors state in their report:

> There was at least a 14-day washout interval from the last dose of anacetrapib (or matching placebo) in between the treatment periods.

Nevertheless, cross-over trials are conducted without a wash-out included. One such example is that of Allan, Hays, Jensen, et al. (2008) who compared transdermal fentanyl with sustained release oral morphine, each used for four weeks, for treating chronic non-cancer pain. In this case, the patients recruited could not be denied active treatment during a wash-out period, as this would cause unethical suffering. It is unclear from the results of this trial how the presence (almost inevitable) of a carry-over effect influenced the conclusions.

Drop-out is a major problem in cross-over trials, because considerable cooperation from the subjects is required. A subject who misses the second period effectively nullifies their contribution in the first period. One way of reducing drop-out rates is to ensure the trial is as short as possible and so a balance has to be struck between this and extending the wash-out to ensure that Period II is free of carry-over. Clearly the addition of a run-in period compounds the difficulties. In the trial of Krishna, Anderson, Bergman, *et al.* (2007) there was a run-in period of 4 days then a 10-day Period I treatment, a wash-out of a minimum of 14 days, and then a final 10-day Period II on the other treatment. The minimum time for the trial was therefore 38 days.

Further, if the 1 : 1 randomization between sequences is either not used or not achieved, then the statistical properties of the cross-over design are compromised.

12.1.3   Analysis and trial size

In a two-period cross-over trial comparing two treatments *A* and *B*, patients will be randomized in equal numbers of *m* per sequence. For a continuous variable, a full analysis consists of three separate two-sample *t*-tests. The first is to test the possibility of a period effect and the second a treatment-period interaction (details are given by Senn, 2002). Assuming these two analyses indicate no period effect and no treatment-period interaction, then a paired analysis ignoring the sequence ordering is appropriate for testing the difference between treatments.

12.1.3.1   Difference in means

For a continuous endpoint measure, using the notation of Elbourne, Altman, Higgins, *et al.* (2002), if we let the outcomes on individual *i* be x_i^A and x_i^B for treatments *A* and *B*, then the within-patient difference is

$$d_i = x_i^A - x_i^B$$

We then have

$$\bar{d} = \sum_{i=1}^{2m} d_i/2m = \bar{x}^A - \bar{x}^B$$

and

$$SE(\bar{d}) = SD(d_i)/\sqrt{2m},$$

where

$$SD(d_i) = \sum_{i=0}^{i=2m} (d_i - \bar{d})^2/(2m - 1)$$

with degrees of freedom $df = 2m - 1$. The corresponding paired t-test for testing the null hypothesis of no difference between treatments is

$$t = \frac{\bar{d}}{SE(\bar{d})}. \tag{12.1}$$

However, this and the following analyses should not be taken as representing the results of the original trial.

Using Equation (12.1) with these values gives $t = 0.6/0.6214 = 0.97$ and, from Table T1, the p-value $= 2(1 - 0.83398) = 0.33$. In this example, the degrees of freedom $df = 39$, implies a relatively large sample situation so that Table T1 rather than Table T4 for the Student's t-distribution can be used.

The associated analysis using a statistical package is summarized in Figure 12.2(a) using the command (**ttest**) followed by the hypothesis that it is wished to test (**Diff==0**), closely mirroring our previous calculations.

Example 12.2   Intraocular pressure with bimatoprost or latanoprost

Quaranta, Pizzolante, Riva, *et al.* (2008) randomized 40 patients with normal-tension glaucoma in a two-period cross-over trial to either latanoprost or bimatoprost for 8 weeks, and then to the opposite medicine for 8 weeks. There appears to be no wash-out period within the design, but since the endpoint measures are taken 8 weeks post commencement of therapy, this may be of little consequence. At the end of each treatment period they evaluated the intraocular pressure and obtained mean values for one particular assessment time of 13.7 and 14.3 mmHg for latanoprost and bimatoprost, respectively. From the corresponding confidence intervals of each mean quoted, it is possible to deduce these had standard deviations of 2.74 and 3.22 mmHg. The corresponding paired difference of the $2m = 40$ means was $\bar{d} = 0.6$. The corresponding standard error of this is not given and cannot be calculated without access to the individual data items; the authors do not appear to have analyzed their trial making full use of the cross-over design.

As the individual data items are understandably not given by Quaranta, Pizzolante, Riva, *et al.* (2008), we have mimicked their analysis by generating simulated data with the same means and standard deviations as the two treatment group values concerned. This was done by drawing 40 random samples from Normal distributions with the reported means and standard deviations. From these we have simulated, ignoring the period when observed, the individual differences d_i to obtain a $SD = 3.93$ and hence a standard error

$$SE(\bar{d}) = 3.93/\sqrt{40} = 0.6214.$$

Example 12.2   *(Continued)*

(a)
Commands

```
ttest Diff == 0
```

Output
```
One-sample t test
-----------------------------------------------------------------
Variable  |  Obs   Mean   Std. Err.    [95% Conf. Interval]
+----------------------------------------------------------------
    Diff  |  40    0.60   0.6214        -0.6569 to 1.8569
-----------------------------------------------------------------
        mean = mean(Diff) t = 0.9656
                  Ho:  mean = 0     degrees of freedom = 39
Ha: mean != 0 Pr(|T| > |t|) = 0.3402
-----------------------------------------------------------------
```

(b)
Alternative command

```
regress Diff
```

Alternative output

Analysis of Variance (ANOVA)

```
-----------------------------------------------------------------
  Source  |   SS       df    MS            Number of obs = 40
-----------------------------------------    F(0, 39) = 0.00
   Model  |   0        0
Residual  | 602.3637  39   15.4452
-----------------------------------------------------------------
   Total  | 602.3637  39   15.4452    Root MSE = 3.93
-----------------------------------------------------------------
    Diff  | Coef.   Std. Err.   t    P>|t|   [95% Conf. Interval]
-----------------------------------------------------------------
   _cons  | 0.6000   0.6214    0.97  0.340   -0.6569 to 1.8569
-----------------------------------------------------------------
```

Figure 12.2   Edited commands and output from a statistical package for analyzing a cross-over trial comparing treatments for intraocular pressure in patients with normal-tension glaucoma (from simulated data mimicking the trial of Quaranta, Pizzolante, Riva, *et al.*, 2008)

Example 12.3   Fuel metabolism during exercise

Small cross-over trials are sometimes conducted such as that described by Jenni, Oetliker, Allemann, *et al.* (2008) who studied fuel metabolism during exercise in euglycaemia and hyperglycaemia in only seven patients with type-1 diabetes mellitus. Their trial is essentially a laboratory-based study rather than a therapeutic trial. In the corresponding analysis, $df = 6$ so that Table T4 would need to be

Example 12.3 *(Continued)*

used in this case. To be statistically significant at the 5% level, the test statistic t would therefore need to exceed 2.447 rather than 1.96 (the value from Table T1) and at the 1% level 3.707 rather than 2.576 (from Table T1). The advantage of a statistical package is that it automatically takes due account of the sample size through the *df* in calculating the precise *p*-values. The authors do not appear to have analyzed their trial making full use of the cross-over design.

An alternative approach to the analysis of a cross-over trial is to fit a linear model using a regression command (see Figure 8.9). In this case, there is no dependent variable but only Diff (the *y* variable), so the command is simply (**regress Diff**). The final row of Figure 12.2(b) gives the corresponding output which replicates the earlier analysis. We comment on other sections of the output below.

Although the regression command of Figure 12.2 provides no new insight, it has the potential to adjust the comparison between the treatments in the cross-over trial to allow for patient characteristics which are thought to be importantly prognostic for outcome. In our illustrative example we have also added, at random on a 1 : 1 basis, whether each of the subjects is male or female. Further, we assume that males and females are *known* to differ in their likely responses to treatment, so that if we do not take gender into account we may obtain a false impression of the magnitude of any treatment differences observed. To adjust for gender, we can extend the regression model previously described. We write Diff as *y* for convenience, from $y = \beta_0$ alone to $y = \beta_0 + \beta_{\text{Gender}}(\text{Gender})$, where Gender $= 0$ for males and 1 for females. This second model is fitted using the command (**regress Diff Gender**). The corresponding command and output are described in Figure 12.3.

Commands

```
table Gender, contents (n Diff mean Diff sd Diff) row
regress Diff Gender
```

Output

```
--------+------------------------------------------
Gender | N(Diff)   mean(Diff)    sd(Diff)
--------+------------------------------------------
 Male  |    25        0.6393        4.0877
Female |    15        0.5345        3.7914
--------+------------------------------------------
 Total |    40        0.6000        3.9300
--------+------------------------------------------
```

Analysis of Variance (ANOVA)

```
---------+------------------------------------------------
 Source  |    SS      df      MS        Number of obs = 40
---------+----------------------------   F(1, 38) = 0.01
 Model   |   0.1031    1     0.1031      Prob > F = 0.9361
Residual | 602.2606   38    15.8490
---------+------------------------------------------------
 Total   | 602.3637   39    15.4452      Root MSE = 3.9811
---------+------------------------------------------------
```

Example 12.3 *(Continued)*

```
--------+--------------------------------------------------------
 Diff  |  Coef.     Std. Err.    t     P>|t|   [95% Conf. Interval]
--------+--------------------------------------------------------
Gender |  -0.1049    1.3002    -0.08   0.936    -2.7370 to 2.5273
 _cons |   0.6393    0.7962     0.80   0.427    -0.9725 to 2.2512
--------+--------------------------------------------------------
```

Figure 12.3   Commands and output from a statistical package for analyzing a cross-over trial comparing treatments, adjusted for gender, for intraocular pressure in patients with normal-tension glaucoma (based on Quaranta, Pizzolante, Riva, et al., 2008)

The regression coefficient estimates are now $b_0 = 0.6393$ (which differs from our earlier estimate of 0.6000) and $b_{Gender} = -0.1049$. The latter is not statistically significant since $t = -0.1049/1.3002 = -0.08$ based on $df = 38$ and has p-value $= 0.936$. We therefore conclude that gender has little influence on the comparison between treatments, so that the earlier (and simpler) model with $b_0 = 0.60$ alone is adequate. However, since the null hypothesis was not rejected, we are essentially concluding that the null model $\beta_0 = 0$ describes the data adequately. We therefore find little evidence for a difference in intraocular pressure between the two treatment groups.

The ANOVA tables of Figures 12.2 and 12.3, although not essential features of the analyses just described, are very useful in situations when comparing more than two interventions such as in the designs we will describe in Chapter 13. ANOVA essentially partitions the total variation between individual observations into component parts, individual parts being attributed to the influence of the variables under consideration (only Gender in Figure 12.3) and the remainder to the residual or random error variation. In the *ANOVA* of Figure 12.3, the total variation of 602.3637 is split into 0.1031 due to gender and the remainder 602.2606 is termed residual which, in this example, is the most substantial part. The corresponding variances are calculated by dividing these by the respective degrees of freedom, $df = 1$ and 38 respectively, to give 0.1031 and $602.2606/38 = 15.8490$. The Fisher F-test then compares these by their ratio, so that $F(1, 38) = 0.1031/15.8490 = 0.0065$. If this is substantially greater than unity (which is clearly not the case here) the null hypothesis of no effect of gender (on the observed differences between the treatments included in the cross-over trial) would be rejected, and Gender would be retained in the model describing the trial results. In this case, the difference between the treatments would differ in the males and the females.

The same format of *ANOVA* is given in Figure 12.2 but for this model $df = 0$ so that the total variation of 602.3637 cannot be partitioned in this case. Essentially, all the variation is then regarded as residual or random error.

When designing a cross-over trial we need to estimate the patient numbers required. This in turn implies specifying a planning standardized effect size, which involves both the anticipated difference between the treatments and the anticipated standard deviation of the individual within patient differences, $SD(d_i)$. For simplicity, this is assumed to be the same for every participant. The within-subject standard deviation quantifies the anticipated variation among measurements on the same individual, irrespective of the treatment received. It is a compound of true variation in the individual and any measurement error. The between-subject standard deviation quantifies the anticipated variation between subjects. Elbourne, Altman, Higgins, *et al.* (2002) provide the following relationship between the standard deviations of observations made on a patients receiving *A* then *B*, and that of their difference as

$$\sigma_{\text{Within}}^2 [SD(d_i)]^2 = [SD(x_i^A)]^2 + [SD(x_i^B)]^2 - 2\rho[SD(x_i^A)SD(x_i^B)]. \qquad (12.2)$$

Here ρ, which must take a value between -1 and $+1$, is the correlation between *A* and *B* outcomes calculated from all the 2*m* subject pairs. In the common case, where $SD(x_i^A)$ and $SD(x_i^B)$ are assumed to be equal, we label these σ_{Between} and Equation (12.2) becomes

$$\sigma_{\text{Within}}^2 = \sigma_{\text{Between}}^2 + \sigma_{\text{Between}}^2 - 2\rho\sigma_{\text{Between}}^2 = 2(1-\rho)\sigma_{\text{Between}}^2. \qquad (12.3)$$

A pragmatic way to obtain σ_{Within} for planning purposes is to postulate the range of values which the differences d_i are likely to take, and divide this range by four. Alternatively, if an anticipated value of σ_{Between} is available, then Equation (12.3) can be used for a given ρ. We note that Equation (12.3) implies that $\sigma_{\text{Within}} < \sigma_{\text{between}}$ provided $\rho > 0.5$; this will usually be the case as experience suggests that ρ is often between 0.60 and 0.75 in this type of trial. Very different values are anticipated in the split-mouth designs discussed in Section 12.2 below.

In this situation, the anticipated standardized effect size still takes the familiar form of $\Delta_{\text{Plan}} = \delta_{\text{Plan}}/\sigma_{\text{Within-Plan}}$ and the number of patients required for a cross-over design is estimated using an adaption of Equation (9.5) to give

$$N = \frac{(z_{1-\alpha/2} + z_{1-\beta})^2}{\Delta_{\text{Plan}}^2} + \frac{z_{1-\alpha/2}^2}{2}. \qquad (12.4)$$

Example 12.4   Cross-over trial size – ambulatory blood pressure

At the planning stage of the trial of Figure 12.1 which was eventually conducted by Krishna, Anderson, Bergmann, *et al.* (2002), they assumed a within-subject standard deviation for average 24-hour systolic blood pressure of $\sigma_{\text{Within-Plan}} = 5.7$ mmHg and an anticipated difference of $\delta_{\text{Plan}} = 6$ mmHg between that of placebo and anacetrapib. As a consequence, $\Delta_{\text{Plan}} = 6/5.7 \approx 1.0$ which, by the Cohen (1988) criteria, is a large effect. Assuming a two-sided test size of 5% and a power of 95%, use of Table T2 and Equation (12.4) leads to

$$N = \frac{2(1.96 + 1.6449)^2}{1^2} + \frac{1.96^2}{2} = 27.91.$$

This suggests 28 healthy volunteers should be recruited, 14 randomized to each treatment sequence. In fact, the investigators used a one-sided test so that Equation (12.4) then gives $N = 23.57$, implying 12 per sequence and not the 11 as obtained by the authors. This discrepancy is caused by their omission of the last term of Equation (12.4) which is a small sample correction that should have been used here.

12.1.3.2 Difference in proportions

If the endpoint is binary rather than continuous in nature, then the cross-over trial results can be summarized in the format of Table 12.1. In this example, culture specimens from the patients are judged as to whether they are negative or positive with respect to growth of *Pseudomonas aeruginosa* during the two treatment periods.

In Table 12.1 the letter e, for example, represents the number of patients whose culture was negative with both aziththromycin (A) and placebo (P). The difference between the proportions that are culture positive with A and with P is estimated by

Table 12.1   Results and notation for a two-period cross-over trial comparing the numbers of patients with cystic fibrosis whose cultures grew *P. aeruginosa* when receiving placebo (*P*) or azithromycin (*A*) (data from Equi, Balfour-Lynn, Bush and Rosenthal, *et al.*, 2002)

Grew *P. aeruginosa* culture with placebo	Grew *P. aeruginosa* culture with Azithromycin			Anticipated proportions
	Negative	Positive	Total	
Negative	17 (e)	6 (f)	23 ($e + f$)	π_P
Positive	7 (g)	11 (h)	18 ($g + h$)	$1 - \pi_P$
Total	24 ($e + g$)	17 ($f + h$)	41 ($N_{\text{Sequences}}$)	
Anticipated proportions	π_A	$1 - \pi_A$		

$$d = \frac{f+h}{N_{\text{Sequences}}} - \frac{g+h}{N_{\text{Sequences}}} = \frac{f-g}{N_{\text{Sequences}}}. \tag{12.5}$$

Alternatively, the data arising from the cross-over designs are sometimes summarized using the odds ratio, calculated as $\psi = f/g$. Thus ψ is therefore a measure of how much more likely it is that a patient will be culture positive with P as opposed to when receiving A. We note that the $(e+h)$ patients who respond to both P and A in the same way (i.e. they are either negative with both treatments or positive with both treatments) do not enter this calculation. The corresponding expressions for the exact confidence intervals for ψ are complex but are usually an integral part of the output of the statistical packages used for the analysis.

The test of the null hypothesis of no difference between the two treatments, and assuming any carryover effect is minimal, is the McNemar test. The null hypothesis implies that f and g are expected to be equal given that there are a total of $f + g$ discordant pairs. In large samples, this leads to a test of the null hypothesis by considering the value of

$$z = \frac{f-g}{\sqrt{f+g}}. \tag{12.6}$$

Example 12.5   Crossover trial – culture of P. aerugenosa in cystic fibrosis

We use the data from Equi, Balfour-Lynn, Bush and Rosenthal, *et al.* (2002) summarized in Table 12.1, from which

$$d = \frac{f-g}{N_{\text{Sequences}}} = \frac{6-7}{41} = -0.0244$$

and $\psi = 6/7 = 0.86$. Equation (12.6) gives

$$z = \frac{6-7}{\sqrt{6+7}} = -0.28.$$

Use of Table T1 gives the p-value $= 2(1 - 0.61026) = 0.78$ which would not be regarded as statistically significant. We should note that $N = 41$ is not an even number. In fact, 20 were assigned the sequence AP but 21 were assigned PA.

The corresponding command (**mcc Placebo Azithromycin**) and the edited output from a statistical package are given in Figure 12.4. We stated that Equation (12.6) was really only for large samples, which this example is clearly not. This accounts for the discrepancy between the p-value $= 0.78$ obtained in our calculation and that of the 'exact' result with a value of 1. For small samples, a

Example 12.5   *(Continued)*

modification to Equation (12.6) can be made by reducing the absolute value of the numerator by 0.5. In our example, this leads to $z = -0.5/\sqrt{13} = -0.14$ and then Table T1 gives the p-value $= 2(1 - 0.55567) = 0.89$, which is then closer to the exact value of 0.78.

Command

```
tabulate Placebo Azithromycin
mcc Placebo Azithromycin
```

Edited Output

```
-------------------------------------------------
         |      Azithromycin        |
 Placebo |   Negative    Positive   |  Total
-------------------------------------------------
Negative |     17            6      |    23
Positive |      7           11      |    18
-------------------------------------------------
   Total |     24           17      |    41
-------------------------------------------------
```

```
McNemar's chi2 (1) = 0.08    Prob > chi2 = 0.7815
Exact McNemar significance probability = 1.0000

Proportion with factor
   Placebo        0.4390
   Azithromycin  0.4146
-------------------------------------------------
                    [95% Conf. Interval]
-------------------------------------------------
difference   0.0244     -0.1722 to 0.2210
odds ratio   1.1667      0.3357 to 4.2020   (exact)
-------------------------------------------------
```

Figure 12.4   Edited commands and output from a statistical package for analyzing a cross-over trial comparing treatments for patients with cystic fibrosis (data from Equi, Balfour-Lynn, Bush and Rosenthal, *et al.*, 2002).

For a 1 : 1 randomized two-period two-treatment cross-over trial with two-sided test size α and power $1 - \beta$, the number of sequences required is

$$N_{\text{Sequences}} = \frac{\left(z_{1-\alpha/2}(\psi + 1) + z_{1-\beta}\sqrt{[(\psi + 1)^2 - (\psi - 1)^2\pi_{\text{Discordant}}]}\right)^2}{(\psi - 1)^2\pi_{\text{Discordant}}}. \quad (12.7)$$

In order to calculate the required sample size $N_{\text{Sequences}}$, we need to specify the anticipated values of ψ and $\pi_{\text{Discordant}}$ or alternatively f and g. However, an investigating team may find it difficult to anticipate the discordant values f and g. They may find it easier to specify the anticipated planning proportions, π_A and π_B, which represent the marginal probabilities of response to treatments (say) A and B. In this case, $\pi_A(1 - \pi_B)$ is an estimate of the anticipated value of

$$\frac{f}{N_{\text{Sequences}}}$$

and $\pi_B(1 - \pi_A)$ the value of

$$\frac{g}{N_{\text{Sequences}}}$$

From these, the anticipated values for

$$\pi_{\text{Discordant}} = \frac{f + g}{N_{\text{Sequences}}} = \pi_A(1 - \pi_B) + \pi_B(1 - \pi_A)$$

and

$$\psi = \frac{f}{g} = \frac{\pi_A(1 - \pi_B)}{\pi_B(1 - \pi_A)}$$

can be obtained.

These calculations assume that the response to treatment A is *independent* of the response to treatment B in each subject. Although this is not likely to be truly the case, we have to make assumptions of some kind for sample size calculation purposes.

Example 12.6   Crossover trial – sample size

Suppose the trial of Equi, Balfour-Lynn, Bush and Rosenthal, *et al.* (2002) was repeated, but with a different formulation of azithromycin thought to be much more effective. The investigators assume that $\psi_{\text{Plan}} = 2.5$ and the proportion of discordant pairs is set at approximately the same as for the previous trial at $\pi_{\text{Discordant}} = 0.3$. Assuming a two-sided test size of 5%, power 80%, use of Table T2 and Equation (12.7) give:

$$N_{\text{Sequences}} = \frac{\left[1.96(2.5 + 1) + 0.8416\sqrt{[(2.5 + 1)^2 - (2.5 - 1)^2 \times 0.3]}\right]^2}{(2.5 - 1)^2 \times 0.3}$$

$$= 140.06$$

or approximately 150 sequences (75 *AB* and 75 *BA*).

Example 12.6   *(Continued)*

Had $\psi_{\text{Plan}} = 2$ been used for planning purposes, but $\pi_{\text{Discordant}} = 0.3$ retained, then $N_{\text{Sequences}} = 234 \approx 240$. In contrast, retaining $\psi_{\text{Plan}} = 2.5$ but with $\pi_{\text{Discordant}} = 0.4$ yields $N_{\text{Sequences}} = 105 \approx 110$. This illustrates how sensitive the calculations are to the planning assumptions made and once again underlines the need to study a range of possibilities before a final decision on the eventual trial size is made.

Further aspects of design and analysis of cross-over trials can be found in Senn (2002). In particular, it is described how temporal changes across periods may be accounted for during analysis. We should not underestimate the importance of these designs in the special circumstances in which they arise and are particularly suitable. Jones (2008) gives a short review of why these designs are so important in certain contexts.

12.2 Split-mouth designs

12.2.1 Design

In a split-mouth design, although not confined to dental applications alone, one side of the mouth receives one of the interventions and the other side the alternative. In a sense, the left and right sides of the mouth replace Periods I and II in the cross-over design, although there is now no temporal component. The usual situation is to find an eligible tooth on one side and match it with an equally eligible tooth on the other. The unit for analysis and hence planning is the difference in outcome measure between the two paired teeth. In certain applications, there may be several suitable matched pairs within an individual's mouth. The corresponding randomization essentially allocates one of the interventions (say the standard restorative approach) to the left or right side and then the other intervention (the test) is given to the designated tooth on the opposite side of the mouth. We might expect the allocation to left and right to be blocked so that a 1 : 1 ratio over all the patients eventually recruited to the trial is maintained. We described the trial of Lo, Luo, Fan and Wei (2001) in Example 1.5, who used the split-mouth design when comparing two glass ionomer restoratives. This design is evidently very similar to that of the cross-over trial, except there is no equivalent to the periods or to the wash-out although a carry-over (now termed carry-across) effect is likely to be present.

12.2.2 Difficulties

In principle, split-mouth designs could be applied to the clinical situation of oral lichen planus described by Poon, Goh, Kim, *et al.* (2006) of Example 2.1. However, with topical treatments being applied to each side of the mouth serious problems with carry-across effects would certainly ensue. This possibility would clearly have excluded this design option for that trial.

The difficulties concerned with the use of split-mouth designs have been set out very clearly by Hujoel (1998) and we have based this section closely on that article. The author points out that the four major difficulties are associated with recruitment, possible bias, statistical efficiency and complexity of subsequent analysis.

Clearly whatever design is chosen, no clinical trial can be conducted without finding suitable patients with the condition in question. This requires precise eligibility criteria to be applied so that in the situation of dentition, eligible teeth have to be identified. However, for the split-mouth design, if one tooth is identified with the necessary characteristics then a second (on the other side of the mouth) of similar condition also has to be found. For a patient to be eligible, a pair of matched teeth therefore has to be identified.

Example 12.7   Restoratives for dental caries

In the trial conducted by Lo, Luo, Fan and Wei (2001) of Example 1.5 comparing two restoratives for dental treatment, they targeted school children in the age range 6–14 inclusive. However, among the 1327 pupils identified who had one or two bilateral matched pairs of carious posterior teeth that required either class I or II restorations, only 89 were selected as eligible for the trial. Thus 93% of the children examined were *not* eligible for the trial. In this case, identifying the children to examine would be straightforward, but determining which of these are eligible for the trial and which not must have been a very time-consuming and resource-intensive business. As Hujoel (1998) states:

> The more complex the entry criteria, the more difficult the recruitment, and the more questions regarding generalizability (of the results) may arise.

The bias in the design arises as the effects of the treatments given to one side of the mouth have the potential to carry-across to the other side. The final comparison within the mouth is of A (with B given in the other side) versus B (with A given on the other side). So the comparison is eventually $A(B) - B(A)$ which may give a biased view of the true difference $A - B$. Such a bias may magnify, have no effect on or reduce the apparent difference, but which of these occurs is impossible to determine. This means that even if the difficulties of recruitment can be overcome, there still remains an assessment by the design team of whether or not the carry-across effect can be ignored or at least be regarded as minimal.

The random allocation of within-patient units does have the potential to increase the precision of the estimate of the difference between interventions. However, the increase in precision is directly related to the within-patient correlation coefficient ρ_{Within} of the intervention specific responses within patients. If ρ_{Within} is large and positive then this leads to fewer patients being required than if the same planning values were used for a randomized two-group (independent) parallel design. Conversely if ρ_{Within} is small, then it is the split-mouth design that requires the most patients. Hujoel and Moulton (1988) suggest that, when only a few sites per mouth are studied, low within-patient correlation coefficients are common in periodontal research. This contrasts with applications for cross-over trials discussed earlier, where the correlations tend to be higher. They also suggest, using evidence from a caries prevention trial, values of ρ_{Within} between -0.17 and $+0.02$ are likely. Such low values provide a strong indication that a split-mouth design would not be useful in such a context.

Hujoel (1998) also points out that the statistical analysis can be more complex although, in our view, should not be regarded as a major obstacle to their use. Care at the analysis stage is certainly required so that, for example, due account is taken of the fact that the 101 bilateral matched pairs included within the trial of Lo, Luo, Fan and Wei (2001) were identified from only 89 children, 77 with a single pair and 12 with two sets of matched pairs. Nevertheless a complex analysis may obscure the clarity of the clinical message intended, which is obviously not a good thing.

12.2.3   Analysis and trial size

The form of analysis of the split-mouth design and the basics of sample size calculation of, for example, one matched pair of teeth per mouth, follow that of the cross-over trial. In this case, however, the left and right hand cavities (if appropriate) would replace the period but wash-out cannot be used to prevent contamination.

Example 12.8   Split-mouth design – caries prevention

The results of a split-mouth design conducted by Arrow and Riordan (1995) which compared glass-ionomer cement (GIC) and a resin-based fissure sealant for caries prevention in 352 cases are summarized in Table 12.2. For this example we have, using Equation (12.6), $z = (77 - 40)/\sqrt{(77 + 40)} = 3.42$ and from Table T1 the p-value $= 2(1 - 0.99969) = 0.0006$. The corresponding estimate of the odds ratio is $OR = f/g = 77/40 = 1.925$, implying that children are almost twice as likely to be caries free with the resin-based approach.

Table 12.3   Results from a split-mouth design comparing treatments for caries prevention (data from Arrow and Riordan, 1995)

GIC (Standard)	Resin-based fissure sealant (Test)		
	Caries	No caries	Total
Caries	9 (e)	77 (f)	86
No Caries	40 (g)	226 (h)	266
Total	49	303	352

Example 12.8 *(Continued)*

The associated analysis using a statistical package is given in Figure 12.5 using the command (**mcc GIC resin**). The output indicates two alternative measures for summarizing the results with the associated confidence intervals. One is the difference in proportions with caries indicating 10.51% (95% *CI* 4.3–16.7%) fewer with the resin-based fissure sealant and the odds ratio of 1.925 (95% *CI* 1.30–2.90%) that we calculated earlier. We also note that the *p*-value obtained from the McNemar test of 0.0006 is increased to 0.0008 using the more sensitive methods of calculation used by the statistical package. In this case, this change makes no material difference to the interpretation.

Command

```
tabulate GIC Resin
mcc GIC Resin
```

Output

```
-----------------------------------------------------
          |  Resin-based  fissure sealant  |
    GIC   |    Caries       No caries      |   Total
-----------------------------------------------------
  Caries  |      9             77          |    86
No caries |     40            226          |   266
-----------------------------------------------------
   Total  |     49            303          |   352
-----------------------------------------------------
```

McNemar's chi2 (1) = 11.70 Prob > chi2 = 0.0006
Exact McNemar significance probability = 0.0008

Proportion with factor
    GIC   0.2443 (86/352)
   Resin   0.1392 (49/352)   [95% Conf. Int]
----
difference   0.1051   0.0431 to 0.1672
odds ratio   1.925   1.2974 to 2.8956 (exact)

Figure 12.5 Edited commands and output from a statistical package for analyzing a split-mouth design comparing treatments for caries prevention (data from Arrow and Riordan, 1995)

To estimate the size of a clinical trial using the split-mouth design, use can be made of expressions (12.4) and (12.7) given for the cross-over trial.

Example 12.9 Split-mouth design – caries prevention

Suppose we wished to replicate the trial described in Table 12.1 in another geographical location, but using the information from the earlier trial $\pi_{Discordant} = (40 + 77)/352 = 0.33$ for planning purposes. However, the design team are sceptical of attaining such a high odds ratio of $\psi = 1.9$, and so set $\psi_{Plan} = 1.5$. Use of Table T2 with a two-sided test size, $\alpha = 0.05$, gives $z_{0.975} = 1.96$ and, for a power of 90%, a one-sided $1 - \beta = 0.90$ gives $z_{0.90} = 1.2816$. Thus from Equation (12.7)

$$N_{Mouths} = \frac{\left[1.96(1.5 + 1) + 1.2816\sqrt{[(1.5 + 1)^2 - (1.5 - 1)^2 \times 0.33]}\right]^2}{(1.5 - 1)^2 \times 0.33}$$

$$= 791.9$$

or 800 mouths with suitably matched teeth on each side of the oral cavity.

Thus 400 children, with one tooth on each side of the oral cavity, would be randomized to receive GIC to the left side and resin-based to the right, with the other 400 children receiving the complementary allocation. Were the power to be reduced to 80%, then 330 children would be required while if the anticipated ψ_{Plan} was increased to 2, but retaining 90% power, then 280 children would be needed. However, the latter implies that the very large treatment effect would be observed and caution dictates that this option is an unlikely possibility.

Example 12.10 Split-mouth design – restorative treatment

Lo, Luo, Fan and Wei et al. (2001) of Example 1.5 report the net occlusive wear values of ChemFlex and Fuji IX Gp at 2 years in permanent teeth as 75 and 79 μm, respectively, with corresponding standard deviations of 23 and 20 μm. If the trial were to be repeated, how many children would need to be randomized?

The standard deviations quoted are for between subjects so that using the larger of these as the value for planning we have, using Equation (12.3),

$$\sigma_{Within\text{-}Plan} = \sqrt{2(1 - \rho_{Plan})} \times 23 = 32.53\sqrt{1 - \rho_{Plan}}$$

Thus, with $\delta_{Plan} = (79 - 75) = 4$ μm, the anticipated standardized effect size is

$$\Delta_{Plan} = \frac{4}{32.53\sqrt{1 - \rho_{Plan}}} = \frac{0.123}{\sqrt{1 - \rho_{Plan}}}$$

This provides a wide range of possibilities for the eventual sample size depending on the value of ρ_{Plan} chosen. Without knowledge of a specific value for ρ_{Plan} a

Example 12.10 *(Continued)*

range of values such as 0 (no correlation), 0.25, 0.5 and 0.75 may be investigated. The corresponding values for Δ_{Plan} are 0.12, 0.14, 0.17 and 0.25, which are all small by the Cohen (1988) criteria.

Assuming a two-sided test size of 5% and a power of 80%, then using Table T2 and Equation (12.4) suggests for the largest $\Delta_{\text{Plan}} = 0.25$,

$$N = \frac{(1.96 + 0.8416)^2}{0.25^2} + \frac{1.96^2}{2} = 127.50$$

or approximately 130 children with suitable target teeth on the left and right sides of the oral cavity. For the smaller values of Δ_{Plan} of 0.12, 0.14 and 0.17, the corresponding values of N are 550, 400 and 280 respectively. This range of values for the possible trial size illustrate that an appropriate choice for the value of ρ_{Plan} is very critical.

12.3 Paired organs

12.3.1 Design

In discussing split-mouth designs it is important to recognize that the observations made on teeth within the same oral cavity, even when on opposite sides of the mouth or from the upper and lower jaw, are to some extent correlated. The strength of this association will need to be taken into account at the design and analysis stages of any corresponding trial. This extends to other situations such as, for example, a patient presenting with multiple burns in the trial conducted by Ang, Lee, Gan, *et al.* (2001) of Example 2.2 and those with eczema in the trial of Meggitt, Gray and Reynolds (2006) of Example 1.2. This will also be the case in trials concerned with paired organs, such as the eyes and kidneys.

To take eyes as one example, if both eyes are affected by the condition of concern then (assuming the same treatment is given to each eye) the patient may respond to treatment in neither eye, one eye or both eyes. In this case, the outcome variable can be regarded as ordered categorical, taking possible values 0, 1 or 2. Each patient response therefore contributes a single observation and no new issues arise from the paired nature of the eyes.

On the other hand, suppose both eyes have the same condition but each eye receives a different treatment, then the response information cannot be collated into a single (patient) variable but the information on each eye needs to remain distinct. Although each eye is scored 0 or 1 as before, the 'eyes' are now the unit for analysis. However if the eyes behave quite independently of each other, each patient contributes two observations so that, for example, the trial size is now $N = E$, i.e. the number of eyes rather than the number of patients P. In most circumstances, $P = E/2$. In contrast, if the correlation is unity both eyes will either respond or both will not respond. In this case, the second eye provides no additional information over the first so the trial size will be $N = P$, the number of patients. Between these two extremes there may be some correlation so that, as discussed below, we will require the chosen trial size N_{Plan} to be between the two extremes, that is, $P < N_{\text{Plan}} < E$.

12.3.2   Analysis and trial size

12.3.2.1   Ordered categorical variable

What follows for an ordered categorical variable with $\kappa = 3$ levels (0, 1 and 2) is a special case of that discussed in Chapter 9. Some details are repeated here however as the context is rather different. The form of analysis required uses the Wilcoxon rank-sum test which, as pointed out in Chapter 8, is also referred to as the Mann–Whitney test. We illustrate the principles involved by means of an example.

Example 12.11   Comparing treatments

Table 12.3 illustrates the type of outcomes that we may encounter in a small randomized trial comparing Standard (S) and Test (T) treatments in patients with bilateral eye involvement of a particular condition. The same (say) topical treatment is applied to both eyes and the individual responses in each eye are noted. Thus, for example, 6/32 (18.8%) patients respond in both eyes with S but a greater proportion 11/32 (34.4%) with T. These response rates could then be compared using the command **(prtesti 32 6 32 11, count)** as in Figure 8.3. This test results in a p-value $= 0.157$. However the Wilcoxon test, the results of which are summarized in Figure 12.6, makes full use of the information in the three categories rather than first reducing them to a binary variable before comparing groups. The command **ranksum Eyes, by(Treat) porder** results in a p-value $= 0.0248$ which is statistically significant and contrasts markedly with what we might have concluded from the less efficient comparison.

Table 12.5   Illustrative example of the numbers of patients with no, one or both eyes responding according to treatment group (Standard or Test)

Eyes responding (i)	Control (S) r_S	Test (T) r_T	Control (S) p_{Si}	Test (T) p_{Ti}	$(p_{Si}+p_{Ti})/2$	Control (S) q_{Si}	Test (T) q_{Ti}	OR_{Observed}
Neither (0)	16	7	0.5000	0.2188	0.3599	0.5000	0.2188	
								3.570
One (1)	10	14	0.3125	0.4375	0.3750	0.8125	0.6563	
								2.269
Both (2)	6	11	0.1875	0.3438	0.2657	1.0000	1.0000	
Total	$n_S = 32$	$n_T = 32$	1.0000	1.0000				

Example 12.11 *(Continued)*

Command

```
ranksum Eyes, by(Treat) porder
```

Output

```
Two-sample Wilcoxon rank-sum (Mann-Whitney) test

    Treat  |   obs   rank sum    expected
-----------+----------------------------------
 Standard  |    32        883        1040
     Test  |    32       1197        1040
-----------+----------------------------------
 combined  |    64       2080        2080

 unadjusted variance    5546.67
 adjustment for ties    -652.70
                        --------
 adjusted variance      4893.97

Ho: Eyes(Treat==Standard) = Eyes(Treat==Test)
            z = -2.244
    Prob > |z| = 0.0248
```

Figure 12.6   Edited commands and output from a statistical package for analyzing the data of Table 12.3 using the Wilcoxon rank-sum or Mann–Whitney test

To illustrate how a sample size may be determined, we have added the column $(p_{Si} + p_{Ti})/2$ to Table 12.3 and also the cumulative probabilities. For example, $q_{S1} = 0.5000 + 0.3125 = 0.8125$ and $q_{T1} = 0.2188 + 0.4375 = 0.6563$. From these cumulative probabilities we can estimate the odds ratio of Category 0 to Categories 1 and 2 combined, and the odds ratio of the combined Categories 0 and 1 to Category 2. These are calculated using

$$OR_1 = \frac{q_{S1}(1 - q_{T1})}{q_{T1}(1 - q_{S1})} \text{ and } OR_2 = \frac{q_{S2}(1 - q_{T2})}{q_{T2}(1 - q_{S2})}. \tag{12.8}$$

From these,

$$OR_1 = \frac{0.5000(1 - 0.2188)}{0.2188(1 - 0.5000)} = 3.570 \text{ and } OR_2 = \frac{0.8125(1 - 0.6563)}{0.6563(1 - 0.8125)} = 2.269$$

and the average of these odds ratios is $OR = (3.570 + 2.269)/2 = 2.92$ or approximately 3.

The first requirement for determining trial size is to specify the planning values for the anticipated proportion of patients responding in each category, 0, 1 or 2 for the standard treatment, S. We denote these as $\pi_{S0}, \pi_{S1}, \pi_{S2}$ with $\pi_{S0} + \pi_{S1} + \pi_{S2} = 1$. We define Q_{S0}, Q_{S1}, Q_{S2} to be the corresponding cumulative proportions, so that $Q_{S0} = \pi_{S0}$,

$Q_{S1} = \pi_{S0} + \pi_{S1}$ and $Q_{S2} = \pi_{S0} + \pi_{S1} + \pi_{S2} = 1$. The notation is essentially the same as for Table 12.3 with π replacing p and Q replacing q. The next requirement is to specify a planning value for the common odds ratio, OR_{Plan}. Once this is defined we can use the following expressions to obtain the planning values for the cumulative proportions responding in each category in the test group, T. Thus

$$Q_{T1} = \frac{OR_{Plan} \times Q_{S1}}{[1 - Q_{S1} + (OR_{Plan} \times Q_{S1})]} \text{ and } Q_{T2} = \frac{OR_{Plan} \times Q_{S2}}{[1 - Q_{S2} + (OR_{Plan} \times Q_{S2})]} \qquad (12.9)$$

Once these are determined, then planning values for π_{T0}, π_{T1} and π_{T2} can be obtained. The penultimate step in this rather complex process is to determine

$$\overline{\pi}_0 = (\pi_{S0} + \pi_{T0})/2, \overline{\pi}_1 = (\pi_{S1} + \pi_{T1})/2 \text{ and } \overline{\pi}_2 = (\pi_{S2} + \pi_{T2})/2.$$

Finally, the trial size is then given by

$$m_3 = \frac{6(z_{1-\alpha/2} + z_{1-\beta})^2}{\Gamma(\log OR_{Plan})^2}. \qquad (12.10)$$

where $\Gamma = [1 - (\overline{\pi}_0^3 + \overline{\pi}_1^3 + \overline{\pi}_2^3)]$. This is precisely the same as Equation (9.8) but for the special case of $\kappa = 3$. When the mean proportions $\overline{\pi}_i$ in each category are approximately equal to 1/3, we have $\Gamma \approx 8/9$.

Example 12.12   Comparing two groups – odds ratio

Suppose the results of Table 12.3 are to be used to plan a confirmatory trial. We assume the distribution of the number of eyes responding in group S approximate those observed there. The observed mean $OR = 3$ indicated a rather large difference between treatment groups, but the new investigating team are somewhat cautious in their planning and adopt $OR_{Plan} = 2.5$. They also note that determining Γ in Equation (12.10) is rather a tedious business. Instead, we assume that the respective mean planning proportions are approximately equal and take $\Gamma = 8/9 = 0.88889$.

Using Table T2 with a 5% two-sided test size, $\alpha = 0.05$ gives $z_{0.975} = 1.96$ and for a power of 80% a one-sided $1 - \beta = 0.80$ gives $z_{0.80} = 0.8416$. From Equation (12.10), the number of patients to include in one treatment group is

$$m_3 = \frac{6 \times (1.96 + 0.8416)^2}{0.88889 \times (\log 2.5)^2} = 63.10,$$

or approximately 70. The planned total trial size is therefore $N = 2 \times 70 = 140$ patients involving 280 eyes. In this case, for patients to be eligible both eyes have to meet the inclusion criteria.

More precise calculations using the software of Machin, Campbell, Tan and Tan (2009) calculates Γ, as opposed to using the approximate value, and gives $m = 75$ leading to approximately $N = 150$ patients to be recruited.

12.3.2.2 *Continuous measure*

In the situation in which the endpoint measure is a continuous variable and can be measured on both eyes, we can think of the patient as a cluster from which $k = 2$ observations are made. Cluster designs for trials were discussed in Chapter 11. Here we have a special case of Table 11.3 but now with many clusters (the patients) each with two eyes randomly assigned (one to receiving one intervention and one the other) to treatment. The corresponding analysis command, taking exactly the same format, is: **regress Endpoint Intervention, vce(cluster Patient)**. Here **Endpoint** represents the measure we are using, perhaps inter-ocular pressure (IOP), **Intervention** the two treatment groups and **Patient** the cluster, while **vce** indicates that because of correlation within each cluster the standard errors have to be calculated to take this into account.

To determine sample size, the design effect (DE) of Equation (11.8) has to be used with $k = 2$, so that $DE = 1 + \rho_{\text{Eyes}}$. If the trial size m is calculated (e.g. from Equation (9.5)) as though the eyes were 'individual entities' instead of 'paired entities', then this number would need to be inflated to $m_{\text{Eyes}} = m(1 + \rho_{\text{Eyes}})$ eyes per intervention group to take account of the correlation between eyes.

CHAPTER 13

More Than Two Interventions

In this chapter we consider extensions of the basic parallel two-group randomized trial. These include parallel designs of three or more groups, including those comparing each of several interventions with a standard which may be a placebo, those comprising different doses of the compound and those with no structure in the groups to be compared. The specific situation of the factorial design in which more than one type of intervention comparison can be included in the same trial is also described. Methods of analysis and for estimating the numbers of subjects to be recruited to such trials are outlined.

13.1   Introduction

Although the two-arm parallel group design is perhaps the most common, there are many situations demanding alternatives. This includes where there is more than one alternative to the standard, where there is the prospect of investigating a dose response relation or when more than one component of therapy can be given simultaneously with or without the other in a factorial design structure. These designs can also be concerned with questions of superiority or non-inferiority. These designs are generally more difficult to conduct, for example, by needing a more complex protocol, by making the informed consent process more involved and lengthy and by having to be larger in terms of patient numbers. Nevertheless, these disadvantages may be compensated by the additional insights that results from such designs may bring.

13.2   Unstructured comparisons

13.2.1   Design

In an unstructured design of $g > 2$ groups, sometimes the interventions being compared are unrelated. For example, perhaps they are using totally different approaches to the treatment of a disease or condition and for which no standard approach has been established. In this case, assuming the outcome will be summarized by the mean value for each group, then the null hypothesis is H_0: $\mu_1 = \mu_2 = \cdots = \mu_g$ (although there is a whole range of possible alternative hypotheses). For example, for $g = 3$ these are H_{A1}: $\mu_1 = \mu_2 \neq \mu_3$; H_{A2}: $\mu_1 \neq \mu_2 = \mu_3$; H_{A3}: $\mu_1 = \mu_3 \neq \mu_2$ and H_{A4}: $\mu_1 \neq \mu_2 \neq \mu_3$. Despite these numerous alternatives, the context of the trial under consideration may suggest that only one or two of these are appropriate.

Example 13.1   Newly diagnosed patients treated for type-2 diabetes

Weng, Li, Xu, *et al.* (2008) were interested in determining whether the disease modifying effect in newly diagnosed patients treated for type-2 diabetes was due to the insulin therapy itself, or due to the effects of simply eliminating glucotoxicity by achieving excellent glycaemic control. Further, if the latter was the case, then they wished to determine which of two early intensive therapies would be more beneficial. Thus the trial compares two short-term insulin therapies, multiple daily insulin injections (MDI) and continuous subcutaneous insulin infusion (CSII), both of which target overall glycaemic control with an oral hypoglycaemic agent (OHA). The outcome of interest is the remission proportion at 1 year in those who achieved glycaemic control.

13.2.2   Trial size

In Example 13.1 of Weng, Li, Xu, *et al.* (2008), the endpoint measure is a binary variable as the objective of the trial is to estimate the respective treatment remission proportions, π_{OHA}, π_{MDI} and π_{CSII}. However, the authors identified two specific comparisons they wished to make which imply testing the following two hypotheses: H_{01}: $\pi_{OHA} = (\pi_{MDI} + \pi_{CSII})/2$ and H_{02}: $\pi_{MDI} = \pi_{CSII}$. In planning such a trial, the investigators would therefore need to specify two planning effect sizes: δ_{Plan1} and δ_{Plan2}.

The authors anticipated that the proportions in long-term remission with OHA would be 25% while in those who received insulin treatment (CSII or MDI) it would be 45%. For testing H_{01}, with two-sided significance level of 5% and power 80%, use of Equation (9.6) with allocation ratio $\lambda = 1$ implies approximately 90 patients to receive OHA and consequently 45 to receive CSII and 45 MDI. An alternative strategy may be to use a 1 : 2 ratio ($\lambda = 2$) as the investigators know another hypothesis is also under consideration. This scenario suggests 70 patients for OHA, and twice that number to be allocated either CSII or MDI (compared to 45 each earlier). This gives more power to testing H_{01} and hence the fewer patient numbers required in the OHA group.

However, this number of patients would be insufficient to test H_{02}: $\pi_{MDI} = \pi_{CSII}$ unless the anticipated difference between CSII and MDI is greater than 20%. The authors worked on the basis of 90 patients for each of the three groups, and this is sufficient to test for a 20% difference between CSII and MDI. However, now that 90 are also to be assigned to OHA, this implies a power increase from 80% to 90% for testing H_{01}. An increase in power is often a good thing but nevertheless increases the duration and raises the cost of the clinical trial.

In simplistic terms, designing on the basis of H_{01} provided insufficient patient numbers to test H_{02}, whereas designing on H_{02} yields more than sufficient patient numbers for H_{01}. Clearly the investigating team have to decide on the relative priorities of the two questions posed. In general, it is this kind of dilemma that makes such trials difficult to design as some compromise with respect to the final sample size will have to be found.

13.2.3   Analysis

In the example discussed, the analysis for testing of the two null hypotheses amounts to two separate two-sample tests as in Section 9.4, the form of which will depend on the type of endpoint variable under consideration. These tests are not independent of each other as they each use, at least in part, the same patient observations.

Example 13.2   Newly diagnosed patients treated for type-2 diabetes

In the trial of Example 1.10, Weng, Li, Xu, *et al.* (2008) observed that remission rates at 1 year in those who achieved glycaemic control were 51.1% (68/133) with CSII, 44.9% (53/118) with MDI and 26.7% (27/101) with OHA. The analysis is illustrated using a statistical package and follows the approach of regression Equation (8.13) and the **logit** and **logistic** commands of Figure 8.10. It is summarized in Figure 13.1.

Commands – First hypothesis

```
tabulate Type Remission
logit Remission Type
logistic Remission Type
```

Output – First hypothesis

```
------------+----------------------+--------
            |       Remission      |
    Type    |    No    Yes    (%)  |  Total
------------+----------------------+--------
CSII or MDI |   130    121  (48.2) |   251
       OHA  |    74     27  (26.7) |   101
------------+----------------------+--------
     Total  | Difference   (21.5)  |   352
------------+----------------------+--------

Logistic regression
Number of obs = 352 LR chi2(1) = 14.11 Prob > chi2 = 0.0002
Log likelihood = -232.45731
-----------------------------------------------------------------
```

Example 13.2   *(Continued)*

```
---------------------------------------------------------------------
Remission  |   Coef.      Std. Err.     z       P>|z|  [95% Conf. Interval]
-----------+---------------------------------------------------------
      Type | -0.9365       0.2579     -3.63    0.001   -1.4419 to -0.4310
     _cons |  0.8647       0.3382
---------------------------------------------------------------------


---------------------------------------------------------------------
Remission  |    OR        Std. Err.     z       P>|z|   [95% Conf. Interval]
-----------+---------------------------------------------------------
Type       | 0.3920        0.1011     -3.63    0.001    0.2365 to 0.6498
---------------------------------------------------------------------
```

Commands – Second hypothesis

```
tabulate Treat Remission if Treat!=3
logit Remission Treat if Treat!=3
logistic Remission Treat if Treat!=3
```

Output – Second hypothesis

```
-------+----------------------+--------
       |       Remission      |
Treat  |   No    Yes   (%)    |  Total
-------+----------------------+--------
 CSII  |   65     68   (51.1) |   133
  MDI  |   65     53   (44.9) |   118
-------+----------------------+--------
Total  |    Difference (6.2)  |
-------+----------------------+--------
```

```
Logistic regression
Number of obs = 251 LR chi2 (1) = 0.97 Prob > chi2 = 0.3253
Log likelihood = -173.33488


---------------------------------------------------------------------
Remission  |   Coef.      Std. Err.    z       P>|z|  [95% Conf. Interval]
-----------+---------------------------------------------------------
     Treat | -0.2492       0.2537    -0.98    0.326   -0.7464 to 0.2479
     _cons |  0.2943       0.3932
---------------------------------------------------------------------


---------------------------------------------------------------------
Remission  |    OR        Std. Err.    z       P>|z|  [95% Conf. Interval]
-----------+---------------------------------------------------------
     Treat | 0.7794        0.1977    -0.98    0.326    0.4741 to 1.2814
---------------------------------------------------------------------
```

Figure 13.1   Edited commands and output from a statistical package for analyzing a parallel group trial comparing three treatments for diabetes mellitus (data from Weng, Li, Xu, *et al.*, 2008)

Example 13.2 *(Continued)*

From the analysis of Figure 13.1 we might conclude that there is a difference in remission rates between the treatment types used (OHA versus insulin), which is estimated as 21.5% and $OR = 0.39$ (95% CI 0.24 to 0.65). However, the difference between the use of CSII and MDI is not proven, with an estimated difference of only 6.2% and $OR = 0.78$ (95% CI 0.47 to 1.28).

As we noted in Chapter 8, in circumstances where there is repeat statistical testing within the same dataset, then this can cause the single significance level set at the design stage of the trial to be no longer applicable. The way in which the significance level changes depends in a complex way on how many and what comparisons are to be made, and usually this cannot be quantified readily. One method used is to apply the Bonferroni correction to each of the p-values obtained. This simply multiplies each of these by the number of statistical tests undertaken. From the analysis of Figure 13.1, the two p-values are therefore 0.001 and 0.326 which are then modified to become 0.002 and 0.652, respectively. In this example, these changes have little influence on the interpretation.

13.3 Comparisons with placebo (or standard)

13.3.1 Design

In certain situations there may be several potentially active treatments under consideration, each of which it would be desirable to test against a placebo. The treatments considered may be entirely different formulations (not different doses of the same compound), and we may simply be trying to determine which, if any, are active relative to placebo rather than to make a comparison between them. This can be expressed for a binary outcome in terms of testing the null hypothesis, H_0: $\pi_{Standard} - \pi_{Testi} = 0$ against each of the alternative hypotheses $H_{Alternativei}$: $\pi_{Standard} - \pi_{Testi} \neq 0$, where i corresponds to each of the $g - 1$ alternative (non-standard) treatment options. Alternatively, in such cases a common minimum effect size to be demonstrated may be set by the clinical team for all the comparisons. Any treatment that demonstrates this minimum level would then be considered as 'sufficiently active' and perhaps evaluated further in subsequent trials. The conventional parallel group design would be to randomize these treatments and placebo (g options) equally, perhaps in blocks of size $b = g$ or $2g$.

Example 13.3 Comparison of second-generation antipsychotic drugs with first-generation haloperidol

Kahn, Fleischhacker, Boter, *et al.* (2008) describe a randomized trial comparing four second-generation antipsychotic drugs: Amisulpride (*A*), Olanzapine (*O*), Quetiapine (*Q*) and Ziprasidone (*Z*), with the first-generation drug Haloperidol

---

Example 13.3   *(Continued)*

(H) in patients with first-episode schizophrenia and schizophreniform disorder. In this example, the comparison is not with a placebo but with the first generation drug, H. A total of 498 patients were randomized with a $1 : 1 : 1 : 1 : 1$ allocation ratio using a minimization procedure. The endpoint was the time from randomization to discontinuation of the treatment allocated (the event) and the Kaplan–Meier estimates of the 12-month discontinuation rates were A: 40%, O: 33%, Q: 53% and Z: 45%, compared to H: 72%.

13.3.2   Trial size

Fleiss (1986, pp 95–96) has shown that in this situation it is better to have a larger number of patients receiving placebo (or standard) than each of the other interventions. This is because every one of the $g-1$ comparisons is made against placebo, so that its effect needs to be well established. Accordingly, the placebo group should have $\sqrt{(g-1)}$ patients for every one patient of the other treatment options. For example, if $g = 5$, then $\sqrt{(g-1)} = \sqrt{4} = 2$, thus the recommended randomization is $2 : 1 : 1 : 1 : 1$ which can be conducted in blocks of size $b = 6$ or 12. However, if $g = 6$ for example, then $\sqrt{6} = 2.45$ which is not an integer but, with convenient rounding, this leads to a randomization ratio of $2.5 : 1 : 1 : 1 : 1 : 1$ or equivalently $5 : 2 : 2 : 2 : 2 : 2$. The options can then be randomized in blocks of size $b = 15$ or 30.

If the variable being measured is continuous and can be assumed to have a Normal distribution then the number of subjects m for the non-placebo treatment groups can be calculated by suitably adapting Equation (9.5) to give

$$m = \left(1 + \frac{1}{\sqrt{g-1}}\right)\left[\frac{(z_{1-\alpha/2} + z_{1-\beta})^2}{\Delta_{\mathrm{Plan}}^2} + \frac{z_{1-\alpha/2}^2}{4}\right], \quad g \geq 2. \qquad (13.1)$$

The corresponding number for the placebo group is $n = \sqrt{(g-1)} \times m$. This implies a total trial size of $N = n + (g-1) \times m = m\,[\sqrt{(g-1)} + (g-1)]$ patients.

A similar adjustment is made in the cases of binary, ordered categorical and time-to-event outcomes of Equations (9.6), (9.8) and (9.11).

Example 13.4   Maintenance treatments for heroin dependence

Schottenfeld, Charwarski and Mazlan (2008) designed a three-arm trial of buprenorphine, naltrexone and placebo to investigate alternative maintenance treatments to reduce problems associated with heroin dependence. On the basis of earlier studies, they anticipated that the Kaplan–Meier estimates of the proportion abstinent at 6-months would be $\pi_{\mathrm{N}} = 0.72$ and $\pi_{\mathrm{B}} = 0.42$ for naltrexone and

---

Example 13.4 *(Continued)*

buprenorphine, respectively, and for placebo π_P would range from 0.12 to 0.24. A conservative planning value would take $\pi_P = 0.24$.

Using Equation (9.9) this leads to the anticipated effect size for naltrexone versus placebo as $HR_{N-P} = \log 0.72/\log 0.24 = 0.23$ and that for buprenorphine versus placebo as $HR_{B-P} = \log 0.42/\log 0.24 = 0.61$. On this basis, the investigators specified what they termed a 'medium effect size' equivalent to $HR_{Plan} = 0.5$, which is a compromise between $HR_{N-P} = 0.23$ and $HR_{B-P} = 0.61$. This implies that the design comparison used is that between $\pi_P = 0.24$ and $\pi_{Active} = \exp(HR_{Plan} \times \pi_P) = \exp[0.5 \times \log(0.24)] = 0.49$.

Use of Equation (9.11) with $\lambda = 1$ and Table T2 for two-sided test size of 5% and power 80% gives

$$m = \left(\frac{1+0.5}{1-0.5}\right)^2 \frac{(1.96 + 0.8416)^2}{[(1 - 0.24) + (1 - 0.49)]} = 55.6 \approx 60.$$

This implies, as the investigators had planned, recruiting 180 patients and then randomizing these equally to the 3 arms in blocks of possible size $b = 3$, 6 or 9. However, the approach of Fleiss (1986) with $g = 3$ suggests that a better design would be to recruit $m\sqrt{(g-1)} = 55.6 \times \sqrt{2} = 78.6$ or 80 to the placebo group, and 60 to each of naltrexone and buprenorphine or a total of 200 heroin users in all. This alternative would imply a randomization ratio of $4 : 3 : 3$ which could be organized in blocks of $b = 10$ or 20.

13.3.3 Analysis

The analysis of such a design involves comparing each test option against the placebo using, for a continuous endpoint variable, the t-test based on Equation (8.2) but with the pooled standard error of Equation (8.5) based on data from all g groups. For the Fleiss (1986) design, the corresponding degrees of freedom will be $df = m\,[\sqrt{(g-1)} + g] - g$ and

$$SE_0(d) = \sqrt{s_{Pool}^2 \left(\frac{1}{m\sqrt{g-1}} + \frac{1}{m}\right)}.$$

Example 13.5   Aggressive challenging behaviour in patients with intellectual disability

Tyrer, Oliver-Africano, Ahmed, *et al.* (2008) give the median and range of quality of life scores of Table 13.1 following 4 weeks of treatment with placebo,

Example 13.5   *(Continued)*

risperidone or haloperidol for aggressive challenging behaviour in patients with intellectual disability. The authors concluded that patients given placebo showed no evidence at any time of worse response than those assigned to either of the antipsychotic drugs. They therefore recommended that:

> Antipsychotic drugs should no longer be regarded as acceptable routine treatment for aggressive challenging behaviour in people with intellectual disability.

Table 13.1   Median and range of quality of life scores at 4 weeks (data from Tyrer, Oliver-Africano, Ahmed, *et al.*, 2008) together with simulated data based on these to mimic a trial using the Fleiss (1986) design

	Placebo	Risperidone	Haloperidol	
	Actual data of Tyrer, Oliver-Africano, Ahmed, *et al.* (2008)			
Number of patients	29	29	28	
Median	72	70	66	
Range	65.7–77.75	60–78	59.5–75.5	
	Simulated data for the Fleiss (1986) design			
Number of patients	42	29	28	
Mean	72.12	70.73	65.95	Pooled
Standard deviation	2.56	4.01	4.31	3.57
Difference from placebo		1.39	6.18	
	t-statistic	1.62	7.10	
	p-value	0.109	0.001	

As we do not have access to the data, and indeed the trial design was not of the form suggested by Fleiss (1986), we have produced simulated trial data summarized in the lower panel of Table 13.1. As will therefore be clear, our analysis summarized in Figure 13.2 cannot be taken as any guide to the relative merits of the treatments concerned.

Commands

```
table GROUP, contents(n QoL mean QoL sd QoL) row
anova QoL GROUP
xi: regress QoL i.GROUP
```

Output

```
------------+------------------------------------
     GROUP |  N(QoL)   mean(QoL)   sd(QoL)
------------+------------------------------------
   Placebo |    42       72.13       2.56
Risperidone |   29       70.73       4.01
Haloperidol |   28       65.95       4.31
------------+------------------------------------
```

Example 13.5 *(Continued)*

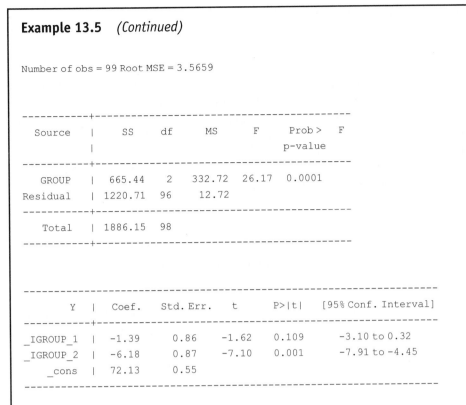

Number of obs = 99 Root MSE = 3.5659

```
----------+-------------------------------------------
  Source  |    SS      df     MS      F    Prob >   F
          |                                 p-value
----------+-------------------------------------------
  GROUP   |  665.44    2    332.72  26.17  0.0001
Residual  | 1220.71   96     12.72
----------+-------------------------------------------
  Total   | 1886.15   98
----------+-------------------------------------------
```

```
----------+--------------------------------------------------------------
    Y     |  Coef.   Std. Err.    t     P>|t|   [95% Conf. Interval]
----------+--------------------------------------------------------------
_IGROUP_1 |  -1.39     0.86     -1.62   0.109     -3.10 to 0.32
_IGROUP_2 |  -6.18     0.87     -7.10   0.001     -7.91 to -4.45
   _cons  |  72.13     0.55
----------+--------------------------------------------------------------
```

Figure 13.2 Edited commands and output for the analysis of quality of life scores using the simulated data of the lower section of Table 13.1 (based on the trial of Tyrer, Oliver-Africano, Ahmed, *et al.*, 2008)

An overall comparison of the differences between groups can be conducted using ANOVA which is implemented in Figure 13.2 using the command (**anova QoL GROUP**). This gives a test of the null hypothesis: H_0: $\mu_{\text{Placebo}} = \mu_{\text{Risperidone}} = \mu_{\text{Haloperidol}} = 0$ and gives a p-value $= 0.0001$ suggesting a statistically significant difference between groups. This same analysis can be made using a regression model by means of (**xi: regress QoL i.GROUP**). Here the **xi** indicates that a categorical variable is anticipated and **i.GROUP** identifies the variable in the model. In general, there can be more than one such variable in a model.

The regression coefficients of -1.39, -6.18 correspond to the differences in means between haloperidol and placebo, and risperidone and placebo, respectively. They suggest that QoL may be statistically significantly lower (p-value $= 0.001$) with haloperidol but not with risperidone (p-value $= 0.109$). The corresponding means are calculated as: placebo (_cons $= 72.13$), risperidone (_cons + _IGROUP_1 $= 72.13 - 1.39 = 70.73$) and haloperidol (_cons + _IGROUP_2 $= 72.13 - 6.18 = 65.94$) which, apart from some small rounding errors, are those of the lower panel of Table 13.1.

13.4 Dose response designs

13.4.1 Design

In contrast to the trial of Example 13.3 of Kahn, Fleischhacker, Boter, *et al.* (2008), in which four different drugs were compared against a standard, the trial of Example 1.9 by Stevinson, Devaraj, Fountain-Barber, *et al.* (2003) compared two doses of homeopathic arnica with placebo to examine any dose response relation. The report of their trial suggested that, irrespective of dose, there was no advantage to homeopathic arnica over placebo in the prevention of pain and bruising following hand surgery. However, in the analysis no consideration of the increasing dose, 0, 6 and 30 of homeopathic arnica appears to have been taken.

Example 13.6   Tocilizumab in rheumatoid arthritis

Smolen, Beaulieu, Rubbert-Roth, *et al.* (2008) compare tocilizumab in two doses of 4 and 8 mg/kg against placebo to test the therapeutic effect of blocking interleukin in patients with rheumatoid arthritis. They recruited a total of 623 patients randomized equally to the three arms. Their trial results suggest a dose response in favour of tocilizumab with respect to several American College of Rheumatology (ACR) criteria. The primary efficacy endpoint was the proportion of patients with 20% improvement in rheumatoid arthritis signs and symptoms (ACR20), although many secondary endpoints were also included.

13.4.2 Trial size

In the simplest design situation, the design of such a trial would have g equally spaced dose levels, with levels labelled d_i where $i = 0, 1, 2, \ldots, g - 1$. If the dose response is linear and the endpoint of interest is a continuous measure, this situation can be summarized by the following (linear regression) model:

$$y_{ij} = \beta_0 + \beta_{\text{Dose}} d_i + \varepsilon_{ij}. \tag{13.2}$$

Here y_{ij} is the outcome measure for patient j receiving dose i and ε_{ij} is the corresponding random error term. In this equation, β_{Dose} represents the slope of the linear dose-response relation and replaces β_1 or β_{Treat} of Equation (2.1) as the main focus for the statistical analysis. For expository purposes we assume the same number of subjects m will receive the g different doses and the standard deviation σ is constant within all dose groups.

Once the trial is completed, the slope of the fitted linear regression equation is estimated by

$$b_{\text{Dose}} = \frac{\sum\limits_{i=0}^{g-1} \sum\limits_{j=1}^{m} (d_i - \bar{d}) y_{ij}}{m \sum\limits_{i=0}^{g-1} (d_i - \bar{d})^2}. \tag{13.3}$$

The corresponding standard error of b_{Dose} is

$$SE(b_{\text{Dose}}) = \frac{\sigma}{\sqrt{m}} \frac{1}{\sqrt{\sum\limits_{i=0}^{g-1} (d_i - \bar{d})^2}}. \tag{13.4}$$

This can then be used in the fundamental Equation (9.3) by replacing $2\sigma^2$ by $\sigma^2 / \sum\limits_{i=0}^{g} (d_i - \bar{d})^2$ and δ by β_{Dose} to give

$$m = \frac{\sigma^2}{\sum\limits_{i=0}^{g} (d_i - \bar{d})^2} \frac{(z_{1-\alpha/2} + z_{1-\beta})^2}{\beta_{\text{Dose}}^2}. \tag{13.5}$$

For specified dose levels β_{DosePlan} and σ_{Plan}, the total trial size will then be $N = gm$ with m patients being randomized to each of the g dose groups.

We should note that β_{DosePlan} is the planning regression slope which might be anticipated in practice as the difference between the anticipated endpoint measures at the lowest dose (often 0) and the highest dose, divided by the range ($d_{\text{Maximum}} - d_{\text{Minimum}}$) of the doses to be included in the design.

Example 13.7 Sample size – ISA247 in plaque psoriasis

Papp, Bissonnette, Rosoph, *et al.* (2008) compare ISA247 in three doses of 0.2, 0.3 and 0.4 mg/kg against placebo in patients with moderate to severe psoriasis. They concluded that the highest dose provided the best efficacy. In this example, the doses are not equally spaced so that Equation (13.5) has to be used for sample size purposes. Suppose we wish to repeat this trial and to detect a 'moderate' effect change of $\Delta_{\text{Cohen}} = 0.5$. In terms of the regression slope from the lowest dose 0 to the highest 0.4 mg/kg, this implies $\Delta_{\text{Plan}} = 0.5/(0.4 - 0) = 1.25$. Further, with these four doses

$$\sum_{i=0}^{3} (d_i - \bar{d})^2 = 0.0875.$$

Example 13.7   *(Continued)*

Finally, with a two-sided test size of $\alpha = 0.05$ and power $1 - \beta = 0.9$, use of Table T2 and Equation (13.5) give

$$m = \frac{1}{0.0875} \times \frac{(1.96 + 1.2816)^2}{1.25^2} = 76.86 \approx 80 \text{ patients per dose.}$$

This gives a planned trial size of $N = 4 \times 80$ or 320 in total. Although not directly comparable, this is fewer than the 451 recruited to the published trial.

In the special case where the doses are equally spaced, they can then be coded as 0, 1, 2, $\cdots$, $g - 1$, so that

$$SE(b_{\text{Dose}}) = \frac{\sigma}{\sqrt{m}} \sqrt{\frac{12}{g(g^2 - 1)}}.$$

and

$$m = \frac{12\sigma^2_{\text{Plan}}}{g(g^2 - 1)} \frac{(z_{1-\alpha/2} + z_{1-\beta})^2}{\beta^2_{\text{DosePlan}}} = \frac{6}{g(g^2 - 1)} \times \frac{2(z_{1-\alpha/2} + z_{1-\beta})^2}{\Delta^2_{\text{Plan}}}. \qquad (13.6)$$

As anticipated, for the case $g = 2$ Equation (13.5) becomes the fundamental Equation (9.3) as does Equation (13.6), since in this case $6/[g(g^2 - 1)] = 1$.

Example 13.8   Sample size – tocilizumab in rheumatoid arthritis

In the trial of Smolen, Beaulieu, Rubbert-Roth, *et al.* (2008) of Example 13.6, which has equally spaced doses, we can deduce from their Tables 1 and 4 that the mean pain levels assessed by visual analogue scale (VAS) (mm) at 24 weeks were approximately 45, 36 and 30 mm for doses 0, 4 and 8 mg/kg of tocilizumab. If a repeat trial was planned, then a reasonable value for the regression slope, β_{DosePlan}, might be the observed change between 0 and 8 mg/kg from this trial or $\beta_{\text{DosePlan}} = (30 - 45)/(8 - 0) = -15/8 = -1.875$. From their Table 1, the corresponding standard deviation is approximately $\sigma_{\text{Plan}} = 22$ leading to $\Delta_{\text{Plan}} = 1.875/22 = 0.085$. However, to use Equation (13.6) we have to recode the dose 0, 4 and 8 to 0, 1 and 2, respectively. This necessitates multiplying the standardized effect size by 4; we therefore have $\Delta_{\text{Plan}} = 4 \times 0.085 = 0.34$. Using a two-sided test size of $\alpha = 0.05$ and power $1 - \beta = 0.9$, use of Table T2 and Equation (13.6) gives

$$m = \frac{6}{3(3^2 - 1)} \left[\frac{2(1.96 + 1.2816)^2}{0.34^2} \right] = 45.45 \approx 46 \text{ patients per dose.}$$

This gives a planned trial size of $N = 3 \times 46$ or 138 patients in total.

13.4.3 Analysis

As in all circumstances, the form of the analysis will depend on the type of endpoint variable concerned. However for a binary outcome, the principle hypothesis to test will often be one of linearity on the logit scale of the dose response relation. Alternatively if a non-linear response is anticipated, then careful thought is required to determine the associated regression model to describe the relationship.

Example 13.9   Sample size – ISA247 in plaque psoriasis

Papp, Bissonnette, Rosoph, *et al.* (2008, Table 3) summarize one aspect of their trial by the number of patients with 75% reduction in psoriasis at week 12. Their results are summarized in Table 13.2.

Table 13.2   Number of patients with 75% reduction in psoriasis at week 12 by dose of ISA247 (data from Papp, Bissonnette, Rosoph, *et al.*, 2008, Table 3)

	Dose of ISA247 (mg/kg)				
	0	0.2	0.3	0.4	All
Number of patients	113	105	111	113	442
Number with 75% reduction (%)	4 (3.5)	14 (13.3)	26 (23.4)	44 (38.9)	88 (19.5)

The corresponding logistic regression based on the individual data from the 442 patients with the variable (**response**) taking the value 1 for a response and 0 for failure to respond. The command (**logit response Dose**) and the results of such an analysis are given in Figure 13.3.

Command

```
logit response Dose
```

Edited output

```
Logistic regression                        number of obs = 442
---------------------------------------------------------------
     r |   Coef.    Std. Err.    z    P >|z|   [95% Conf. Interval]
-------+-------------------------------------------------------
  Dose |  6.7293    1.1226     5.99   0.001    4.5291 to 8.9295
 _cons | -3.1552    0.3604    -8.75
---------------------------------------------------------------
```

Figure 13.3   Edited command and output for the analysis of the proportion of patients achieving a 75% reduction in psoriasis at 12 weeks of Table 13.2 (based on the trial of Papp, Bissonnette, Rosoph, *et al.*, 2008)

Example 13.9   *(Continued)*

This output results in the estimated model logit$(p) = -3.1552 + 6.7293 \times$ Dose which corresponds, on the logit proportion-who-respond scale, to

$$p_{\text{Estimate}} = 1/[1 + \exp(3.1552 + 6.7293 \text{ Dose})]$$

which is plotted in Figure 13.4 along with the proportions observed from Table 13.2. In this example the model describes the data very closely, although this will not always be the case.

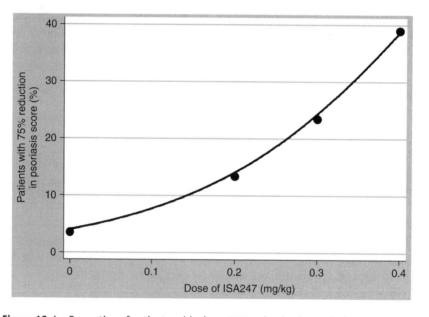

Figure 13.4   Proportion of patients achieving a 75% reduction in psoriasis at 12 weeks by dose of ISA247 (mg/kg) (data from Papp, Bissonnette, Rosoph, *et al.*, 2008, Table 3)

13.4.4   Reporting

Although it may seem obvious, tabular presentation of the results for a dose response design should reflect the increasing (or decreasing) order of the doses included in the trial. Although Papp, Bissonnette, Rosoph, *et al.* (2008) tabulate in columns in the order 0 (placebo), 0.2, 0.3 and 0.4 mg/kg, Stevinson, Devaraj, Fountain-Barber, *et al.* (2003) choose the column order Arnica 6c, Placebo and Arnica 30C, while Smolen, Beaulieu, Rubbert-Roth, *et al.* (2008) uses 4, 8 and then 0 mg/kg (placebo). The latter two tabulations make it difficult for a reader to identify patterns along the rows of any of the variables within these tables. The rule for columns in tables should follow that for graphs, by plotting smallest to largest (here dose) values from left to right on the horizontal scale. This ordering (or the reverse) is also necessary if a statistical test for trend is to be conducted.

13.5 Factorial trials

13.5.1 Design

In some circumstances there may be two distinct therapeutic questions that are posed and, in some such cases, both questions may be answered within a single trial by use of a factorial design. In a 2×2 factorial design, the two intervention types or factors A and B are each studied at two levels.

Example 13.10 2×2 factorial design – patients with low back pain

In a trial conducted by Hancock, Maher, Latimer, *et al.* (2007), patients with low back pain were given advice, including the suggested use of paracetemol, by their general practitioner. They were then randomized to receive either diclofenac or placebo diclofenac (the two levels of diclofenac), and also to receive either manipulative therapy or placebo manipulative therapy (the two levels of manipulative therapy). An important feature of this trial was their use of a placebo controlled double-blind design. This included placebo diclofenac (a placebo to 'blind' a drug is not unusual) but also placebo spinal manipulative therapy which must have been more difficult to make 'blind'. The four possible combinations are illustrated in Figure 13.5 and the endpoint chosen was patient recovery or not at 12-weeks post randomization.

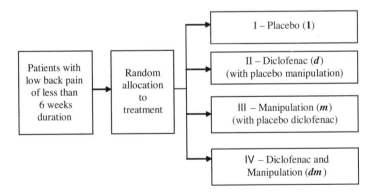

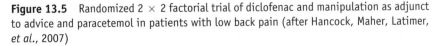

Figure 13.5   Randomized 2×2 factorial trial of diclofenac and manipulation as adjunct to advice and paracetemol in patients with low back pain (after Hancock, Maher, Latimer, *et al.*, 2007)

Example 13.10   *(Continued)*

The two questions posed simultaneously are the value of diclofenac (termed the main effect of diclofenac) and the value of manipulative therapy (similarly termed the main effect of manipulative therapy). In addition, this factorial design allows an estimate of the diclofenac by manipulative therapy interaction; that is, for example, whether the effect of diclofenac remains the same in the presence and absence of manipulative therapy.

As we illustrate in Figure 13.5, the 2 × 2 factorial design options are often summarized on similar lines to: neither diclofenac nor manipulation (double-placebo) (**1**), diclofenac (with placebo manipulation) (**d**), manipulation (with placebo diclofenac) (**m**) or both diclofenac and manipulation (**dm**).

13.5.2   Randomization

Patients eligible for 2 × 2 factorial trials are randomized to one of the four treatment options in equal numbers. The reason for equal allocation being chosen is that this enables the most statistically efficient analysis to be undertaken. It is particularly important that the four treatment options are kept approximately balanced through-out the progress of the trial. This is often done using blocks of size $b = 4$, 8 or 12. The randomization methods of Chapter 5 extend relatively easily to this more complex design situation. For example, if the design involves the four combinations labelled for convenience A, B, C and D, then each of these could be allocated the successive digit pairs: $0-1 : 2-3 : 4-5$ and $6-7$, respectively. If an 8 or 9 occur in the random sequence chosen, these are ignored as there is no associated intervention for these digits. Using this approach of simple randomization, the sequence 534 554 25 would ascribe the first 8 trial recruits to *CBC CCC BC* respectively. In this sequence, the first 8 subjects of the allocation would receive: A 0, B 2, C 6 and D 0. This is clearly not a desirable outcome, as no subject is allocated to either of the interventions A or D.

An alternative way, when there are four groups, is first to divide those members of the random sequence equal to four or more by four, and replace these digits by their corresponding remainder part. The first number of the above sequence of 8 digits is 5, which once divided by 4 gives remainder 1, the second 3 remains as it is, while the third 4 becomes 0, and so on. The new sequence is now 130 110 21. In technical terms, this is the same sequence as previously but each integer reduced modulo 4 (mod 4). If the interventions in the experiment are numbered 1–4 rather than 0–3, then for convenience we add 1 to each member of the sequence to obtain 241 221 32. The randomization for the first 8 units for the 4 interventions then generates *BDA BBA CB* so, once completed for eight subjects, 2 receive A, 4 B, 1 C and 1 D. It is essential to choose the details of the method to be used before the randomization process takes place.

A more satisfactory method is to first generate all 24 possible sequences for the order of the four treatments ranging from *ABCD* to *DCBA* as in Table 13.3. Once

Table 13.3 All possible permuted blocks of size 4

00	ABCD	06	BACD	12	CABD	18	DABC
01	ABDC	07	BADC	13	CADB	19	DACB
02	ACBD	08	BCAD	14	CBAD	20	DBAC
03	ACDB	09	BCDA	15	CBDA	21	DBCA
04	ADBC	10	BDAC	16	CDAB	22	DCAB
05	ADCB	11	BDCA	17	CDBA	23	DCBA

achieved, each pair of the chosen sequence 53 45 54 25 can be reduced modulo 24 to obtain 05, 21, 06 and 01. As the sequences are numbered from 00 to 23, this generates for the first 16 patients the randomization sequence: *ADCB DBCA BACD ABCD*. This clearly produces equal numbers in each group after every 4, 8, 12, 16 patients and so on.

Randomization was carried out with randomly permuted blocks of 4, 8 and 12 for the 240 patients recruited to the trial of Hancock, Maher, Latimer, *et al.* (2007). However they do not detail how many blocks of the different sizes were utilized, although this additional piece of information is necessary for a satisfactory description of the processes involved.

In Section 2.7 it was emphasized that the interventions should be initiated as soon after randomization as possible, although this may not be possible in all cases.

Example 13.11   Timing of randomization – surgery for cleft palate repair

We referred briefly to a trial reported by Yeow, Lee, Cheng, *et al.* (2007) in Section 2.6 which has a 2 × 2 factorial design. One factor is the comparison of two alternative forms of surgery for cleft palette, while the other is whether this should be performed at 6 or 12 months of age. In this trial, randomization is at 6 months of age. For one group the surgery is immediate, while for the other it is delayed by 6 months. If a child is allocated to the immediate surgery group, there is little opportunity either to withdraw from the trial or to request the other surgical procedure. In contrast, if allocated to surgery at 12 months then this allows a long period (6 months) for the patient (essentially the parent in this case) to consider withdrawal from the trial or to request the other surgical option. It is therefore likely that there will be different withdrawal and compliance rates among these two groups. A strategy for randomization in these circumstances is to randomize first to surgery at 6 or 12 months. Then, if 6 months is allocated, immediately initiate the second randomization to type of surgery. In contrast, if 12 months is allocated, delay randomizing the type of surgery until immediately before it is due at 12 months. This example illustrates that great care should always be taken when selecting a suitable randomization strategy for the design in question.

13.5.3   Analysis

Example 13.12   2 × 2 factorial design – chronic obstructive pulmonary disease

Calverley, Pauwels, Vestbo, *et al.* (2003) used a 2 × 2 factorial design to investigate the combination of salmeterol and flucticasone for patients with chronic obstructive pulmonary disease. The four treatment groups were placebo (**1**), salmeterol (**s**), flucticasone (**f**) and the combination salmeterol and flucticasone (**sf**). The endpoint was forced expiratory volume assessed 1 year from randomization (FEV$_1$). The authors report mean values for (**1**), (**s**), (**f**) and (**sf**) as 1264, 1323 1302 and 1396 mL, based on information from approximately 360 patients per group. From the reported confidence intervals it can be deduced that the SD is approximately 265 mL.

From this information, the main effect of salmeterol can be estimated by subtracting from the mean value of those combinations of which salmeterol is a member the mean of those for which salmeterol is not a member; hence

$$S = \left[\frac{1323 + 1396}{2}\right] - \left[\frac{1264 + 1302}{2}\right] = 1359.5 - 1283.0 = 76.5 \text{ ml.}$$

Since each mean in this calculation has an approximate standard error $SD/\sqrt{360}$, the standard error of the mean effect S is approximately

$$SE(S) = \sqrt{\frac{1}{2^2}\left[\frac{265^2}{360} + \frac{265^2}{360}\right] + \frac{1}{2^2}\left[\frac{265^2}{360} + \frac{265^2}{360}\right]} = 265/\sqrt{360} = 13.97.$$

The z-test for the main effect of salmeterol is therefore $z = S/SE(S) = 76.5/13.97 = 5.47$. This is very large and has a very small p-value < 0.0001. Similarly, the main effect of flucticasone is

$$F = \left[\frac{1302 + 1396}{2}\right] - \left[\frac{1264 + 1323}{2}\right] = 55.5,$$

with the same standard error $SE(F) = 13.97$ so that $z = S/SE(F) = 55.5/13.97 = 3.97$. From Table T1, this has a p-value $= 2(1 - 0.99996) = 0.0008$. Both salmeterol and flucticasone therefore have a statistically significant effect but that of salmeterol would appear to be the most important clinically.

To test if there is an interaction, it is necessary to calculate $SF = [1264 + 1396] - [1323 + 1302] = 35.0$, which has standard error

$$SE(SF) = \sqrt{\left[\frac{265^2}{360} + \frac{265^2}{360}\right] + \left[\frac{265^2}{360} + \frac{265^2}{360}\right]} = (2 \times 265)/\sqrt{360} = 27.93.$$

Example 13.12 *(Continued)*

Thus the z-test for the interaction is $z = SF/SE(SF) = 35.5/27.93 = 1.27$, which from Table T1 has a p-value $= 2(1 - 0.89796) = 0.204$. This is not statistically significant at the 5% level. The magnitude of the interaction is small relative to the main effects and is therefore unlikely to be of any clinical consequence.

Analysis of a factorial design is best conducted using the regression model approach, which for the situation we have just described may be written as

$$y = \beta_0 + \beta_S x_S + \beta_F x_F, \tag{13.7}$$

where y is FEV_1, $x_S = 1$ if salmeterol given (otherwise $x_S = 0$), $x_F = 1$ if flucticasone given (otherwise $x_F = 0$) and β_0, β_S, β_F are the corresponding regression coefficients. To test for the presence of an interaction, the above model is expanded to

$$y = \beta_0 + \beta_S x_S + \beta_F x_F + \beta_{SF} x_S x_F. \tag{13.8}$$

Here the extra variable is merely the product of x_S and x_F, and the interaction is assessed by testing the null hypothesis that $\beta_{SF} = 0$.

Once again, the advantage of the regression approach is that further terms can be added to Equations (13.7) or (13.8) to allow for other variables that possibly influence outcome; in this example a covariate of whether or not the patient is a current smoker can be added.

13.5.4 Trial size

In a 2×2 factorial trial there are four means to be estimated, each from m subjects within the respective group. However, when estimating the influence of each factor (the main effect), we are comparing two means each based on $2m$ observations. These two analyses (since there are two factors) make the assumption that there is no interaction between them, that is, the effect of factor A (say) is the same irrespective of which level of factor B (say) is also given to the patient.

Suppose the 2×2 factorial trial compares two factors, D and M. As in the trial involving patients with low back pain, we recommend planning in several stages. The first step would be to consider the sample size for factor D. The second step would be to consider the sample size for factor M which may have an effect size, test size and power that are different from those in the factor D comparison.

Clearly, if the sample sizes are similar then there is no difficulty in choosing the larger as the required sample size. If the sample sizes are disparate, then a discussion would ensue as to the most important comparison and perhaps a reasonable compromise reached.

Example 13.13   2 × 2 factorial design – chronic obstructive pulmonary disease

Calverley, Pauwels, Vestbo, *et al.* (2003) used a planning difference of $\delta_{\mathrm{Plan}} = 0.1$ L with $SD_{\mathrm{Plan}} = 0.35$ L, giving a standardized effect size of $\Delta_{\mathrm{Plan}} = 0.1/0.35 = 0.29$. For a two-sided test size of 5% and power 90%, Equation (9.5) gives approximately 260 patients in each of two (not four) equal-sized groups. This implies that 130 patients will be allocated to each of the four treatment groups.

If we were concerned with estimating the interaction (if any) between salmeterol and flucticasone reliably, then this is equivalent to estimating the interaction $SF = 35.0$ L which has $SD(SF) = \sqrt{4} \times 265 = 530$, giving a standardized effects size of $\Delta_{\mathrm{Plan}} = 35.0/530 = 0.07$. This is very small and would require a large trial of approximately 9000 participants to investigate in detail. Assessing interaction effects usually requires substantial increases to the sample size.

13.5.5   Practical issues

The factorial design may be particularly useful in circumstances where (say) factor *A* addresses a major therapeutic question while factor *B* poses a secondary one. For example, *A* might be the addition of a further drug to an established combination-chemotherapy for a cancer while *B* may the comparison of anti-emetics delivered with the drugs. However, the concern over the estimation of any interaction between the two factors remains, although its very presence could not be detected if the two questions are not posed simultaneously.

As we emphasized when describing Figure 1.2, in some cases, the best experimental design may not be a practical option for the trial. For example, in the context of a planned 2 × 2 factorial trial of (say) two drugs *A* and *B*, against a placebo for each, there are four combinations: (**1**), *a*, *b* and *ab*. With these combinations there is the intention that one in four of the patients receive both placebos, therefore with no chance of activity. In an adjuvant treatment setting, this may turn out to be the best option if tested. Equally, patients may receive both *A* and *B*, perhaps associated with unacceptably high toxicity. These considerations may reduce the optimal four-group parallel design to a practical three-group design of either [(**1**), *a*, *b*] or [*a*, *b*, *ab*] configuration, depending on the circumstances. Both these designs are statistically less efficient than the full factorial, and so may require more patients than the full design to answer the less complete range of questions.

Example 13.14   Malignant pleural mesothelioma

The trial conducted by Muers, Stephens, Fisher, *et al.* (2008) investigated the role of adjuvant chemotherapy using a combination of mitomycin, vinblastine and cisplatinin (MVP) and single-agent V in patients with malignant pleural mesothelioma. All patients received active symptom control (ASC) for their disease. The patients were randomized on a 1 : 1 : 1 basis to receive No chemotherapy (**1**), V (*v*) or the combination MVP (*mvp*). The potential fourth arm comprising the two-drug combination of mitomycin and cisplatin (*mp*) to complete a 2×2 factorial design was presumably not considered appropriate in this situation.

13.5.6   Reporting

Although no new principles for reporting are raised with factorial designs, it is nevertheless important to describe the steps in arriving at the sample size chosen very carefully. Care is also needed in describing the randomization processes, particularly the block size and also whether or not both factors were randomized at the same point in time.

CHAPTER 14

Further Topics

This chapter describes trial design options which have the potential to reduce the numbers of participants required, either by adopting sequential recruitment or adaptive strategies. We also suggest a design that can roll on continually by introducing new treatment options from the evidence accumulated, dropping those of either proven efficacy or if found not to be effective. These designs make use of intermediate endpoints, which may replace traditionally used endpoints that require longer patient follow-up. We introduce circumstances where very large but simple trials are warranted. Bayesian statistical methodology is briefly described. Its potential for use in aiding the design and interim analysis of very small trials is explored. Designs which modify the informed consent process to facilitate patient recruitment are introduced. Finally, there is a brief description of the methodology and role of systematic overviews of clinical trials.

14.1   Introduction

The clinical trial designs we have described in earlier chapters (e.g. the parallel group, factorial and cross-over designs) have a relatively long history, been used extensively and become established mechanisms by which clinical trial questions can be addressed. We have not, however, explored the full potential of the two-period cross-over design, which can be adapted by adding a third period that then overcomes some of the shortcomings of the basic design. This and many other developments with respect to the cross-over design are discussed in careful detail by Senn (2002).

In general, those conducting clinical trials are always seeking alternative design options and design-related strategies that may answer the questions posed more effectively. Any such developments would be attractive if they could involve fewer patients and/or shorten the clinical trial process. Possible strategies include the use of surrogate endpoints. These are designed not necessarily to replace traditional endpoints, but to indicate the same level of benefit or lack of more rapidly than otherwise possible. The aim is to inject any improvement in therapy into clinical practice as soon as possible.

Randomized Clinical Trials: Design, Practice and Reporting   David Machin and Peter M Fayers
© 2010 John Wiley & Sons, Ltd

We also discuss the special situations in which very large trials are appropriate, and how these can be accommodated. The possibility of using Bayesian statistical approaches is discussed, including use of these techniques for interim analysis or when sample sizes are very restricted as in trials in rare diseases or conditions. Prior information from systematic reviews of the literature and other sources form an integral part of these latter approaches. In addition, we suggest that systematic reviews be routinely carried out *before* launching new clinical trials as a means of confirming the need to carry out the planned clinical trial in question. Reviews should be updated *during* the trial for interim analysis purposes, and updated again *after* completing trials although the later updates may not reveal many new developments. By this means, a full synthesis of the current knowledge on the topic of interest will be obtained.

Also included in this chapter is a discussion of designs for which the consent process differs according to the allocated intervention.

We stress, however, that we are only attempting to discuss a flavour of some other possibilities for design, rather than providing a comprehensive review. In general, implementation of these designs requires experienced clinical investigators with a strong statistical team preferably located within a well-organized trial office.

14.2   Adaptive approaches

14.2.1   Introduction

The calculation of sample size using the methods of Chapter 9 requires a pre-specified allocation ratio, effect size, significance level and power. Arriving at an appropriate sample size cannot be achieved by simply plugging these values into standard formulae, but involves a debate within the protocol development team who will discuss several (if not many) strategies before a final trial size N_{Fixed} is determined. Once all the relevant stages have been completed and the trial opened to recruitment, then the objective is to recruit this fixed number of patients in as short a time as is practical. In this section we explore some situations in which the sample size is not fixed in advance, but in which the accumulating data is used to determine the final trial size.

14.2.2   Sequential designs

In contrast to a fixed sample size design, the book by Whitehead (1997) and the associated statistical software PEST (2004) describe and implement different sequential designs. In general, these designs do not incorporate a fixed sample size N_{Fixed} which, once achieved, will then close the trial to recruitment. Rather, a strategy by which the accumulating data are examined sequentially against boundaries set by the design is suggested. This may enable the trial to close before the fixed recruitment target is attained.

Example 14.1 Sequential design – mattress types for operative procedures

Brown, McElvenny, Nixon, *et al.* (2000, Figure 1) provide one example of a sequential design in the (two-sided test) double triangular design of Figure 14.1. The aim of the trial was to reduce the incidence of pressure sores developing during operative procedures by comparing a standard mattress with a gel pad mattress. A measure of the difference between the two interventions Z is continually updated as the data from the trial accumulates. Since more patients are continually being recruited, the reliability of the estimate of Z improves. This ever-increasing amount of information is measured by V. As the trial progresses, the pair (V, Z) are plotted on Figure 14.1 until such time as the plotting point falls outside the 'continue' areas. Depending on which boundary is crossed, either efficacy is claimed for one of the interventions under test, or there is no statistically significant difference between them. Whenever and whichever boundary is crossed, the trial is then closed to further recruitment. The properties of the designs are such that the actual number of patients recruited may be less than or greater than N_{Fixed}, that is, the size of a fixed-size trial with the same planning characteristics of Δ_{Plan}, α and $1 - \beta$. It is hoped that efficacy or otherwise is demonstrated with fewer patients than with a fixed sample size design, although in some circumstances a larger number might be required. The trial will usually be more rapidly completed and consume fewer resources.

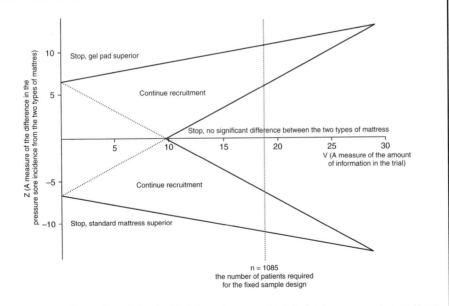

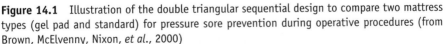

Figure 14.1 Illustration of the double triangular sequential design to compare two mattress types (gel pad and standard) for pressure sore prevention during operative procedures (from Brown, McElvenny, Nixon, *et al.*, 2000)

In the trial that Brown, McElvenny, Nixon, *et al.* (2000) are describing, the primary endpoint was determined as a success (no pressure sore) or failure (pressure sore) at one or more of the five susceptible skin sites (sacrum, buttocks and heels) assessed at four stages during the operative day and on the hospital ward the following day. If we denote the anticipated planning proportions of pressure sores developing as π_{Gel} and $\pi_{Standard}$ with the corresponding mattress types, then for design purposes the log-odds ratio

$$\theta_{Plan} = \log \left(\frac{\pi_{Gel}(1 - \pi_{Standard})}{\pi_{Standard}(1 - \pi_{Gel})} \right)$$

has to be specified. The corresponding null hypothesis is H_0: $\theta = 0$ and the alternative is: H_A: $\theta \neq 0$. Once the trial is underway, if the number of patients randomized and assessed by a particular calendar time during the trial's progress are $n_{Standard}$ and n_{Gel} of which $f_{Standard}$ and f_{Gel} are found to have pressure sores, then

$$Z = \frac{n_{Gel}f_{Standard} - n_{Standard}f_{Gel}}{n} \text{ and } V = \frac{n_{Gel}n_{Standard}f(1-f)}{n^3},$$

where $f = f_{Standard} + f_{Gel}$ and $n = n_{Standard} + n_{Gel}$.

There are variations from the (single) observation-by-observation plotting of (V, Z), in that information can be accumulated in predefined groups of patients of a convenient size and (V, Z) only plotted after information on each group is accumulated. This is then termed a group sequential design. However, use of a group sequential design changes the linear boundaries of Figure 14.1 into a Christmas-tree shape within these boundaries. The form of these new boundaries depends on the group sizes at each successive interim analysis.

Example 14.2   Pressure sore prevention trial

Figure 14.2, taken from Brown, McElvenny, Nixon, *et al.* (2000), illustrates the progress of the double triangular sequential design during the course of the trial conducted by Nixon, McElvenny, Mason, *et al.* (1998). There were three interim looks at the accumulating data and we can see that the third cross ($V = 11.6$, $Z = 9.9$) is clearly outside the boundary favouring Gel; at that point, the trial was closed to patient recruitment.

However, more patients had been recruited in the intervening period from when the data for the third analysis was recorded in the hospitals, passed to the trial office for processing, analysis completed and reported to an independent DMC and then considering it before recommending closure of the trial. The fourth cross, which corresponded to ($V = 12.9$, $Z = 10.2$), summarizes the analysis which includes these later patients. As this too is outside the boundary it confirms the earlier conclusion of a reduced risk of pressure sores with the Gel mattress although, in general, there may be trials when this may not be the case. Such a possibility raises real concerns, so it is very important that any lag between the receipt of data and analysis is kept to a minimum. The final estimate of θ, the odds ratio, is $OR = 0.50$ (95% CI 0.28 to 0.90) and this was based on a total of 446 randomized patients. This

Example 14.2 *(Continued)*

turns out to be far less than would have been recruited using the same design criteria for a fixed sample size design. Thus with $\pi_{\text{Standard}} = 0.10$, $\pi_{\text{Gel}} = 0.05$, $OR_{\text{Plan}} = [0.10 (1 - 0.10)]/[0.05/(1 - 0.95)] = 0.4737$, $\theta_{\text{Plan}} = \log(0.47) = -0.75$, (two-sided) $\alpha = 0.05$ and $1 - \beta = 0.9$, Equation (9.8) with $\kappa = 2$ gives $m_2 = 541$ or $N = 1082$ which is close to that indicated by $n = 1085$ in Figure 14.1.

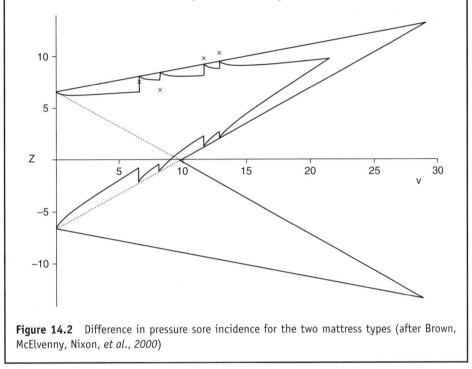

Figure 14.2   Difference in pressure sore incidence for the two mattress types (after Brown, McElvenny, Nixon, *et al.*, 2000)

In this example, the group sequential design resulted in a recruitment of less than half that of the equivalent fixed sample size design, bringing considerable savings yet still answering the question posed. Now that the trial is over, we know that this advantage has indeed accrued. However, when planning the trial there was some concern as to what the final sample size would be. To this end Brown, McElvenny, Nixon, *et al.* (2000) state:

> For this sequential design, randomization was to occur until a stopping boundary was crossed which was almost certain to occur by the time 1700 patients had been recruited and very likely to occur considerably sooner.

This possible number of 1700 is 600 patients more than that of the corresponding fixed sample size design and 1200 more than that actually accrued. Such uncertainty makes the logistics of planning for a sequential trial very troublesome as the resources (often funding) required and the duration of the trial cannot be stipulated in advance.

In this example, the endpoint of pressure sore development or not was determined within two days of patient randomization, so that the information necessary for monitoring this trial became quickly available to the monitoring team. Nevertheless, additional patients were accrued while the information was being processed and it is likely that this overrun could be much more extensive if the endpoint had required a lengthier follow-up of patients. These and other issues are discussed by Brown, McElvenny, Nixon, *et al.* (2000), who provide a very useful case study of some practical consequences when faced with conducting a trial using a sequential design.

Example 14.3   Unresectable hepatocellular carcinoma (HCC)

Llovet, Real, Montaňa, *et al.* (2002) describe a three-arm randomized trial using a sequential design, but of a single triangular type which would correspond to the upward sloping triangle in Figure 14.3. In fact, two such identical triangular designs were constructed, one for the comparison of chemoembolization with conservative treatment (control) and a second for the comparison of arterial embolization with the same control. Patients were randomized within defined strata into the three groups using equal allocation. The design(s) anticipated a 2-year survival of 40% in the control group and in each of the test groups, 65%. These correspond to $HR_{Plan} = \log 0.65/\log 0.40 = 0.47$ in both cases. This is a very large anticipated benefit for these treatments over control. The investigators set a

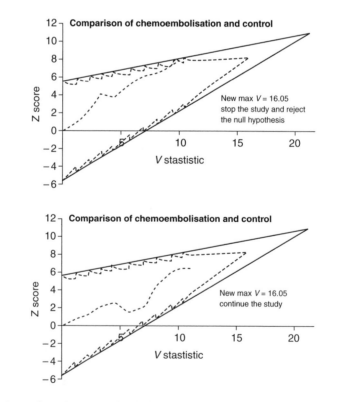

Figure 14.3   Design of sequential analyses of chemoembolization vs control (upper) and embolization vs control (lower) (after Llovet, Real, Montaňa, *et al., 2002*)

Example 14.3 *(Continued)*

two-sided $\alpha = 0.05$ and $1 - \beta = 0.8$. No comparison between the two test treatments was intended.

The authors include a footnote to their Figure 2 explaining details of the boundaries chosen and a summary of their conclusions drawn. This is reproduced in the following where the emphasis has been added:

> A positive z value indicates that treatment was better than control, whereas a negative indicates the opposite. The slope of the upper boundary of the triangle was 0.26 (treatment better than control) and the lower was 0.79 (treatment worse than or equal to control). The V statistic represents the sample size. After the ninth inspection, the upper triangular boundary was crossed, favouring chemoembolisation vs control, with a hazard ratio of death of 0.47 (95% CI 0.25 − 0.91, p = 0.025; upper). Conversely in the lower diagram, comparing embolisation with control, the plot lines remain within the boundaries, *indicating the need to recruit additional patients to achieve a valid conclusion.*

The total number of patients recruited was 112, with 35 allocated to control, 37 arterial embolization and 40 chemoembolization with 25, 25 and 21 being the corresponding numbers of deaths observed by the time of the final analysis. Despite equal allocation being part of the design, patient numbers are not entirely balanced. This was probably due to having eight different strata, each balanced for the three treatment groups, which is far too many categories for what turned out to be a small trial. Had a fixed-sample size trial been planned with the same design parameters, then for a time-to-event endpoint Equation (9.11) gives the numbers per group needed as 66 in order to observe 33 deaths. Hence the total trial size would be $3 \times 66 = 198$ in order to observe the required 99 deaths. This is almost twice the size of the sequential trial conducted, although one might argue that this trial was prematurely closed as one of the questions posed had not been answered. However, as we have shown in Section 13.3, Fleiss (1986) suggested that the allocation ratio in trials where $g - 1$ groups are compared with control should be weighted towards the control group. In this case, a better allocation ratio would be $\sqrt{(3-1)} : 1 : 1$ or approximately $3 : 2 : 2$ in favour of symptomatic treatment, in which case 96 would be randomized to control, 57 to each of the embolization groups, or a total of 210 patients to observe 106 deaths. There seems no reason why this strategy could not have been adopted here.

14.2.3 Other adaptive designs

In Section 9.6, we introduced the idea of an internal pilot study whose purpose was to reassess if the trial size had been appropriately determined at the design stage. The rationale is that at the planning stage, although it may be possible to agree the anticipated absolute benefit, judging the likely value of the associated standard deviation of a continuous outcome variable can be problematical. The pilot data allow the estimate of the standard deviation to become more firmly established. This can then be used with the (initial) planning effect size to revise Δ_{Plan}. If Δ_{Plan} becomes revised downwards, the standard sample size calculations are repeated to obtain the revised (and increased) sample size. Hence the initial N_{Fixed} is revised to the larger $N_{\text{FixedRevised}}$ and the trial continues to recruit until this new target is achieved. We emphasized that this adjustment should take no account of the newly observed trial data relating to the difference between the intervention groups. Nevertheless, just as with the sequential designs described, there are designs which do indeed make use of information on this difference and 'adapt' the design accordingly.

Example 14.4   Acute myeloid leukaemia

Giles, Kantarjian, Cortes, *et al.* (2003) use an adaptive design in a randomized trial to compare three combination treatments: Idarubicin and Ara-C (IA), Troxacitabine and Ara-C (TA) and Troxacitabine and Idarubicin (TI) in patients with adverse karyotype acute myeloid leukaemia (AML). The primary (compound) endpoint was defined as complete remission, with no grade 4 toxicity (apart from haematological) by day 50. Initially the allocation was balanced between the three groups with a probability of 1/3 of allocation to each. However, as the data on activity of each combination accrued, the assignment probabilities shifted in favour of the arms that were doing better. An extract of their detailed data on the patient-by-patient allocation probabilities, the treatment actually received and whether or not the patient responded is summarized in Table 14.1. The trial commenced with randomization to the three options, dropped TI after patient 24, and finally concluded after patient 34 that TA was the best option.

Table 14.1 Extract from the data generated by the adaptive design of Giles, Kantarjian, Cortes, *et al.* (2003, Table 2)

Patient	Allocation probabilities			Treatment Assigned	CR	CR rates		
	Control IA	TA	TI			Control IA	TA	TI
0	0.333	0.333	0.333					
—	—	—	—			—	—	—
10				TA	Yes	2/5	1/1	1/4
11	0.333	0.498	0.169	TA	Yes			
—	—	—	—	—	—	—	—	—
20				IA	Yes	3/7	4/8	1/5
21	0.333	0.490	0.177	IA	Yes			
—	—	—	—	—	—	—	—	—
30				IA	Yes	9/15	5/10	1/5
31	0.957	0.043	0.000	IA	No			
—	—	—	—	—	—	—	—	—
34				IA	Yes	10/18	5/11	1/5

The adaptive design can be thought of as a 'race' between the three options under test; we are looking for the 'winner' but the margin of the win is not considered. For example, although TI was dropped from the comparison after

---

Example 14.4 *(Continued)*

Patient 25 was recruited, the response rate of 1/5 (20%) has a 95% confidence interval from 5 to 57% so there remains considerable uncertainty about the true value of this combination.

Exactly how the changing allocation probabilities are calculated is described. The rationale for not changing the probability for IA from 0.333 until Patient 25 when it jumps to 0.871, while that for TI simultaneously drops to 0.000, is explained in an exceedingly complex statistical methods section of the publication which will leave most readers baffled. As a consequence of this, and the very small numbers of patients in the trial, we wonder if the results are convincing enough to investigators outside the institution concerned. In this kind of situation, with 34 patients recruited in 7 months (and hence not such a rare patient type), we would strongly recommend multicentre involvement to increase the potential pool of patients and then consider an appropriate design in these circumstances.

In contrast to the sequential designs with a 1 : 1 allocation ratio, with this design the allocation ratio constantly changes and eventually becomes very extreme. This may raise difficulties with the informed consent procedures. How would patients react to being told of a 90% chance of allocation to one treatment versus 10% to the other? However, Giles, Kantarjian, Cortes, *et al.* (2003) make it clear that the protocol was appropriately approved by their institutional review board and all patients gave signed informed consent. They also state:

> This randomization process was used in an attempt to align two somewhat conflicting major issues (i.e. the reluctance of investigators to randomly assign patients to standard or control regimens that were known to be highly unsatisfactory and the demand for truly randomized studies to generate plausible data) . . .

Phillips (2006) and Day and Småstuen (2008) provide topical comments on such designs.

Gerb and Köpcke (2007) note that designs of the type conducted by Giles, Kantarjian, Cortes, *et al.* (2003) are considered in the EMEA (2005) guidelines for clinical trials in small populations. However, as we have previously indicated, we would contend this example does not consider a 'small' population, but is just a small trial. Nevertheless, the principle of having a number (more than two, possibly many) of alternatives under test and dropping some of these as the trial progresses has application in larger trial situations. Thus Parmar, Barthel, Sydes, *et al.* (2008) have explored the possibility of designs for randomized trials with several arms in which, as information accumulates, a rolling process of dropping one or more of these and (possibly) replacing them by new options is initiated.

An example of this type of design is given in Figure 14.4 in which patients are initially (Stage I) randomized to three options, one of which is regarded as the standard or control. Sometime later, a comparison between these arms is then made using an intermediate endpoint, in this case progression free survival (PFS), rather than using the endpoint of primary concern which is overall survival (OS). At this point, Option 2 appears to be doing no better than Option 1 (Control) whereas Option 3 appears to be better. Consequently

Option 2 is dropped from the design, Option 3 continues and, in this case, a new option (Option 4) is introduced. Randomization continues in Stage II between Option 1, Option 3 and Option 4.

Example 14.5   Rolling design – advancing metastatic prostate cancer

James, Sydes, Clarke, *et al.* (2008) describe an ongoing trial using ideas encapsulated in Figure 14.4 but involving six options for systemic therapy for patients with advancing metastatic prostate cancer. They point out that the design, approval process, launch and recruitment were all major challenges; the eventual outcome will be of considerable interest.

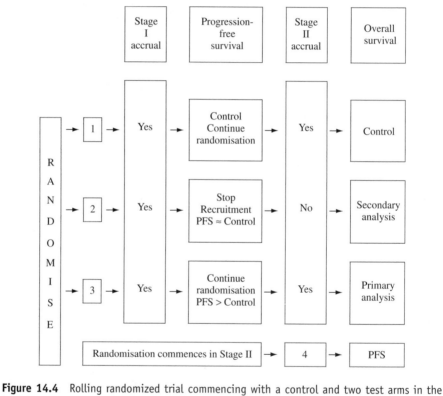

Figure 14.4   Rolling randomized trial commencing with a control and two test arms in the initial stage, one test dropping after stage I accrual and a new test arm replacing this in stage II (adapted from Parmar, Barthel, Sydes, *et al.*, 2008)

14.3   Large simple trials

In some situations, investigators may be concerned with questions that have considerable public health impact even if the advantage demonstrated to one intervention over the other is numerically small. This is particularly relevant in the fields of cardiovascular disease and the more common types of cancer, where even a small increase in cure or survival rates will bring major benefits to many patients. As we have seen in terms of trial size, the smaller the potential benefit, and hence the effect size, then the larger the trial must be in order to be reasonably confident that the benefit envisaged really exists at all. To be specific, with a 1 : 1 allocation ratio, two-sided $\alpha = 0.05$ and $1 - \beta = 0.9$, then a decrease of Δ_{Cohen} in Equation (9.5) from 0.2 to 0.1 increases the required trial size from approximately 1000 to more than 4000. One extreme example of 'large' is the trial of Chen, Pan, Chen, *et al.* (2005) which included 45 852 patients with acute myocardial infarction who were randomized to receive, in addition to standard interventions, either metoprolol or matching placebo.

Trials involving many thousands of patients to estimate a small benefit reliably are a major undertaking. To be justified they must be practical. They therefore have to be in common diseases or conditions in order for the required numbers of participants to be available in a reasonable timeframe. Such trials must be testing a treatment or intervention that not only has wide applicability, but can also be easily administered by the clinician teams responsible or even better by the subjects themselves. In most instances, any treatment under test must be readily available across a wide range of health care systems and this tends to imply they need to be low cost. This is especially the case if the trial demonstrates a clinically useful benefit, since putting these results into actual practice will also have future cost implications. The treatments must be relatively non-toxic; otherwise, the small benefit will be outweighed by the side effects.

There will be few circumstances where such trials cannot involve multicentre recruitment, possibly on an international scale. This means that the design team will need to consult a wide range of collaborating teams; obtaining consensus on the final design may not be easy. The trial office will need to be prepared for the organizational consequences. These factors all suggest that these trials should be 'simple' trials – implying minimal imposition on the recruiting centres with respect to the data they record on each subject (albeit on many individuals). This in turn reduces the trial office work to the minimum required, while retaining sufficient information to answer the questions posed.

Example 14.6   Large simple trial – chronic heart failure

In the Candesartan in Heart failure: Assessment of Reduction in Mortality and morbidity (CHARM)-Added trial of McMurray, Östergren, Swedberg, *et al.* (2003), patients with chronic heart failure (CHF) who were being treated with ACE inhibitors were randomized to either placebo or candesartan. The primary outcome was a composite event of the first of either unplanned admission to hospital for the management of worsening CHF or time to cardiovascular death. The authors state:

> The planned sample size of 2300 patients was designed to provide around 80% power to detect a 16% relative reduction in the primary outcome, assuming an annual placebo event rate of 18%.

In the event 2548 patients were enrolled, 1272 received placebo and 1276 candesartan. However, the report of the trial which recruited patients from Canada, Sweden, USA and the UK was based on 538 and 483 events respectively – far fewer than the number of patients randomized. The above disparity is typical of

Example 14.6 *(Continued)*

trials with time-to-event endpoints, as the number to recruit derived from Equation (9.11) is effectively the number needed to recruit 'in order to observe the required number of events'.

The results of the trial are summarized in Figure 14.5. This depicts a lower event rate in those patients receiving candesartan with $HR = 0.85$ (95% CI 0.75 to 0.95, p-value $= 0.011$), which remains essentially unchanged after adjusting for prognostic factors such as heart-disease risk factors, medical history and medical treatment prior to randomization. The difference in annual event rates was reported as 2.5% (14.1% with candesartan and 16.6% with placebo). Despite this small difference, the authors concluded that:

'The addition of candesartan . . . leads to a further clinically important reduction in relevant cardiovascular events . . . .'

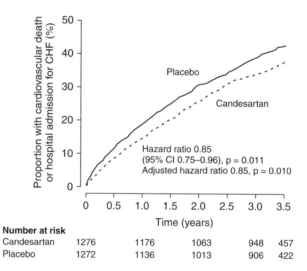

Number at risk

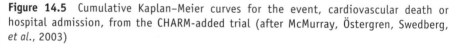

Figure 14.5 Cumulative Kaplan–Meier curves for the event, cardiovascular death or hospital admission, from the CHARM-added trial (after McMurray, Östergren, Swedberg, *et al.*, 2003)

Example 14.7 Large simple trial – early breast cancer

The trial of ATAC (Arimidex, Tamoxifen Alone or in Combination) Trialists' Group (2002), as the group name suggests, was designed to test the combination of tamoxifen (T) and anastrozole (arimidex) (A) as adjuvant treatment for postmenopausal women with early breast cancer. The design had three arms, two of which contained placebo (Figure 14.6). The options included (*t*), (*a*) and (*at*) but omitted the double placebo (1) from what could have potentially been a 2 × 2 factorial design. The trial involved a relatively common disease and used

Example 14.7 *(Continued)*

very simple (and low cost) treatments taken as tablets with very few anticipated side effects. The primary endpoint of disease-free survival was used to assess sample size. For equivalence, stated as 'non-inferiority or superiority' by the authors, 352 events per group were required for a greater than 90% power to be concluded between anastrozole and tamoxifen. This equivalence was defined as the ruling out of a HR greater than 1.25 on the basis of the 90% confidence interval. Also to show a reduction of 20% in event rates by anastrozole alone or the combination versus tamoxifen alone (superiority), 80% power was achievable at a 5% significance level with the same number of events. The trial is essentially posing two questions and the investigators estimated that about 9000 patients would need to be recruited.

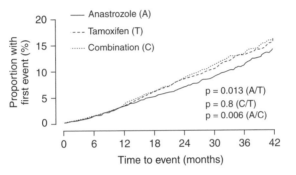

Figure 14.6 Cumulative Kaplan–Meier curves for disease-free survival (i.e. all first events) in the intention to treat population (after ATAC Trialists' Group, 2002)

To replicate equivalence sample size calculation, use is made of Equation (9.10) but with the entries of Table T2 for one-sided $\alpha = 0.1$ and two-sided $1 - \beta = 0.9$, providing $z_{0.9} = 1.2816$ and $z_{0.8} = 0.8416$. Thus with equal allocation, $\lambda = 1$ and $HR_{Plan} = 1.25$, we have the number of events required per group as

$$e_1 = \left(\frac{1 + 1.25}{1 - 1.25}\right)^2 (1.2816 + 0.8416)^2 = 365.2 \approx 370.$$

Thus a total of $3 \times 370 = 1110$ events are required. The trial recruited 9366 women although the preliminary results that they report do not appear to quote the 90% confidence interval on which the equivalence of tamoxifen and anastrozole were to be judged.

Needless to say, such large (although simple) trials are a considerable undertaking and, if nothing else, require a very experienced planning team with substantial resources. Both trials illustrated here were funded by the pharmaceutical industry but with very strong academic involvement.

14.4   Bayesian methods

14.4.1   Introduction

The essence of Bayesian methodology in the context of clinical trials is to incorporate relevant external information concerning the question under consideration into the design, monitoring, analysis and interpretation processes. The object of the approach is not solely to improve the trial design process but also to facilitate decisions with respect to whether or not the trial conclusions should be adopted into routine clinical practice. This all coincides with the opinions of Clarke, Hopewell and Chalmers (2007) who state that clinical trials should begin and end with up-to-date systematic reviews of the other relevant evidence. From a Bayesian perspective, this can begin with summarizing the evidence at the planning stage of the trial which may impact on the final design chosen, summarizing accumulating external evidence as the trial is recruiting and until it closes and then putting all of this alongside the trial evidence to assist in the interpretation.

14.4.2   Mechanics

In broad terms, the usual (or most frequent) approach to the estimation of a parameter such as β_1 or β_{Treat} of Equation (2.1) is to regard the parameter as a fixed value for the population concerned. Once the data are collected from the trial, this is estimated by $b_{\text{TreatData}}$. The corresponding standard error (SE_{Data}) gives a measure of the precision with which β_{Treat} is estimated entirely from the *internal* evidence of the data itself. The distribution of this estimate is assumed to have a Normal form and this is termed the *likelihood* distribution. The Bayesian approach seeks to review the relevant external evidence pertinent to the trial question. This may range from very little to quite extensive, and is also used to estimate β_{Treat}. The information is summarized by $b_{\text{TreatExternal}}$, which is also assumed to have a Normal distribution form with standard error SE_{External}. This is termed the *prior* distribution. Since both the internal and external information is addressing the same question, it seems natural to combine the two. This could be done by taking a simple average of $b_{\text{TreatData}}$ and $b_{\text{TreatExternal}}$ but this ignores the relative precision of the two estimates. For example, if $b_{\text{TreatData}}$ is based on data from a very large randomized trial while the external information is very sparse, it would seem foolish to ignore this fact when calculating the average. One means of taking the precision into account is to estimate β_{Treat} by the weighted mean, i.e.

$$b_{\text{TreatBayes}} = \frac{W_{\text{Data}} b_{\text{Treat}} + W_{\text{External}} b_{\text{TreatExternal}}}{W_{\text{Data}} + W_{\text{External}}}, \qquad (14.1)$$

where $W_{\text{Data}} = 1/SE_{\text{Data}}^2$ and $W_{\text{External}} = 1/SE_{\text{External}}^2$. As both $b_{\text{TreatData}}$ and $b_{\text{TreatExternal}}$ are assumed to have a Normal distribution form, $b_{\text{TreatBayes}}$ also will but with standard error:

$$SE(b_{\text{TreatBayes}}) = \frac{1}{\sqrt{W_{\text{Data}} + W_{\text{External}}}}. \qquad (14.2)$$

The distribution, obtained from a combination of the prior and likelihood distributions, is termed the *posterior* distribution of the parameter from which a probability statement can then be derived concerning the true value of the parameter, β_{Treat}.

Example 14.8 Prior, likelihood and posterior distributions

Tan, Wee, Wong and Machin (2008, Table 5) give an example of the *prior, likelihood and posterior distributions* in Figure 14.7 which might arise if two treatments were being compared with a time-to-event endpoint. In this case, we are interested in estimating *HR*. No difference between treatments corresponds to $HR = 1$ (or equivalently $\log HR = 0$), while an advantage to the test treatment will result in $HR < 1$ or $\log HR < 0$. For the likelihood, the $SE_{\text{Data}}(\log HR)$ depends critically on the number of deaths observed within the trial. Similarly for the prior distribution, its *SE* also depends on the number of 'weighted deaths' in the external information.

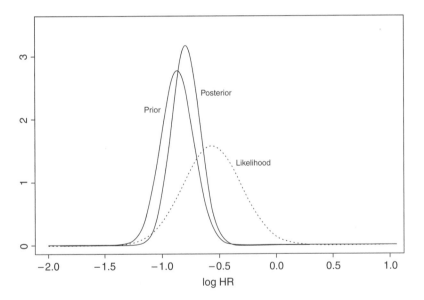

Figure 14.7 Illustration of how an external prior and the likelihood distribution from the trial data are combined into a posterior distribution (based on information from Tan, Wee, Wong and Machin, 2008)

In Figure 14.7, the prior distribution has a mean of approximately $\log HR = -0.9$ (or $HR = 0.4$) suggesting that the external information indicates a substantial benefit to the test treatment. This prior also has a relatively sharp peak indicating a small *SE* and hence a relatively large number of 'weighted deaths' associated with it. The trial, once conducted, gave a likelihood distribution

---

Example 14.8 *(Continued)*

centred on log $HR = -0.55$ (or $HR = 0.58$), which indicates a benefit but not as large as the prior distribution had suggested. In addition, the likelihood is not so peaked indicating fewer 'real' deaths than 'weighted deaths'. Finally the combination of these two distributions to obtain the posterior takes a more central position. This synthesis suggests log $HR = -0.7$ (or $HR = 0.50$).

In the above explanation, we have used the terms 'real' and 'weighted' deaths. 'Real' corresponds to the actual numbers of deaths that are observed during the course of the randomized clinical trial. In summarizing the external evidence, if this were to include a randomized trial of the exact same design which the investigators are planning, then the reported deaths D within that trial would be 'real'. However, what is more likely is that the external information will be in some sense tangential to the exact trial question posed. For example suppose that, rather than a randomized comparison, two single-arm studies had been conducted using exactly the same arms as those proposed in the trial in planning. Between them, the number of deaths reported was also D. In this case, the evidence is not so reliable so the external summary down-weights D to a reduced value d. The number d now describes the 'weighted' number of deaths from these two studies.

14.4.3 Constructing the priors

The information available, and pertinent to the trial in question, has to be summarized in a prior distribution. An integral part of the process of constructing the priors is to perform a thorough and ongoing literature search using the standard approaches adopted by any systematic overview. Such a search may reveal a whole range of studies including, for example, randomized trials using the same regimens as those proposed for the new trial but in a different patient group, non-randomized comparative studies, single-arm studies of one or other of the intended arms and case series. Tan, Bruzzi, Dear and Machin (2003) have suggested how each such disparate study may be judged within the context of the intended trial, and then appropriately weighted before being merged into a single prior distribution such as that of Figure 14.7. The mean of such a distribution would correspond to the planning effect size, which can then be assessed by the design team as clinically worthwhile in their context and, if regarded as reasonable, used as a basis for sample size estimation purposes.

Example 14.9 Nasopharyngeal cancer

At the calendar time of the design of the trial SQNP01 (Wee, Tan, Tai, *et al.*, 2005), comparing chemo-radiation (CRT) and radiotherapy alone (RT) in patients with nasopharyngeal cancer, information in the literature was available on nine publications relevant to the trial design. These were not amalgamated into a

> **Example 14.9**   *(Continued)*
>
> prior distribution for the effect size, however. Once the trial was closed and reported, a case study was undertaken using the suggested approach of Tan, Bruzzi, Dear and Machin (2003). Omitting details (given by Tan, Wee, Wong and Machin, 2008), this synthesis resulted in a prior distribution with mean $\log HR = -0.9$ ($HR \approx 0.4$) and $SE = 0.2$. This is the prior distribution of Figure 14.7 and clearly indicates a considerable advantage of CRT over RT. The prior therefore summarized what turned out to be rather strong information regarding the true effect size.

In contrast to this situation, in other cases there may be little external evidence available. In such circumstances one approach is to elicit clinical opinion about the likely benefit (of test over control) from a wide range of individuals knowledgeable about both the disease in question and the alternative approaches to therapy. This information can then be collated and an 'elicited prior distribution' obtained.

> **Example 14.9   Hepatocellular carcinoma**
>
> Although information was available from one randomized trial which had perhaps been prematurely closed, Tan, Chung, Tai, *et al.* (2003) sought the opinions of 14 different investigators experienced in the treatment of hepatocellular carcinoma to develop an elicited prior distribution. Following the methodology suggested by Spiegelhalter, Freedman and Parmar (1994), this resulted in a prior with $\log HR = -0.47$ ($HR = 0.6$) and $SE = 0.43$ derived from their opinions with respect to the advantage in 2-year recurrence-free survival of iodine-131-lipiodol as adjuvant treatment over surgery alone. This information was then used to inform the planning of a confirmatory trial that was then conducted.

14.4.4   Interim and final analyses

The prior obtained for planning purposes, or that prior updated from new external evidence accumulated during the course of a trial, may be used in monitoring trial progress. As well as providing an independent DMC with evidence from the accumulating data in the trial, this external information may assist them when making their recommendation with respect to the future course of the trial. Early closure of the trial could be recommended if the current data or the (updated) prior (or the combination of these) indicate strong evidence of benefit to patients receiving one intervention arm. Alternatively at this stage the DMC may recommend an increase in the trial size as appropriate. Finally, once the trial data is complete, the continually updated prior can be combined with the likelihood distribution from the data to give the posterior distribution, from which estimates of the treatment effect can be obtained. Fayers, Ashby and Parmar (1997) illustrate how a Bayesian approach using different prior distributions was used in interim analyses of a trial in which patients with oesophageal cancer were randomized to receive or not pre-operative chemotherapy.

14.4.5   Very small trials

For those designing trials in rare tumour types or small disease subgroups, standard approaches to determining trial size for given anticipated effect size, test size and power will lead to a suggested value far beyond what is feasible (whatever the duration of the recruitment period and extent of multicentre collaboration). Before deciding on a strategy for very small trials we have to have some idea of what is meant by 'very small'. Thus Tan, Dear, Bruzzi and Machin (2003) define this as less than 50 possible patients recruited in 5 years with multicentre/multinational recruitment. Under this definition, a single centre can never conduct a *very small* trial – it must be multicentre. This was a criticism we made in commenting on the *single* institution and *small* adaptive trial of Giles, Kantarjian, Cortes, *et al.* (2003) in patients with adverse karyotype AML.

If the anticipated effect size is large, for example an improvement in survival rates in a cancer from 40% to 80%, then with two-sided $\alpha = 0.05$, $1 - \beta = 0.8$, Equation (9.11) leads to a trial size of just over 50. In these circumstances, such a trial would be feasible. However, in most situations the true effect size is likely to be very much smaller than this so any randomized trials should be correspondingly larger. This difficulty has often lead investigators to conduct single-arm trials with all the available patients. The argument is that all patients will be available to receive the test option, that is twice as many as would be the case in a randomized controlled trial, and hence would provide more information. Treatment comparisons are then made with previous experience of similar patients. However, by not conducting a randomized comparison, we are left with all the difficulties of interpretation whatever the outcome; this is therefore not an approach we would recommend.

As we have pointed out, Gerb and Köpcke (2007) have stated that adaptive designs may be appropriate in these circumstances but also suggest, without describing them, that Bayesian approaches are also possible. The suggestion that Tan, Dear, Bruzzi and Machin (2003) make is to construct a prior from pertinent information available and/or expert opinion, then to randomize equally to the (two) intervention groups as many patients as possible in an agreed timeframe. The effect size and corresponding confidence interval can be estimated from the patient data that is accumulated. This likelihood distribution information is then combined with the updated prior distribution to form the posterior distribution that is then used to help with the final interpretation.

We must recognize that conclusions drawn from this evidence, although the best possible given the circumstances, are seldom likely to be conclusive but will provide a firm basis for rational decision making.

14.4.6   Comment

The approach outlined is highly relevant for rare diseases and conditions, while the formal synthesis of the accumulating external evidence component of this process is a valuable exercise in itself in all circumstances (whatever the ultimate size of the trial concerned). However, there is a need for formal standards and conventions to be established, including guidelines for the reporting of Bayesian designs for clinical trials.

14.5 Zelen randomized-consent designs

In view of difficulties associated with obtaining informed patient consent to join a trial, various options have been proposed to minimize these difficulties. One suggestion is a Zelen (1992) design in which eligible patients are randomized to one of the two treatment groups before they are informed about the details of the trial. Once randomized, then those who are allocated to the standard treatment are all treated with it and no consent to take part in the trial is sought. This is the Standard (G_1) arm of Figure 14.8. The ethical argument is that this is the treatment they would have received in the absence of the trial, so no permission is needed. On the other hand, those who are randomized to the experimental treatment (New, G_2) are asked for their consent. If they agree they are treated with the experimental treatment; if they disagree they are treated with the standard treatment. This is known as Zelen's single-consent design.

An alternative to the single-consent design is that those randomized to the standard treatment may also be asked if they are willing to accept the treatment chosen for them. This is the Zelen double-consent design of Figure 14.9. What they actually go on to receive, Standard or New, is then left to their choice. Whichever intervention they are randomized to receive, they are made aware of the other option under test. However,

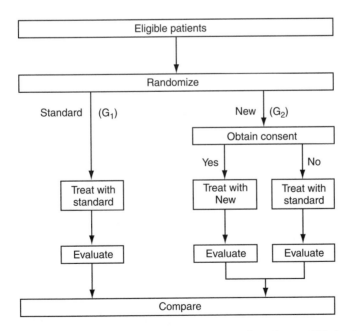

Figure 14.8 The Zelen single-randomized consent design (after Altman, Whitehead, Parmar, et al., 1995)

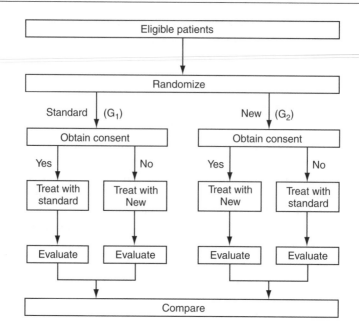

Figure 14.9 The Zelen double-randomized consent design (after Altman, Whitehead, Parmar, *et al.*, 1995)

Huibers, Bleijenberg, Beurkens, *et al.* (2004) propose a modification to this design in which, although patients are randomized before being approached and consent is then sought from both arms in the same way, neither arm is told of the existence of the alternative therapy. This design was used successfully in an occupational health trial in which fatigued employees absent from work were randomly assigned to receive cognitive behavioural therapy or no intervention.

Whatever type of Zelen design chosen, the analysis must be made using the intention-to-treat principle, that is, it is based on the treatment to which patients were randomized, not the treatment they actually received if it differs from this.

The chief difficulty is that these designs each involve some deception and, although carried out with the best of intent, this is difficult to describe as ethical. Most trials also require additional assessments to be made on patients, even those in the control group, and so consent is required for this and an explanation of why these are being made has to be provided. This process clearly nullifies the advantage of a Zelen approach in avoiding seeking consent from some of the patients.

The properties of these designs have been examined in some detail by Altman, Whitehead, Parmar, *et al.* (1995) from a perspective of conducting clinical trials in cancer. They concluded that:

> 'There are serious statistical arguments against the use of randomized consent designs, which should discourage their use'.

However, Berkowitz (1998) argued for their use in surgical trials to repair cleft palate on the grounds of alleged difficulties of obtaining consent by conventional methods. This point of view was rebutted by Machin and Lee (2000); who counter argued that during the whole reconstruction process, which usually takes several years, many procedures will be undertaken in the surgical management of the cleft that are regarded as standard and some will be used for which there is considerable uncertainty as to the correct approach. Under these circumstances a patient, or more realistically parents, could be guided through the entire reconstruction process before any intervention takes place. This therefore sensitizes the potential consent-giver from the very beginning that, although certain procedures are standard, there are others in which the best approach is not clear. Once at that (unclear) stage of the reconstruction process, a choice will have to be made. A brief description of the future trial the child may enter, although distant in time for the child concerned, could therefore be introduced and reference made to the randomization requirement. As care of the child proceeds stage by stage, more and more information about the trial can be provided. At the crucial point in time, the consent-giver, who may change from the proxy to the young adult concerned, will be truly informed of available options. Finally, Machin and Lee (2000) contrast this with the very difficult situation when a newly diagnosed cancer patient who, having been told of their life-threatening condition, is simultaneously asked to be randomized into a clinical trial. It was for this latter type of circumstance that the Zelen approach was formulated.

Despite the criticism of its proposed use in the context of cleft lip repair and cancer, the Zelen design has been found to be very useful in other situations.

Example 14.10   Vaginal cuff infections following hysterectomy

Larsson and Carlsson (2002) conducted a randomized clinical trial to investigate the role of metronidazole compared to a no-treatment control in lowering vaginal cuff infection after hysterectomy among women presenting for surgery with bacterial vaginosis. In total, 213 women were randomized and the process was described as follows (our emphasis):

> Randomization was done according to Zelen (1979), using sealed envelopes in blocks of ten patients and carried out *before* informed consent. The nurse asked patients at pre-operative registration if they wanted to join the study, before the patients met the operating doctor at the final examination. Thus, women randomized to the *non-treatment* group were not asked to join the study, as no antibiotic treatment is the normal procedure at the clinic. Women randomized to the treatment group were asked to join the study and receive treatment.

The authors also state that the trial had approval from both the regional ethics committee and the Swedish Medical Products Agency.

Whether or not Zelen designs are appropriate is very context dependent and, although Larsson and colleagues have successfully used this approach, there are not many examples in the literature for individual-patient randomized trials. However, Piaggio, Carolli, Villar, *et al.* (2001) argue for their use in the context of trials using a cluster design of Chapter 12 and give an important example when comparing standard with new antenatal care; care which could only be implemented on a clinic-by-clinic basis. Clearly Zelen designs cannot be double-blind or employ placebos.

14.6 Systematic overviews

14.6.1 Introduction

Systematic reviews of the literature and other sources of information form an integral part of the design process for any proposed clinical trial. These reviews should encompass all pertinent information and not just, for example, earlier randomized trials. As we have stated, such a process is very useful if routinely applied *before* launching a new clinical trial (as a means of confirming the need to carry out the planned clinical trial in question), *during* the trial (for interim analysis purposes) and *after* completion of the trial (as a means of synthesizing and summarizing the current knowledge on the research question of interest). In this section, however, we restrict our attention to combining information available from randomized trials.

In many instances, randomized trials may have been conducted addressing the same or similar questions. Although possibly none of these provides convincing evidence for a particular approach, taken together they may be firmly suggestive of a benefit. A systematic overview is the process of finding all the randomized trials that are pertinent to a particular question and extracting the necessary details of these. Meta-analysis is the method by which these individual trial results are then combined into an overall synthesis. Many aspects of their application to problems in health care are described by Egger, Davey-Smith and Altman (2001).

A systematic review combines the evidence from the individual trials identified to give a more powerful analysis of any treatment effect. However, it is important to realize that a review can only be as good as its component parts. If the trials being reviewed are of poor quality, then inferences drawn from an overview will have to be made with extreme caution. In contrast, if the basic information is of high quality then their collective and systematic review and synthesis clearly adds substantially to the evidence base for clinical medicine.

Although we will only give a brief introduction to the whole process, the principal stages of a systematic overview and meta-analysis are (i) the systematic identification of all trials that addressed the outcome of interest; (ii) the evaluation of the quality of these trials; (iii) the extraction of the relevant data; and (iv) the statistical combining and analyzing of the collective results. A pivotal feature of the systematic review programme is the Cochrane Collaboration which, as Clarke (2006) describes,

> . . . is an international organisation dedicated to helping people to make well-informed decisions about health care.

An invaluable guide to the whole process of conducting such reviews and full details of the Cochrane Collaboration and Library can be found in Higgins and Green (2005). Indeed, accessing this library is one obvious starting point before embarking on a systematic review. An overview of the methodology pertinent to Health Related Quality of Life (HRQoL) outcomes in clinical trials is given by Fayers and Machin (2007, Chapter 19). Moher, Cook, Eastwood, *et al.* (1999) make suggestions as to how reports of meta-analyses of randomized controlled trials should be presented.

14.6.2 The protocol

As with a clinical trial, an important part of the systematic overview process is to prepare a protocol outlining the procedures that are to be followed. This will mirror most of the components of a trial protocol outlined in Chapter 3. For example, the objectives, particular intervention types to be compared, eligible patient groups and statistical methods all need to be specified. However, there are at least two sections that need to be added. One relates to the process of *literature searching* and the second to *assessing quality* of the trials so identified.

14.6.3 Literature searching

A major part of any systematic review is the literature search, to ensure that all available trials have been identified and included. It is usually the literature search that takes the greatest amount of time. Searching should address published and unpublished literature, trials that were opened but never completed and trials still in progress.

A starting point is to search bibliographic databases, and obtain abstracts of all potentially relevant articles. A key point at this stage is to ensure that a full range of applicable terms is included in the searching strategy. After a relevant publication has been found, the list of references it contains should be scrutinized for any citations of trials not yet identified. In most publications, clues about the value of the citations may be obtained from the introduction and the discussion sections. This searching process refers to completed and published trials. Ongoing trials can often be identified by accessing registers of clinical trials.

Publication bias is a well-known problem in the reporting of clinical trials. Journals are more likely to publish trials that obtain 'interesting' and positive results. This is especially the case if the trials are small, when those without such positive findings may fail to be published. Other means therefore have to be found to track down such unpublished information. A major justification for the compulsory registration of all clinical trials has been the countering of publication bias; it is becoming increasingly possible to establish at least the existence of unpublished and possibly negative trials.

14.6.4 Assessing quality

Full information, such as copies of publications, should be obtained for each potentially usable trial. These can be graded for eligibility and overall quality. Pointers to assessing the quality of trials are provided by Jüni, Altman and Egger (2001).

It is usually recommended that each trial is reviewed by more than one person. This is partly to spread the workload, but mainly to ensure that the ratings are consistent and of a reliable standard. It is therefore important that there should be a formal and pre-specified procedure both for making the ratings and for resolving disagreements between reviewers.

14.6.5 Combining trial results

If there are k trials to be combined, then the process is an extension of that described in Equation (14.1) which is confined to combining information from $k = 2$ sources. In general there will be $W_1, W_2, \ldots, W_k$ weights involved and each trial will provide an estimate of the treatment effect, say, $d_1, d_2, \ldots, d_k$. The latter replace, for example, $b_{\text{TreatData}}$ and $b_{\text{TreatExternal}}$ in Equation (14.1). The result of the calculation from the pooling the trials is denoted $\bar{d}_{\text{Overview}}$, the estimate of the true treatment effect δ. Similarly, the standard error is derived by extending Equation (14.2) which we denote by $SE(\bar{d}_{\text{Overview}})$. From these, the 95% confidence interval for δ, which takes the same form as Equation (8.1), is

$$\bar{d}_{\text{Overview}} - 1.96 \times SE(\bar{d}_{\text{Overview}}) \text{ to } \bar{d}_{\text{Overview}} + 1.96 \times SE(\bar{d}_{\text{Overview}}). \quad (14.3)$$

14.6.6   Forest plot

The standard way to present the results of a meta-analysis is a forest plot. This displays the point estimates for the separate trials and also for the overall effect, together with their associated confidence intervals. The weights for each trial are also shown graphically as a square block. The area of the block and the confidence interval convey similar information, but both make different contributions to the graphic. The confidence intervals depict the range of treatment effects compatible with the results of each trial, and indicate whether each was individually statistically significant. The size of the block draws the eye towards those trials with larger weight (narrower confidence intervals), which dominate the calculation of the pooled result. The pooled confidence interval is also shown, together with a lozenge indicating the value of the overall estimate.

Example 14.11   Ovarian cancer

The Advanced Ovarian Trialist Group (1991) sought to investigate the role of chemotherapy in advanced ovarian cancer. To this end, they identified three single agent trials and eight combination therapy trials in which they were able to compare carboplatin with cisplatin. One of the trials was unpublished, and an important feature of this overview is that additional follow-up was obtained on the trial patients. The synthesis was therefore more up-to-date and was not merely a collation of the evidence that had appeared in the literature. Their overview is summarized in the forest plot of Figure 14.10 with a summary (unshaded) lozenge for the Single agent and Combination groups separately, together with an overall (shaded) lozenge for the two groups combined. The overview favoured carboplatin over cisplatin and, importantly, led to the launch of a new trial comparing cisplatin, doxorubicin and cyclophosphamide (CAP) with carboplatin alone.

14.6.7 Heterogeneity

The bottom left-hand corner of Figure 14.10 contains the statement: '*Test for hetero-geneity*: $\chi^2_{10} = 7.11$; $p = 0.715$' and this highlights one of the complications of meta-analysis. In brief, the methods we have referred to make the assumption that the true effect sizes for each trial are the same or homogeneous. In other words, it is assumed that if all trials had enrolled huge numbers of patients they would all have given the same effect size. In terms of forest plots, homogeneity implies that the confidence intervals of the trials should be largely overlapping. A visual inspection of the forest plot in this example shows that this is clearly the case.

Homogeneity may not be a reasonable assumption, especially when trials have varying entry criteria, for example, in age or severity of disease. Another frequent cause of heterogeneity is that of trials apply treatments using varying dosage levels when there may be corresponding variations in the response rates. In such cases, the association between the presumed factors (age, disease severity or dosage) and the reported individual-trial effect sizes can be investigated.

The presence of heterogeneity may be explored by calculating the statistic

$$Q = \sum_j W_j \times \left(d_j - \bar{d}_{\text{Overview}} \right)^2. \tag{14.4}$$

There is statistically significant heterogeneity if Q exceeds the value from a χ^2 distribution with degrees of freedom, $df = k - 1$, where k is the number of trials concerned.

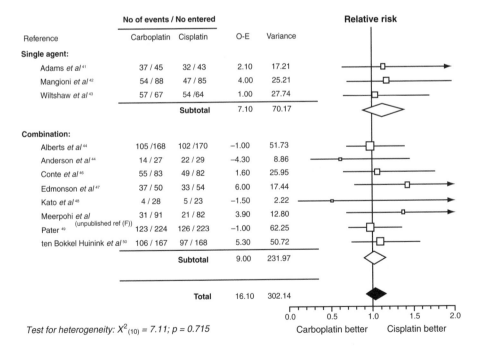

Test for heterogeneity: $\chi^2_{(10)} = 7.11$; $p = 0.715$

Figure 14.10 Forest plot following an overview and meta-analysis of 11 randomized trials in ovarian cancer (after Advanced Ovarian Trialist Group, 1991)

As indicated in the case of Figure 14.10, Equation (14.4) gives $Q = 7.11$ and p-value $= 0.715$, suggesting no statistically significant departure from the assumption of homogeneity. On the other hand, had heterogeneity been established then it would have been inappropriate to summarize the conclusions by the final (shaded) summary lozenge.

14.7   Conclusion

We have shown that the design, conduct and reporting of clinical trials pose many challenges, but good reliable clinical trials are necessary to establish therapeutic efficacy and effectiveness. Only well-conducted randomized clinical trials provide bias-free evidence. Systematic overviews and meta-analyses then synthesize existing knowledge from clinical trials, resulting in truly evidence-based medicine.

Statistical Tables

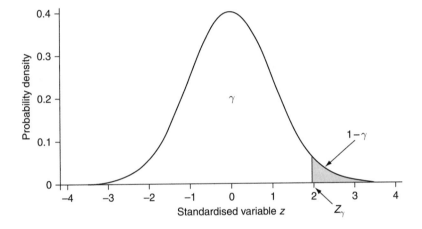

Figure T1   The probability density function of a standardized Normal distribution

Randomized Clinical Trials: Design, Practice and Reporting   David Machin and Peter M Fayers
© 2010 John Wiley & Sons, Ltd

Table T1 The Normal distribution function i.e. probability that a normally distributed variable is less than z_γ

z_γ	0.00	0.01	0.02	0.03	0.04	0.05	0.06	0.07	0.08	0.09
0.0	0.500 00	0.503 99	0.507 98	0.511 97	0.515 95	0.519 94	0.523 92	0.527 90	0.531 88	0.535 86
0.1	0.539 83	0.543 80	0.547 76	0.551 72	0.555 67	0.559 62	0.563 56	0.567 49	0.571 42	0.575 35
0.2	0.579 26	0.583 17	0.587 06	0.590 95	0.594 83	0.598 71	0.602 57	0.606 42	0.610 26	0.614 09
0.3	0.617 91	0.621 72	0.625 52	0.629 30	0.633 07	0.636 83	0.640 58	0.644 31	0.648 03	0.651 73
0.4	0.655 42	0.659 10	0.662 76	0.666 40	0.670 03	0.673 64	0.677 24	0.680 82	0.684 39	0.687 93
0.5	0.691 46	0.694 97	0.698 47	0.701 94	0.705 40	0.708 84	0.712 26	0.715 66	0.719 04	0.722 40
0.6	0.725 75	0.729 07	0.732 37	0.735 65	0.738 91	0.742 15	0.745 37	0.748 57	0.751 75	0.754 90
0.7	0.758 04	0.761 15	0.764 24	0.767 30	0.770 35	0.773 37	0.776 37	0.779 35	0.782 30	0.785 24
0.8	0.788 14	0.791 03	0.793 89	0.796 73	0.799 55	0.802 34	0.805 11	0.807 85	0.810 57	0.813 27
0.9	0.815 94	0.818 59	0.821 21	0.823 81	0.826 39	0.828 94	0.831 47	0.833 98	0.836 46	0.838 91
1.0	0.841 34	0.843 75	0.846 14	0.848 49	0.850 83	0.853 14	0.855 43	0.857 69	0.859 93	0.862 14
1.1	0.864 33	0.866 50	0.868 64	0.870 76	0.872 86	0.874 93	0.876 98	0.879 00	0.881 00	0.882 98
1.2	0.884 93	0.886 86	0.888 77	0.890 65	0.892 51	0.894 35	0.896 17	0.897 96	0.899 73	0.901 47
1.3	0.903 20	0.904 90	0.906 58	0.908 24	0.909 88	0.911 49	0.913 08	0.914 66	0.916 21	0.917 74
1.4	0.919 24	0.920 73	0.922 20	0.923 64	0.925 07	0.926 47	0.927 85	0.929 22	0.930 56	0.931 89
1.5	0.933 19	0.934 48	0.935 74	0.936 99	0.938 22	0.939 43	0.940 62	0.941 79	0.942 95	0.944 08
1.6	0.945 20	0.946 30	0.947 38	0.948 45	0.949 50	0.950 53	0.951 54	0.952 54	0.953 52	0.954 49
1.7	0.955 43	0.956 37	0.957 28	0.958 18	0.959 07	0.959 94	0.960 80	0.961 64	0.962 46	0.963 27
1.8	0.964 07	0.964 85	0.965 62	0.966 38	0.967 12	0.967 84	0.968 56	0.969 26	0.969 95	0.970 62
1.9	0.971 28	0.971 93	0.972 57	0.973 20	0.973 81	0.974 41	**0.975 00**	0.975 58	0.976 15	0.976 70
z_γ	0.00	0.01	0.02	0.03	0.04	0.05	0.06	0.07	0.08	0.09

Table T1 *(Continued)*

z_γ	0.00	0.01	0.02	0.03	0.04	0.05	0.06	0.07	0.08	0.09
2.0	0.977 25	0.977 78	0.978 31	0.978 82	0.979 32	0.979 82	0.980 30	0.980 77	0.981 24	0.981 69
2.1	0.982 14	0.982 57	0.983 00	0.983 41	0.983 82	0.984 22	0.984 61	0.985 00	0.985 37	0.985 74
2.2	0.986 10	0.986 45	0.986 79	0.987 13	0.987 45	0.987 78	0.988 09	0.988 40	0.988 70	0.988 99
2.3	0.989 28	0.989 56	0.989 83	0.990 10	0.990 36	0.990 61	0.990 86	0.991 11	0.991 34	0.991 58
2.4	0.991 80	0.992 02	0.992 24	0.992 45	0.992 66	0.992 86	0.993 05	0.993 24	0.993 43	0.993 61
2.5	0.993 79	0.993 96	0.994 13	0.994 30	0.994 46	0.994 61	0.994 77	0.994 92	**0.995 06**	0.995 20
2.6	0.995 34	0.995 47	0.995 60	0.995 73	0.995 85	0.995 98	0.996 09	0.996 21	0.996 32	0.996 43
2.7	0.996 53	0.996 64	0.996 74	0.996 83	0.996 93	0.997 02	0.997 11	0.997 20	0.997 28	0.997 36
2.8	0.997 44	0.997 52	0.997 60	0.997 67	0.997 74	0.997 81	0.997 88	0.997 95	0.998 01	0.998 07
2.9	0.998 13	0.998 19	0.998 25	0.998 31	0.998 36	0.998 41	0.998 46	0.998 51	0.998 56	0.998 61
3.0	0.998 65	0.998 69	0.998 74	0.998 78	0.998 82	0.998 86	0.998 89	0.998 93	0.998 96	0.999 00
3.1	0.999 03	0.999 06	0.999 10	0.999 13	0.999 16	0.999 18	0.999 21	0.999 24	0.999 26	0.999 29
3.2	0.999 31	0.999 34	0.999 36	0.999 38	0.999 40	0.999 42	0.999 44	0.999 46	0.999 48	0.999 50
3.3	0.999 52	0.999 53	0.999 55	0.999 57	0.999 58	0.999 60	0.999 61	0.999 62	0.999 64	0.999 65
3.4	0.999 66	0.999 68	0.999 69	0.999 70	0.999 71	0.999 72	0.999 73	0.999 74	0.999 75	0.999 76
3.5	0.999 77	0.999 78	0.999 78	0.999 79	0.999 80	0.999 81	0.999 81	0.999 82	0.999 83	0.999 83
3.6	0.999 84	0.999 85	0.999 85	0.999 86	0.999 86	0.999 87	0.999 87	0.999 88	0.999 88	0.999 89
3.7	0.999 89	0.999 90	0.999 90	0.999 90	0.999 91	0.999 91	0.999 92	0.999 92	0.999 92	0.999 92
3.8	0.999 93	0.999 93	0.999 93	0.999 94	0.999 94	0.999 94	0.999 94	0.999 95	0.999 95	0.999 95
3.9	0.999 95	0.999 95	0.999 96	0.999 96	0.999 96	0.999 96	0.999 96	0.999 96	0.999 97	0.999 97
z_γ	0.00	0.01	0.02	0.03	0.04	0.05	0.06	0.07	0.08	0.09

Table T2 Percentage points of the Normal distribution for given α and one β (some frequently used entries are highlighted)

α		$1 - \beta$	
one-sided	two-sided	one-sided	z
0.0005	0.001	0.9995	3.2905
0.0025	0.005	0.9975	2.8070
0.005	**0.01**	0.995	**2.5758**
0.01	0.02	0.99	2.3263
0.0125	0.025	0.9875	2.2414
0.025	**0.05**	0.975	**1.9600**
0.05	0.1	0.95	1.6449
0.1	0.2	**0.9**	**1.2816**
0.15	0.3	0.85	1.0364
0.2	0.4	**0.8**	**0.8416**
0.25	0.5	0.75	0.6745
0.3	0.6	0.7	0.5244
0.35	0.7	0.65	0.3853
0.4	0.8	0.6	0.2533

Table T3 Percentage points of the Normal distribution (some frequently used entries are highlighted)

α		
two-sided	one-sided	z
0.001	0.0005	3.2905
0.005	0.0025	2.8070
0.010	0.0050	**2.5758**
0.020	0.0100	2.3263
0.025	0.0125	2.2414
0.050	0.0250	**1.9600**
0.100	0.0500	1.6449
0.200	**0.1000**	**1.2816**
0.300	0.1500	1.0364
0.400	**0.2000**	**0.8416**
0.500	0.2500	0.6745
0.600	0.3000	0.5244
0.700	0.3500	0.3853
0.800	0.4000	0.2533

Table T4   Students t-distribution

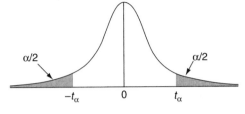

df	0.20	0.10	0.05	0.04	0.03	0.02	0.01	0.001
1	3.078	6.314	12.706	15.895	21.205	31.821	63.657	636.6
2	1.886	2.920	4.303	4.849	5.643	6.965	9.925	31.60
3	1.634	2.353	3.182	3.482	3.896	4.541	5.842	12.92
4	1.530	2.132	2.776	2.999	3.298	3.747	4.604	8.610
5	1.474	2.015	2.571	2.757	3.003	3.365	4.032	6.869
6	1.439	1.943	2.447	2.612	2.829	3.143	3.707	5.959
7	1.414	1.895	2.365	2.517	2.715	2.998	3.499	5.408
8	1.397	1.860	2.306	2.449	2.634	2.896	3.355	5.041
9	1.383	1.833	2.262	2.398	2.574	2.821	3.250	4.781
10	1.372	1.812	2.228	2.359	2.528	2.764	3.169	4.587
11	1.363	1.796	2.201	2.328	2.491	2.718	3.106	4.437
12	1.356	1.782	2.179	2.303	2.461	2.681	3.055	4.318
13	1.350	1.771	2.160	2.282	2.436	2.650	3.012	4.221
14	1.345	1.761	2.145	2.264	2.415	2.624	2.977	4.140
15	1.340	1.753	2.131	2.249	2.397	2.602	2.947	4.073
16	1.337	1.746	2.120	2.235	2.382	2.583	2.921	4.015
17	1.333	1.740	2.110	2.224	2.368	2.567	2.898	3.965
18	1.330	1.734	2.101	2.214	2.356	2.552	2.878	3.922
19	1.328	1.729	2.093	2.205	2.346	2.539	2.861	3.883
20	1.325	1.725	2.086	2.196	2.336	2.528	2.845	3.850
21	1.323	1.721	2.079	2.189	2.327	2.517	2.830	3.819
22	1.321	1.717	2.074	2.183	2.320	2.508	2.818	3.790
23	1.319	1.714	2.069	2.178	2.313	2.499	2.806	3.763
24	1.318	1.711	2.064	2.172	2.307	2.492	2.797	3.744
25	1.316	1.708	2.059	2.166	2.301	2.485	2.787	3.722
26	1.315	1.706	2.056	2.162	2.396	2.479	2.779	3.706
27	1.314	1.703	2.052	2.158	2.291	2.472	2.770	3.687
28	1.313	1.701	2.048	2.154	2.286	2.467	2.763	3.673
29	1.311	1.699	2.045	2.150	2.282	2.462	2.756	3.657
30	1.310	1.697	2.042	2.147	2.278	2.457	2.750	3.646
∞	1.282	1.645	1.960	2.054	2.170	2.326	2.576	3.291

The value tabulated is t_α, such that if X is distributed as Student's t-distribution with f degrees of freedom, then α is the probability that $X \leq -t_\alpha$ or $X \geq t_\alpha$.

Table T5   Random numbers

75 792	78 245	83 270	59 987	75 253	42 729	98 917	83 137	67 588	93 846
80 169	88 847	36 686	36 601	91 654	44 249	52 586	25 702	09 575	18 939
94 071	63 090	23 901	93 268	53 316	87 773	89 260	04 804	99 479	83 909
67 970	29 162	60 224	61 042	98 324	30 425	37 677	90 382	96 230	84 565
91 577	43 019	67 511	28 527	61 750	55 267	07 847	50 165	26 793	80 918
84 334	54 827	51 955	47 256	21 387	28 456	77 296	41 283	01 482	44 494
03 778	05 031	90 146	59 031	96 758	57 420	23 581	38 824	49 592	18 593
58 563	84 810	22 446	80 149	99 676	83 102	35 381	94 030	59 560	32 145
29 068	74 625	90 665	52 747	09 364	57 491	59 049	19 767	83 081	78 441
90 047	44 763	44 **534**	**55 425**	**67** 170	67 937	88 962	49 992	53 583	37 864
54 870	35 009	84 524	32 309	88 815	86 792	89 097	66 600	26 195	88326
23 327	78 957	50 987	77 876	63 960	53 986	46 771	80 998	95 229	59 606
03 876	89 100	66 895	89 468	96 684	95 491	32 222	58 708	34 408	66 930
14 846	86 619	04 238	36 182	05 294	43 791	88 149	22 637	56 775	52 091
94 731	63 786	88 290	60 990	98 407	43 437	74 233	25 880	96 898	52 186
96 046	51 589	84 509	98 162	39 162	59 469	60 563	74 917	02 413	17 967
95 188	25 011	29 947	48 896	83 408	79 684	11 353	13 636	46 380	69 003
67 416	00 626	49 781	77 833	47 073	59 147	50 469	10 807	58 985	98 881
50 002	97 121	26 652	23 667	13 819	54 138	54 173	69 234	28 657	01 031
50 806	62 492	67 131	02 610	43 964	19 528	68 333	69 484	23 527	96 974
43 619	79 413	45 456	31 642	78 162	81 686	73 687	19 751	24 727	98 742
90 476	58 785	15 177	81 377	26 671	70 548	41 383	59 773	59 835	13 719
43 241	22 852	28 915	49 692	75 981	74 215	65 915	36 489	10 233	89 897
57 434	86 821	63 717	54 640	28 782	24 046	84 755	83 021	85 436	29 813
15 731	12 986	03 008	18 739	07 726	75 512	65 295	15 089	81 094	05 260
34 706	04 386	02 945	72 555	97 249	16 798	05 643	42 343	36 106	63 948
16 759	74 867	62 702	32 840	08 565	18 403	10 421	60 687	68 599	78 034
11 895	74 173	72 423	62 838	89 382	57 437	85 314	75 320	01 988	52 518
87 597	21 289	30 904	13 209	04 244	53 651	28 373	90 759	70 286	49 678
63 656	28 328	25 428	38 671	97 372	69 256	49 364	35 398	30 808	59 082
72 414	71 686	65 513	81 236	26 205	10 013	80 610	40 509	50 045	70 530
69 337	19 016	50 420	38 803	55 793	84 035	93 051	57 693	33 673	67 434
64 310	62 819	20 242	08 632	83 905	49 477	29 409	96 563	86 993	91 207
31 243	63 913	66 340	91 169	28 560	69 220	14 730	19 752	51 636	59 434
39 951	83 556	88 718	68 802	06 170	90 451	58 926	50 125	28 532	17 189
57 473	53 613	76 478	82 668	28 315	05 975	96 324	96 135	14 255	29 991
50 259	80 588	94 408	55 754	79 166	20 490	97 112	25 904	20 254	08 781
48 449	97 696	14 321	92 549	95 812	78 371	77 678	56 618	44 769	57 413
50 830	52 921	41 365	46 257	66 889	29 420	95 250	24 080	08 600	04 189
94 646	37 630	50 246	53 925	95 496	82 773	41 021	95 435	83 812	52 558
49 344	07 037	24 221	41 955	47 211	43 418	45 703	78 779	77 215	44 594
49 201	66 377	64 188	50 398	33 157	87 375	55 885	14 174	03 105	85 821
57 221	54 927	59 025	46 847	35 894	14 639	38 452	89 166	72 843	40 954
65 391	57 289	67 771	99 160	08 184	26 262	46 577	32 603	21 677	54 104
01 029	99 783	63 250	39 198	51 042	36 834	40 450	90 864	49 953	61 032
23 218	67 476	45 675	17 299	85 685	57 294	30 847	39 985	44 402	76 665
35 175	51 935	85 800	91 083	97 112	20 865	96 101	83 276	84 149	11 443
28 442	12 188	99 908	51 660	34 350	66 572	43 047	30 217	44 491	79 042
89 327	26 880	83 020	20 428	87 554	33 251	80 684	01 964	04 106	28 243

Each digit 0–9 is equally likely to appear and cannot be predicted from any combination of other digits.

Glossary

The majority of the definitions within this glossary are based on, but are only a selection from, the comprehensive list provided by Day (2007) in the *Dictionary of Clinical Trials*. We have added an explanatory comment to some of the definitions included here, while some are also expanded upon in appropriate sections within the main text.

adaptive design Trial procedures that change as the trial progresses. An example is that of the randomization process changing as the trial progresses and the results become known. Such designs are used so that, if it appears that one intervention is emerging as superior to another, the allocation ratio can be biased in favour of the intervention which seems to be best.

adjust To modify the treatment effect (the adjusted estimate) to account for differences in patient characteristics (usually only when known to be importantly prognostic for outcome) between intervention groups.

allocation ratio The ratio of the number of subjects allocated to one intervention group relative to the number allocated to another in a parallel group trial. Most often the ratio is 1 : 1, or equal allocation.

arm Synonym for group (as in randomized group).

assigned intervention The intervention that a trial participant is due to receive based on a randomization procedure.

attrition Loss, often used to describe loss of patients' data in long-term trials due to patients withdrawing for reasons other than those of meeting the trials' primary endpoint.

audit trail A list of reasons and justifications for all changes that are made to data or documents, and of all procedures that do not comply with agreed trial procedures.
   Such an audit trail particularly applies to information that is entered onto the trial database so that if an item is amended (including deletion) in any way then the original entry is retained, the amendment noted and the date and individual responsible for the change also noted and automatically stored within the database.

autocorrelation Correlation between repeated measurements taken successively in time on the same subject.

baseline characteristic A measurement taken on a subject at the beginning of a trial. Note that 'beginning' is generally taken to be at, or as near as possible to (ideally before), the time of randomization.

Bayesian General statistical methods based around Bayes' theorem which describes a way of moving the thinking about the probability of data, given a hypothesis, to the probability of an hypothesis being true or false.

Randomized Clinical Trials: Design, Practice and Reporting   David Machin and Peter M Fayers
© 2010 John Wiley & Sons, Ltd

posterior distribution   In Bayesian statistics, this is the probability distribution of the treatment effect after combining the prior distribution of the treatment effect with that of the trial data itself.

prior distribution   In Bayesian statistics, this is the probability distribution of the treatment effect (usually obtained before the trial commences) before combining it with the trial data to obtain the posterior distribution.

bias   A process which systematically overestimates or underestimates a **parameter**.

publication bias   The situation where there is a tendency for positive trials to be more widely published (or otherwise reported) than negative trials. This is a particular problem and can cause bias in carrying out overviews and meta-analyses.

recall bias   Any bias in remembering events.

response bias   Any bias that is caused by a systematic difference between those people who respond (typically to a questionnaire) and those who do not respond.

selection bias   The bias caused by the fact that the types of subjects who take part in trials are not a **random sample** of the **population** from which they are drawn.

Specifically, if the random treatment allocation process is not adhered to in that the allocation is known before eligibility is determined (implying that the patients may be selected for the treatment rather than the treatment selected for the patient) then this results in selection bias which may compromise the final evaluation of the alternatives.

blind or mask   Where the investigator, subject (and possibly other people) are not able to distinguish the treatments being compared (by sight, smell, taste, weight, etc.).

single blind   The case when only one party is blind to the treatment allocation. It is usually either the investigator or the subject who is blind, but the term on its own does not differentiate.

double blind   A trial where the subjects and investigators are blind to the treatment or intervention allocation.

triple blind   The situation where the subject is blinded to the trial medication, the investigator is blinded and the data management staff are blinded.

quadruple blind   Subjects are blind to what medication they receive, those administering the treatments are blind to what treatment they are giving each subject, investigators (or those assessing efficacy and safety) are blind to which treatment was given; and data management and statistical personnel are blind as to which treatment each subject received. The only use over that of **triple blind** is when the person who gives the treatment to the subject is not the same as the one who subsequently assesses the effect of the treatment.

It should be noted that these definitions are not consistently adhered to in articles describing randomized trials so that the reader needs to check precisely what is intended by the author's use of these terms.

block randomization   A randomization scheme that uses blocks, each block usually having the same number of treatments (although in random order) as each other block. Commonly, if a trial is comparing two treatments, each block might comprise four patients (two on one treatment and two on the other). In general, block size will depend on the number of interventions within the trial and the corresponding allocation ratio.

Bonferroni correction   An adjustment made when interpreting multiple tests of statistical significance that all address a similar basic question. If two endpoints have been assessed separately, instead of considering whether a p-value is less than (or greater than) 0.05, the calculated p-value would be compared to 0.025. In general, if k p-values have been calculated, the declaration of statistical significance would not be made unless one or more of those p-values is less than $0.05/k$.

An equivalent approach, and one more readily understandable, is to multiply each calculated p-value by k and only declare those adjusted values less than 0.05 as statistically significant.

censored observation   When the time until an event (typically cure, recurrence of symptoms or death) is the data value to be recorded and that event has not yet been observed for a particular subject, then the data value is said to be censored.

cluster design   A design in which individual subjects are not randomized to receive different interventions, but rather groups (or 'clusters') of subjects are randomized. Examples are most common in community intervention trials.

confidence interval (CI)   A range of values for a parameter (such as the difference in means or proportions between two treatment groups) that are all consistent with the observed data. The width of such an interval can vary, depending on how confident we wish to be that the range quoted will truly encompass the value of the parameter. Usually '95% confidence intervals' are quoted. These intervals will, in 95% of repeated cases, include the true value of the parameter of interest. In this case, the confidence level is said to be 95% (or 0.95).

consistency check   An edit check on data to ensure that two (or more) data values could happen in conjunction. Systolic blood pressure measurements must always be at least as great as diastolic measurements so, for any given patient, if the systolic pressure is greater than the diastolic, then the two measures are consistent with each other. It may be that neither is correct – but they are, at least, consistent.

CONSORT   A set of guidelines, adopted by many leading medical journals, describing the way in which clinical trials should be reported. It stands for Consolidation of the Standards of Reporting Trials. Details can be found at www.consort-statement.org.

covariate   A variable that is not of primary interest but which may affect response to treatment. Common examples are subjects' demographic data and baseline assessments of disease severity.

cross-over design   A trial where each subject receives (in a random sequence) each trial medication. After receiving Treatment A, they are 'crossed over' to receive Treatment B (or vice versa). This is the simplest form of cross-over design and is called the two-period cross-over design.

   carryover   A term used mostly in the context of cross-over trials where the effect of the drug is still present after that drug has ceased to be given to a subject, and in particular when that subject is taking another drug.

   period   The intervals of time when a subject is given the first treatment (period 1) or when they are given the second treatment (period 2).

   wash-out   The process of allowing time for drugs to be naturally excreted from the body.

data monitoring committee (DMC)   A group of people who regularly review the accumulating data in a trial with the possibility of stopping the trial or modifying its progress. A trial may be stopped, or changes made to it, if clear evidence of efficacy is seen or if adverse safety is observed in one or more of the intervention groups, or for futility.

dropout or withdrawal   The case where a subject stops participating in a trial before he or she is due according to the trial protocol.

effect   A relative measure such as the extra change in blood pressure produced by one treatment compared to that produced by the comparator treatment.

   effect size or standardized effect size   Strictly, this should simply be the size of an effect but conventionally it is taken to be the size of the effect divided by the standard deviation of the measurement. Thus an effect size of 0.5 indicates a difference between two means equal to half of a standard deviation.

endpoint   A variable that is one of the primary interests in the trial. The variable may relate to efficacy or safety. The term is used almost synonymously with efficacy variable or safety variable.

   composite endpoint   An overall endpoint in a trial made up of more than one component. An example might be the endpoint of 'all cause mortality *or* myocardial infarction'.

intermediate endpoint   An endpoint that does not measure exactly what we want to know but which is a second-best alternative.

primary endpoint   The most important endpoint in a trial.

secondary endpoint   One of (possibly many) less important endpoints in a trial.

surrogate endpoint   A substitute endpoint; a variable that is a substitute for the most clinically meaningful endpoint. In hypertension trials, the most important endpoint would usually be mortality (possibly restricted to cardiovascular reasons) but raised blood pressure would often be the endpoint that is measured. Blood pressure is being used as a surrogate for mortality.

equipoise   The state of having an indifferent opinion about the relative merits of two (or more) alternative treatments. Ethically, a subject should only be randomized into a trial if the treating physician has no clear evidence that one treatment is superior to another. If such evidence does exist then it is considered unethical to randomly choose a treatment. If the physician is in a state of equipoise, then randomization is considered ethical.

equivalence trial   A trial whose primary aim is to demonstrate that interventions are equivalent with regard to certain specified parameters.

equivalence margin   The difference between test treatment and control treatment (in terms of the primary endpoint) that is deemed to be of no clinical importance. Hence, if a new treatment were this much better (or worse) than an old treatment, then the new and old treatments would be considered, in all practical extents, to be just as efficacious.

exclusion criteria   Reasons why a subject should not be enrolled into a trial. These are usually reasons of safety and should not simply be the opposites of inclusion criteria.

factor   Another name for a categorical variable, usually one that is a covariate or a stratification variable, rather than one that is an outcome variable.

factor level   One of the different values that a factor can take. For example, a placebo may be the zero dose (level) of a drug under test in a trial.

factorial design   A trial that compares two (or more) different sets of interventions (factors). The simplest design uses Drug A versus Placebo A and Drug B versus Placebo B. Subject will be randomized to one of four groups: Placebo A + Placebo B, Drug A + Placebo B, Placebo A + Drug B or Drug A + Drug B. This is a very efficient type of design because it not only allows the assessments of Drug A and Drug B in one trial instead of two, but also allows us to investigate the question of whether Drugs A and B show any interaction.

incomplete factorial design   A factorial design where not all combinations of the possible treatments are used.

interaction effect   The difference in the size of the effect caused by two or more factors (treatment types) jointly, compared with the sum of the individual effects of each.

main effect   In factorial trials the main effect of one factor is the size of the effect averaged over all levels of all other factors.

fixed sample size design   A design that determines the number of subjects to be recruited before the trial starts and does not allow the number to be changed. This is the most common type of approach for determining how many subjects should be in a trial.

forest plot   A diagram comprising the individual estimated treatment effects and associated 95% confidence intervals for each trial included in a meta-analysis, together with an overall estimate and confidence interval.

futility analysis   Usually an interim analysis of a trial to determine if the trial objectives are likely to be achieved. Continuation of a trial may be considered futile if there is little chance to detect a clinically useful treatment effect.

Good Clinical Practice (GCP)   A set of principles and guidelines to ensure high quality and high standards in clinical (trials) research.

hypothesis   A statement for which good evidence may not exist but which is to be the subject of a clinical trial.

alternative hypothesis (H_1) This is usually the point of interest in a trial. It is generally phrased in terms of the null hypothesis (of no treatment effect) not being true. If the objective of a trial is to 'compare Drug A with placebo' then the null hypothesis would be that there is no difference between the two treatments and the alternative hypothesis would be that there *is* a difference.

null hypothesis (H_0) The assumption, generally made in statistical significance testing, that there is no difference between groups (in whatever feature is being compared). Evidence (in the form of trial data) is then sought to refute this null hypothesis.

inclusion criteria The requirements that a subject must fulfil to be allowed to enter a trial. These are usually selected to ensure that the subject has the appropriate disease and that he or she is the type of subject that the researchers wish to study. Inclusion criteria should not simply be the opposites of the exclusion criteria.

intention-to-treat (ITT) A strategy for analyzing trial data which (in its simplest form) says that any subject randomized to treatment must be included in the analysis.

    per protocol analysis The analysis of trial data that includes only those subjects from all those randomized who adequately comply with the trial protocol.

interim analysis A formal statistical term indicating an analysis of data part of the way through a trial.

International Conference on Harmonisation (ICH) a group of industry and regulatory representatives from Europe, Japan and the USA who draw up common standards of required test and documentation for drug licensing in these three regions of the world. The web site for ICH is www.ich.org.

large simple trial A trial that enrols many patients (perhaps 20 000 or more) and whose procedures and documentation are kept as simple (and minimal) as possible.

meta-analysis An analysis of the results from two or more similar trials. Such methods are used as a way of synthesizing data from a variety of trials to try to obtain better answers to specific medical questions.

missing data or forms A data value or form that should have been recorded or completed but for some reason was not.

    informative missing The situation where missing data tell us something about the effect of treatment. Usually the 'informative' nature is detrimental to the treatment (e.g. efficacy data missing because a patient has died) but sometimes the information can be more positive (e.g. no further follow-up made as the patient was cured).

    missing at random Missing data where the probability of data being missing may depend on the values of some other measured data but does not depend on the missing values themselves.

model An idealistic description of a real (often uncertain) situation.

    additive model A statistical model where the combined effect of separate variables contributes to the sum of each of their separate effects.

    statistical model Equation including both deterministic and random elements which describes how a process behaves. Examples are regression models and logistic regression. Simple t-tests are based on simple models.

non-inferiority trial A trial whose objective is to show that one intervention 'is not worse than another'. This is subtly different from an **equivalence trial**, which aims to show that two treatments are equivalent, and is obviously different from trying to show that one treatment is different to another (**superiority trial**).

number needed to treat (NNT) The number of patients that a physician would have to treat with a new treatment in order to avoid one event that would otherwise have occurred with a standard treatment.

open trial A trial where the treatments are not blinded.

overview   To look at trial or trial-related data from various sources, considering them as a whole and drawing a conclusion.

paired design   A trial design that involves taking paired observations and usually makes treatment comparisons using paired comparisons, often in the form of cross-over or split-mouth designs.

parallel group design   The most common design for clinical trials, whereby subjects are allocated to receive one of several interventions. All subjects are independently allocated to one of the treatment groups. No subjects receive more than one of the treatments.

parameter   The true (but often unknown) value of some characteristic. The most common parameter that we wish to estimate in clinical trials is the size of the treatment effect.

pilot study   A small study for helping to design a subsequent trial. The main uses of pilot studies are to test practical arrangements (e.g. how long do various activities take? is it possible to do all the things we want to?), to test questionnaires (do the subjects understand the questions in the way intended?) and to investigate variability in data.

> **internal pilot study**   A form of pilot study in which the collected data also form part of the data for the main trial.
>
> *When designing a trial, the sample size determined may hinge on critical assumptions such as the likely response rate in the standard or control arm or, if a continuous outcome measure is under consideration, the likely standard deviation. In such cases an internal pilot study may be conducted, which comprises a predetermined number of the first patients recruited to the trial. Information from these patients is then used to calculate, in our examples, either the response rate or standard deviation. If these are far from those used at the planning stage of the trial they are used to recalculate trial size. However, the trial size is only amended if this new size exceeds the original target.*

placebo   An inert substance usually prepared to look, smell, taste, etc. as similar to the active product being investigated in a trial as possible.

protocol   A document describing all the important details of how a trial will be conducted. It will generally include details of the interventions being used, a rationale for the trial, what procedures will be carried out on the subjects in the trial, how many subjects will be recruited, the design of the trial and how the data will be analyzed.

protocol violation   Something that happens during the trial (usually to one or more of the recruited subjects) that does not fully conform to what was described in the protocol.

QUOROM   A set of guidelines for presenting and publishing the results of meta-analyses and overviews. It stands for QUality Of Reporting Of Meta-analyses. Details can be found at www.consort-statement.org/quorom.pdf.

randomization   The process of allocating subjects to interventions in a manner not happening systematically or predictably.

> **dynamic allocation**   A randomization method that changes the probability of assignment to different treatment groups as a trial progresses.
>
> **minimization**   A pseudo-random method of assigning treatments to subjects to try to balance the distribution of covariates across the treatment groups.
>
> **randomization list**   A list, produced by a random process, that indicates which subjects will receive which intervention in a randomized trial.
>
> **Zelen's randomized consent design**   A design which combines randomization with consent. Subjects are randomized to one of two treatment groups. Those who are randomized to the standard treatment are all treated with it (no consent to take part in the trial is sought). Those who are randomized to the experimental treatment are asked for their consent. If they agree they are treated with the experimental treatment; if they disagree they are treated with the standard treatment. The analysis must be based on the treatment to which patients were randomized, not the treatment they actually receive.

range check   An edit check to identify any data values that fall outside a specified lower limit and upper limit.

repeated measurements design   A trial in which subjects have several measurements of the same variable taken at different times.

seed   A number used to initialize a computerized pseudo-random number generator which is used to create the randomization code to decide which subjects receive which intervention. A pseudo-random number generator provides numbers that appear as if they are completely random but which (technically) are not. Current regulatory requirements specify that the randomization list can be reproduced at any time from knowledge of the seed. Note that tossing a coin is random, but the sequence so generated is not reproducible and so its veracity cannot be confirmed.

sequential design   A general type of trial design, in which subjects are recruited and the accumulating data analyzed after every subject has completed the trial. The analysis does not wait until a fixed number of subjects have completed the trial. The trial continues until to recruit until a positive or negative result becomes evident.

> **closed sequential design**   A sequential trial design where an upper limit on the number of subjects exists (hence 'closed'), but it is possible to draw conclusions and stop the trial before that number of subjects have been recruited.

> **group sequential design**   A form of sequential design where interim analyses are carried out after a number of subjects have been recruited into a trial. Usually only two or three analyses would be planned during such a trial after either half the subjects or one-third and two-thirds of the subjects have completed the trial.

> **open sequential design**   A sequential trial design that does not have any upper limit to the number of subjects that may be recruited.

serious adverse event (SAE)   A regulatory term with a strict meaning. It includes all adverse events that result in death, are life threatening, require patient hospitalization or prolongation of existing hospitalization or result in disability or congenital abnormality. Note some SAEs could be non-serious (and quite routine) in a medical sense.

sham   An alternative term for a placebo but used particularly when the form of the active treatment is not a conventional tablet, capsule, etc.
Examples of sham treatments have included sham acupuncture and even sham surgery.

split-mouth design   A trial where each subject receives each trial medication (Treatment A to one side of the oral cavity and Treatment B to the other).

> **carryacross**   A term used in oral cavity trials where, for example, one side of the mouth receives one drug whose effect may modify (contaminate) the effect of a second drug applied to the other side (and vice versa).

stopping rule   The rule for deciding when to stop recruitment to a trial. This may be based on formal statistical considerations or be more informal.

> **early stopping**   The practice of stopping recruitment to a trial before reaching the target sample size or of stopping follow-up of a trial before the intended final duration. This may be in a sequential trial, after a formal interim analysis or for purely practical reasons that are independent of efficacy or safety concerns.

stratify   To divide those entering a clinical trial into groups according to the values of a categorical variable.

> **stratified randomization**   The use of separate randomization lists for different strata in the sample. This is often done to ensure that possible important prognostic factors are balanced across the intervention groups.

superiority trial   A trial where the objective is to show that one intervention is better than another.

systematic review   A thorough and complete review and assessment of all the published and unpublished literature and information available.

treatment difference or effect   The difference between two treatment groups based on one of the trial endpoints. This might commonly be the difference in mean response, in proportions of responders or in median survival times. It may be expressed through the use of an odds ratio or hazard ratio as appropriate.

    clinically significant difference   A treatment effect that is sufficiently large to be useful for treating patients.

variable   The mathematical term for a characteristic or property of something or someone that is being measured. It may vary from time to time and from subject to subject.

    dependent variable   In a statistical model, the dependent variable is the one we are trying to predict from the independent variable(s).

    design variable   Any variable that contributes to the design of a trial, often because of stratification according to values of the variable.

    independent variable, explanatory variable or covariate   In a regression model, the dependent variable may depend on the independent variables (the most important of which is the assigned treatment group). Other important independent variables are those thought prognostic for outcome. Note, confusingly, that several so-called independent variables may not be independent *of each other*.

    prognostic factor   A factor (often a feature of the patient at diagnosis rather than the treatment received) that is predictive of outcome.

References

Advanced Ovarian Trialist Group (1991) Chemotherapy in advanced ovarian cancer: an overview of randomised clinical trials. *BMJ*, **303**, 884–893. [14]

Allan, L., Hays, H., Jensen, N.-H., de Waroux, B.L.P., Bolt, M., Donald, R. and Kalso, E. (2008) Randomised crossover trial of transdermal fentanyl and sustained release oral morphine for treating chronic non-cancer pain. *BMJ*, **322**, 1–7. [12]

Al-Sarraf, M., Pajak, P.F., Cooper, J.S., Mohiuddin, M., Herskovic, A. and Ager, P.J. (1990) Chemo-radiotherapy in patients with locally advanced nasopharyngeal carcinoma: a radiation therapy oncology group study. *Journal of Clinical Oncology*, **8**, 1342–1351. [2]

Altman, D.G., (1991) Practical Statistics for Medical Research. Chapman and Hall, London. [8]

Altman, D.G., Gore, S.M., Gardner, M.J. and Pocock, S.J. (2000) Statistical guidelines for contributors to medical journals. In Statistics with Confidence, 2nd edn (eds D.G. Altman, D. Machin, T.N. Bryant and M.J. Gardner), British Medical Journal, London, 171–190. [10]

Altman, D.G., Machin, D., Bryant, T.N. and Gardner, M.J. (eds) (2000) Statistics With Confidence, 2nd edn, British Medical Journal, London. [8]

Altman, D.G., Whitehead, J., Parmar, M.K.B., Stenning, S.P., Fayers, P.M., and Machin, D., (1995) Randomised consent designs in cancer clinical trials. *European Journal of Cancer*, **31A**, 1934–1944. [14]

Ang, E.S.-W., Lee, S.-T., Gan, C.S.-G., See, P.G.-J., Chan, Y.-H., Ng, L.-H. and Machin, D., (2001) Evaluating the role of alternative therapy in burn wound management: randomized trial comparing Moist Exposed Burn Ointment with conventional methods in the management of patients with second-degree burns. *Medscape General Medicine*, **3** (2), 3. [2, 7, 12]

Ang, E.S.-W., Lee, S.-T., Gan, C.S.-G., Chan, Y.-H., Cheung, Y.-B. and Machin, D. (2003) Pain control in a randomized controlled trial comparing Moist Exposed Burn Ointment (MEBO) and conventional methods in patients with partial thickness burns. *Journal of Burn Care and Rehabilitation*, **24**, 289–296. [4, 7]

Arrow, P. and Riordan, P.J. (1995) Retention and caries preventive effects of a GIC and a resin-based fissure sealant. *Community Dentistry and Oral Epidemiology*, **23**, 282–285. [12]

ATAC (Arimidex, Tamoxifen Alone or in Combination) Trialists' Group (2002) Anastrozole alone or in combination with tamoxifen versus tamoxifen alone for adjuvant treatment of postmenopausal women with early breast cancer: first results of the ATAC randomised trial. *Lancet*, **359**, 2131–2139. [14]

Begg, C., Cho, M., Eastwood, S., Horton, R., Moher, D., Olkin, I., Pitkin, R., Rennie, D., Schultz, K.F., Simel, D. and Stroup, D.F. (1996) Improving the quality of reporting randomized controlled trials: the CONSORT statement. *Journal of the American Medical Association*, **276**, 637–639. [2, 10]

Bellary, S., O'Hare, J.P., Raymond, N.T., Gumber, A., Mughal, S. , Szczepura, A. , Kumar, S. and Barnett, A.H. (2008) Enhanced diabetes care to patients of south Asian ethnic origin (the United Kingdom Asian Diabetes Study): a cluster randomised trial. *Lancet*, **371**, 1769–1776. [11]

Berkowitz, S. (1998). Prerandomization of clinical trials: a more ethical way for performing cleft palate research. *Plastic and Reconstructive Surgery*, **102**, 1724. [14]

Biostat (2001) Power & precision: release 2.1, Englewood, NJ. [9]

Birkett, M.A. and Day, S.J. (1994) Internal pilot studies for estimating sample size. *Statistics in Medicine*, **13**, 2455–2463. [7]

Bladé, J., Samson, D., Reece, D., Apperley J, Björkstrand, B., Gahrton, G., Gertz, M., Giralt, S., Jagannath, S. and Vesole, D. (1998) Criteria for evaluating disease response and progression in patients with multiple myeloma treated by high-dose therapy and haemopoietic stem cell transplantation. Myeloma Subcommittee of the EBMT. European Group for Blood and Marrow Transplant. *British Journal of Haematology*, **102**, 1115–1123. [4]

BMJ (2006) Editors' checklist, www.bmj.com/advice/checklists.shtml. [10]

Boutron, I., Moher, D., Altman, D.G., Schultz, K.F. and Ravaud, P. (2008) Extending the CONSORT statement to randomized trials of nonpharmacologic treatment: explanation and elaboration. *Annals of Internal Medicine*, **148**, 295–309. [10]

Bradburn, M.J., Clark, T.G., Love, S.B. and Altman, D.G. (2003) Survival analysis part III: multivariate data analysis – choosing a model and assessing its adequacy and fit. *British Journal of Cancer*, **89**, 605–611. [10]

Brandes, A.A., Vastola, F., Basso, U., Berti, F., Inna, G., Rotilio, A., Gardiman, M., Scienza, R., Monfardini, S. and Ermani, M. (2003) A prospective study of glioblastoma in the elderly. *Cancer*, **97**, 657–662. [1]

Brown, J., McElvenny, D., Nixon, J., Bainbridge, J. and Mason, S. (2000) Some practical issues in the design, monitoring and analysis of a sequential randomized trial in pressure sore prevention. *Statistics in Medicine*, **19**, 3389–3400. [4, 14]

Bryant, T.N. (2000) Computer software for calculating confidence intervals (CIA) In Statistics with Confidence, 2nd edn (eds D.G. Altman, D. Machin, T.N. Bryant and M.J. Gardner), British Medical Journal, London, pp. 208–213. [10]

Calverley, P., Pauwels, R., Vestbo, J., Jones, P., Pride, N., Gulsvik, A., Anderson, J. and Maden, C. (2003) Combined salmeterol and flucticasone in the treatment of chronic obstructive pulmonary disease: a randomised controlled trial. *Lancet*, **361**, 449–456. [13]

Campbell, G., Pickles, T. and D'yachkova, Y. (2003) A randomised trial of cranberry versus apple juice in the management of urinary symptoms during external beam radiation therapy for prostate cancer. *Clinical Oncology*, **15**, 322–328. [5]

Campbell, M., Fitzpatrick, R., Haines, A., Kinmonth, A.L., Sandercock, P., Spiegelhalter, D. and Tyrer, P. (2000) Framework for design and evaluation of complex interventions to improve health. *BMJ*, **321**, 694–696. [1]

Campbell, M.J. (2000) Cluster randomized trials in general (family) practice research. *Statistical Methods in Medical Research*, **9**, 81–94. [11]

Campbell, M.J. and Gardner, M.J. (2000) Medians and their differences. In Statistics with Confidence, 2nd edn (eds D.G. Altman, D. Machin, T.N. Bryant and M.J. Gardner), British Medical Journal, London. [8]

Campbell, M.J., Machin, D. and Walters, S.J. (2007) Medical Statistics: a Commonsense Approach: a Text Book for the Health Sciences, 4th edn, John Wiley & Sons, Ltd, Chichester. [8]

Campbell, M.K., Elbourne, D.R. and Altman, D.G. for the CONSORT Group (2004) The CONSORT statement: extension to cluster randomised trials. *British Medical Journal*, **328**, 702–708. [10]

Campbell, M.K., Fayers, P.M. and Grimshaw, J.M. (2005) Determinants of the intracluster correlation coefficient in cluster randomised trials. *Clinical Trials*, **2**, 99–107. [11]

Chen, Z.M., Pan, H.C., Chen, Y.P., Peto, R., Collins, R., Jiang, L.X., Xie, J.X., Liu, L.S. (2005) Early intravenous then oral metoprolol in 45,852 patients with acute myocardial infarction: randomised placebo-controlled trial. *Lancet*, **366**, 1622–1632. [14]

Chow, P.K.-H., Tai, B.-C., Tan, C.-K., Machin, D., Johnson, P.J., Khin, M.-W. and Soo, K.-C. (2002) No role for high-dose tamoxifen in the treatment of inoperable hepatocellular carcinoma: an Asia-Pacific double-blind randomised controlled trial. *Hepatology*, **36**, 1221–1226. [2, 3, 5, 10]

Clarke, M. (2006) The Cochrane Collaboration. In Textbook of Clinical Trials, Chapter 3, 2nd edn (eds D. Machin, S. Day and S. Green), John Wiley & Sons, Ltd, Chichester, pp. 39–46. [14]

Clarke, M., Hopewell, S. and Chalmers, I. (2007) Reports of clinical trials should begin and end with up-to-date systematic reviews of the other relevant evidence: a status report. *Journal of the Royal Society of Medicine*, **100**, 187–190. [14]

Cohen, J. (1988) Statistical Power Analysis for the Behavioral Sciences, 2nd edn, Lawrence Erlbaum, New Jersey. [9, 10, 12, 11, 13]

Comi, G., Pulizzi, A., Rovaris, M., Abramsky, O., Arbizu, T., Boiko, A., Gold, R., Havrdova, E., Komoly, S., Selmaj, K.W., Sharrack, B. and Filippi, M. (2008) Effect of laquinimod on MRI-monitored disease activity in patients with relapsing-remitting multiple sclerosis: a multicentre, randomised, double-blind, placebo-controlled phase IIb study. *Lancet*, **371**, 2085–2092. [4, 10]

Cox, D.R. (1972) Regression models and life tables (with discussion). *Journal of the Royal Statistical Society B*, **34**, 187–220. [1]

CPMP Working Party on Efficacy of Medicinal Products (1995) Biostatistical methodology in clinical trials in applications for marketing authorizations for medicinal products. *Statistics in Medicine*, **14**, 1659–1682. [14]

Craig, P., Dieppe, P.P., Macintyre, S., Mitchie, S., Nazarath, I. and Petticrew, M. (2008) Developing and evaluating complex interventions: the new Medical Research Council guidance. *BMJ*, **337**, 979–983. [2]

Csendes, A., Burdiles, P., Korn, O., Braghetto, I., Huertas, C. and Rojas, J. (2002) Late results of a randomized clinical trial comparing total fundoplication *versus* calibration of the cardia with posterior gastropexy. *British Journal of Surgery*, **87**, 289–297. [5]

Cuschieri, A., Weeden, S., Fielding, J., Bancewicz, J., Craven, J., Joypaul, V., Sydes, M. and Fayers, P. (1999) Patient survival after D1 and D2 resections for gastric cancer: long-term results of the MRC randomized surgical trial. *British Journal of Cancer*, **79**, 1522–1530. [9]

DAMOCLES Study Group (2005) A proposed charter for clinical trial data monitoring committees: helping them to do their job well. *Lancet*, **365**, 711–722. [7]

Day, S. (2007) Dictionary for Clinical Trials, 2nd edn, John Wiley & Sons, Ltd, Chichester. [1, 3, 6]

Day, S. and Småstuen, M. (2008) An open mind on adaptive designs. GCPj, December, Informa UK Ltd, pp. 19–22, www.GCPj.com

De Angelis, C.D., Drazen, J.M., Frizelle, F.A., Haug, C., Hoey, J., Horton, R., Kotzin, S., Laine, C., Marusic, A., Overbeke, A.J.P.M., Schroeder, T.V., Sox, H.C. and Van Der Weyden, M.B. (2004) Clinical trial registration: a statement from the International Committee of Medical Journal Editors. *Annals of Internal Medicine*, **141**, 477–478. [6]

D'Haens, G., Baert, F., van Assche, G., Caenepeel, P., Vergauwe, P., Tuynman, H., De Vos, M., van Deventer, S., Stitt, L., Donner, A., Vermeire, S., Van De Mierop, F.J., Coche, J.-C.R., van der Woude, J., Ochsenkühn, T., van Bodegraven Ad, A., Van Hootengem, P.P., Lambrecht, G.L., Mana, F., Rutgeerts, P., Feagan, B.G. and Hommes, D. (2008) Early combined immunosuppression or conventional management in patients with newly diagnosed Crohn's disease: an open randomised trial. *Lancet*, **371**, 660–667. [10]

Dickersin, K. and Rennie, D. (2003) Registering clinical trials. *Journal of the American Medical Association*, **290**, 516–523. [6, 10]

Donner, A. and Klar, N. (2000) Design and Analysis of Cluster Randomised Trials, Edward Arnold, London. [11]

Drucker, D.J., Buse, J.B., Taylor, K., Kendall, D.M., Trautmann, M. and Zhuang, D., for the DURATION-1 Study Group. (2008) Exenatide once weekly versus twice daily for the treatment of type 2 diabetes: a randomised, open-label, non-inferiority study. *Lancet*, **372**, 1240–1250. [10]

Dupont, W.D. and Plummer, W.D. (1997) PS: power and sample size. *Controlled Clinical Trials*, **18**, 274. [9, 10]

Edwards, S.J.L., Braunholtz, D.A., Lilford, R.J. and Stevens, A.J. (1999) Ethical issues in the design and conduct of cluster randomised controlled trials. *BMJ*, **318**, 1407–1409. [11]

Egger, M., Davey-Smith, G. and Altman, D.G. (eds) (2001) Systematic Reviews in Health Care:Meta-Analysis in Context (2nd edn). BMJ Books, Oxford. [14]

Elbourne, D.R., Altman, D.G., Higgins, J.P.T., Curtin, F., Worthington, H.V. and Vail, A. (2002) Meta-analysis involving cross-over trials: methodological issues. *International Journal of Epidemiology*, **31**, 140–149. [12]

Erbel, R., Di Mario, C., Bartunek, J., Bonnier, J., de Bruyne, B., Eberli, F.R., Erne, P., Haude, M., Heublein, B., Horrigan, M., Ilsley, C., Böse, D., Koolen, J., Lüscher, T.F., Weissman, N. and Waksman, R. (2007). Temporary scaffolding of coronary arteries with bioabsorbable magnesium stents: a prospective, non-randomised multicentre trial. *Lancet*, **369**, 1869–1875. [1, 2, 4, 5, 10]

Equi, A., Balfour-Lynn, I.M., Bush, A. and Rosenthal, M. (2002) Long term azithromycin in children with cystic fibrosis: a randomised, placebo-controlled crossover trial. *Lancet*, **360**, 978–984. [12]

Eron, J., Yeni, P., Gathe, J., Estrada, V., DeJesus, E., Staszewski, S., Lackey, P. and 9 others (2006) The KLEAN study of fosamprenavir-ritonavir versus lopinavir-ritonavir, each in combination with abacavir-lamivudine, for initial treatment of HIV infection over 48 weeks: a randomised non-inferiority trial. *Lancet*, **368**, 476–482. [11]

European Medicines Agency (EMEA), Committee for Medicinal Products for Human Use (CHMP) (2005) Guideline for Clinical Trials in Small Populations, www.emea.eu. int/pdfs/human/ewp/8356105en.pdf. [14]

European Medicines Agency (EMEA). (2009) Procedure for European Union Guidelines and Related Documents within the Pharmaceutical Legislative Framework. EMEA/P/24143/2004 Rev.1, EMEA, Canary Wharf, London. [1]

Fayers, P.M., Ashby, D. and Parmar, M.K.B. (1997) Bayesian data monitoring in clinical trials. *Statistics in Medicine*, **16**, 1413–1430. [14]

Fayers, P.M., Jordhøy, M.S. and Kaasa, S. (2002) Cluster-randomized trials. *Palliative Medicine*, **16**, 69–70. [11]

Fayers, P.M. and King, M. (2008) The baseline characteristics did not differ significantly. *Quality of Life Research*, **17**, 1047–1048. [10]

Fayers, P.M. and Machin, D. (2007) Quality of Life: Assessment, Analysis and Interpretation of Patients-reported Outcomes, 2nd edn, John Wiley & Sons, Ltd, Chichester. [14]

Fitzpatrick, S. (2008a) Clinical Trial Design, ICR Publishing, Marlow, www.icr-global.org. [1]

Fitzpatrick, S. (2008b) The Clinical Trial Protocol, ICR Publishing, Marlow, www.icr-global.org. [1]

Fleiss, J.L. (1986) The Design and Analysis of Clinical Experiments, John Wiley & Sons Ltd, New York.   [13, 14]

Food and Drug Administration (FDA) (1988) Guidelines for the Format and Content of the Clinical and Statistics Section of New Drug Applications. US Department of Health and Human Services, Public Health Service, Food and Drug Administration.   [1]

Frech, S.A., DuPont, H.L., Bourgeois, A.L., McKenzie, R., Blekind-Gerson, J., Figueroa, J.F., Okhuysen, P.C., Geurrero, N.H., Martinez-Sandoval, F.G., Meléndez-Romero, J.H.M., Jiang, Z.-D., Asturias, E.J., Halpern, J., Torres, O.R., Hoffman, A.S., Villar, C.P., Kassem, R.N., Flyer, D.C., Anderson, B.H., Kazempour, K., Breisch, S.A. and Glenn, G.M. (2008) Use of patch containing heat-labile toxin from *Escherichia coli* against travellers' diarrhoea: a phase II, randomised, double-blind, placebo-controlled field trial. *Lancet*, **371**, 2019–2025.   [10]

Freeman, J.V., Walters, S.J. and Campbell, M.J. (2008) How to Display Data. BMJ Books, Oxford.   [1, 8]

Frison, L. and Pocock, S.J. (1992) Repeated measures in clinical trials: analysing mean summary statistics and its implications for design. *Statistics in Medicine*, **11**, 1685–1704.   [10]

Gagnier, J.J., Boon, H., Rochon, P., Moher, D., Barnes, J. and Bombardier, C. (2006) Reporting randomized, controlled trials of herbal interventions: an elaborated CONSORT statement. *Annals of Internal Medicine*, **144**, 364–367.   [10]

Gardner, M.J., Machin, D., Campbell, M.J. and Altman, D.G. (2000) Statistical checklists. In Statistics With Confidence, 2nd edn (eds D.G. Altman, D. Machin, T.N. Bryant and M.J. Gardner), British Medical Journal, London, pp. 191–201.   [10]

Gerb, J. and Köpcke, W. (2007) The new EMEA-CHMP Guideline on Clinical Trials in Small Populations – Methodological and statistical considerations with published examples. *Biocybernetics and Biomedical Engineering*, **27**, 59–66.   [14]

Giles, F.J., Kantarjian, H.M., Cortes, J.E., Garcia-Manero, G., Verstovsek, S., Faderl, S., Thomas, D.A., Ferrajoli, A., O'Brien, S., Wathen, J.K., Xiao, L.-C., Berry, D.A. and Estey, E.H. (2003) Adaptive randomized study of Idarubicin and Cytarabine versus Troxacitabine and Cytarabine versus Troxacitabine and Idarubicin in untreated patients 50 years or older with adverse karyotype acute myeloid leukemia. *Journal of Clinical Oncology*, **21**, 1722–1727.   [14]

Girard, T.D., Kress, J.P., Fuchs, B.D., Thomason J.W.W., Schweickert, W.D., Pun, B.T., Taichman, D.B., Dunn, J.G., Pohlman, A.S., Kinniry, P.A., Jackson, J.C., Canonico, A.E., Light, R.W., Shintani, A.K., Thompson, J.L., Gordon, S.M., Hall, J.B., Ditus, R.S., Bernard, G.R. and Ely, E.W. (2008) Efficacy and safety of a paired sedation and ventilator weaning protocol for mechanically ventilated patients in intensive care (Awakening and Breathing Controlled trial): a randomised controlled trial. *Lancet*, **371**, 126–134.   [10]

Girling, D.J., Parmar, M.K.B., Stenning, S.P., Stephens, R.J. and Stewart, L.A. (2003) Clinical trials in cancer, Oxford University Press, Oxford.   [1]

Glaucoma Laser Trial Research Group (1995) The glaucoma laser trial (GLT): 6. Treatment group differences in visual field changes. *American Journal of Ophthalmology*, **120**, 10–22.   [1]

Grobler, L., Siegfried, N., Askie, L., Hooft, L., Tharyan, P. and Antes, G. (2008) National and multinational prospective trial registers. *Lancet*, **372**, 1201–1202.   [6]

Hancock, M.J., Maher, C.G., Latimer, J., McLachlan, A.J., Cooper, C.W., Day, R.O., Spindler, M.F. and McAuley, J.H. (2007) Assessment of diclofenac or spinal manipulative therapy, or both, in addition to recommended first-line treatment for acute low back pain: a randomised controlled trial. *Lancet*, **370**, 1638–1643.   [10, 13]

Hay, A.D., Costelloe, C., Redmond, N.M., Montgomery, A.A., Fletcher, M., Hollinghurst, S. and Peters, T.J. (2008) Paracetemol plus ibuprofen for the treatment of fever in children (PITCH): randomised controlled trial. *BMJ*, **337**, a1302, doi: 10.1136/bmj.a1302.   [2, 10]

Higgins, J.P.T. and Green, S. (eds) (2005) Cochrane Handbook for Systematic Reviews of Interventions 4.2.4 [updated March 2005]. In The Cochrane Library, Issue 2, John Wiley & Sons, Ltd, Chichester. [1, 14]

Hopewell, S., Clarke, M., Moher, D., Wager, E., Middleton, P. and Altman, D.G. (2008) CONSORT for reporting randomised trials in journal and conferences abstracts. *Lancet*, **371**, 281–283. [10]

Huibers, M.J., Bleijenberg, G., Beurkens, A.J., Kant, I.J., Knottnerus, J.A., van der Windt, D.A., Bazelmans, E. and van Schayck, C.P. (2004) An alternative trial design to overcome validity and recruitment problems in primary care research. *Family Practice*, **21**, 213–218. [14]

Hujoel, P.P. (1998) Design and analysis issues in split mouth clinical trials. *Community Dentistry and Oral Epidemiology*, **26**, 85–86. [12]

Hujoel, P.P. and Moulton, L.H. (1988) Evaluation of test statistics in split mouth clinical trials. *Journal of Periodontal Research*, **23**, 378–386. [12]

ICH E2A (1994) Clinical safety data management: definitions and standards for expedited reporting. CPMP/ICH/377/95, EMEA, Canary Wharf, London, www.emea.eu.int. [6]

ICH E2B(M) (2000) Note for guidance on clinical safety data management: data elements for transmission of individual case safety reports. CPMP/ICH/287/95, EMEA, Canary Wharf, London, www.emea.eu.int. [6]

ICH E3 (1995) Structure and content of clinical study reports. CPMP/ICH/137/95, EMEA, Canary Wharf, London, www.emea.eu.int. [6, 10]

ICH E6 (R1) (1996) Guideline for good clinical practice. CPMP/ICH/135/95, EMEA, Canary Wharf, London, www.emea.eu.int. [1, 3, 4, 5, 6]

ICH E8 (1997) General considerations for clinical trials. CPMP/ICH/291/95, EMEA, Canary Wharf, London, www.emea.eu.int. [6]

ICH E9 (1998) Statistical principles for clinical trials. CPMP/ICH/363/96, EMEA, Canary Wharf, London, www.emea.eu.int. [1, 4, 5, 6]

ICH E9 Expert Working Group (1999) Statistical principles for clinical trials: ICH Harmonised Tripartite Guideline, *Statistics in Medicine*, **18**, 1905–1942. [1, 2, 4, 5, 6, 9]

ICH E10 (2000) Choice of control group in clinical trials. CPMP/ICH/2711/99, EMEA, Canary Wharf, London, www.emea.eu.int. [2, 6]

Institute of Clinical Research (2008) The Fundamental Guidelines for Clinical Research V2.0, ICR Publishing. [1, 2, 3]

Ioannidis, J.P., Evans, S.J., Gotzsche, P.C., O'Neill, R.T., Altman, D.G., Schultz, K. *et al.* (2004) Better reporting of harms in randomized trials: an extension of the CONSORT statement. *Annals of Internal Medicine*, **141**, 781–788. [10]

Jadad, A. (1998) Randomised Controlled Trials, British Medical Journal, London. [1]

James, N.D., Sydes, M.R., Clarke, N.W., Mason, M.D., Dearnaley, D.P., Anderson, J., Popert, R.J., Sanders, K., Morgan, R.C., Stansfeld, J., Dwyer, J., Masters, J. and Parmar, M.K.B. (2008) STAMPEDE: systemic therapy for advancing or metastatic prostate cancer – a multi-arm multi-stage randomized controlled trial. *Clinical Oncology*, **20**, 577–581. [7, 14]

Jenni, S., Oetliker, C., Allemann, S., Ith, M., Tappy, L., Wuerth, S., Egger, A., Boesch, C., Schneiter, Ph., Diem, P., Christ, E. and Stettler, C. (2008) Fuel metabolism during exercise in euglycaemia and hyperglycaemia in patients with type 1 diabetes mellitus – a prospective single-blind randomised crossover trial. *Diabetologia*, **51**, 1457–1465. [12]

Jensen, P.T., Klee, M.C., Thranov, I. and Groenvold, M. (2004) Validation of a questionnaire for self-assessment of sexual function and vaginal changes after gynaecological cancer. *Psycho-Oncology*, **13**, 577–592. [4]

Jones, B. (2008) The cross-over trial: a subtle knife. *Significance*, **5**, 135–137. [12]

Jones, B., Jarvis, P., Lewis, J.A. and Ebbutt, A.F. (1996) Trials to assess equivalence: the importance of rigorous methods. *British Medical Journal*, **313**, 36–39. [11]

Jordhøy, M.S., Fayers, P.M., Ahlner-Elmqvist, M. and Kaasa S. (2002) Lack of concealment may lead to selection bias in cluster randomized trials of palliative care. *Palliative Medicine*, **16**, 43–49. [11]

Jüni, P., Altman, D.G. and Egger, M. (2001). Assessing the quality of controlled clinical trials. *BMJ*, **323**, 42–46. [14]

Kahn, R.S., Fleischhacker, W.W., Boter, H., Davidson, M., Vergouwe, Y., Keet, I.P.M. and 13 others (2008) Effectiveness of antipsychotic drugs in first-episode schizophrenia and schizophreniform disorder: an open randomised clinical trial. *Lancet*, **371**, 1085–1097. [2, 10, 13]

Kaplan, E.L. and Meier, P. (1958) Non parametric estimation from incomplete observations. *Journal of the American Statistical Association*, **53**, 457–481. [1]

Kohler, J.A., Imeson, J., Ellershaw, C. and Lie, S.O. (2000) A randomized trial of 13-cis retinoic acid in children with advanced neuroblastoma after high-dose therapy. *British Journal of Cancer*, **83**, 1124–1127. [8]

Krishna, R., Anderson, M.S., Bergman, A.J., Jin, B., Fallon, M., Cote, J., Rosko, K., Chavez-Eng, C., Lutz, R., Bloomfield, D.M., Gutierrez, M., Doherty, J., Bieberdorf, F., Chodakewitz, J., Gottesdiener, K.M. and Wagner, J.A. (2007) Effect of the cholesteryl ester transfer protein inhibitor, anacetrapib, on lipoproteins in patients with dyslipidaemia and on 24-h ambulatory blood pressure in healthy individuals: two double-blind, randomized placebo-controlled phase I studies. *Lancet*, **370**, 1907–1914. [1, 2, 10, 12]

Larsson, P.-G. and Carlsson, B. (2002) Does pre- and postoperative metronidazole treatment lower vaginal cuff infection rate after abdominal hysterectomy among women with bacterial vaginosis? *Infectious Diseases in Obstetrics and Gynecolgy*, **10**, 133–140. [10, 14]

Lau, W.Y., Lai, E.C.H., Leung, T.W.T. and Yu, S.C.H. (2008) Adjuvant intra-arterial iodine-131-labelled lipiodol for resectable hepatocellular carcinoma: a prospective randomized trial-update on 5-year and 10-year survival. *Annals of Surgery*, **247**, 43–48. [7]

Lau, W.Y., Leung, T.W.T., Ho, S.K.W., Chan, M., Machin, D., Lau, J., Chan, A.T.C., Yeo, W., Mok, T.S.K., Yu, S.C.H., Leung, N.W.Y. and Johnson, P.J. (1999) Adjuvant intra-arterial iodine-131-labelled lipiodol for resectable hepatocellular carcinoma: a prospective randomised trial. *Lancet*, **353**, 797–801. [7, 8, 10]

Lenth, R.V. (2006) Java Applets for Power and Sample Size. www.stat.uiowa.edu/~rlenth/Power. [9]

Levie, K., Gjorup, I., Skinhøj, P. and Stoffel, M. (2002) A 2-dose regimen of recombinant hepatitis B vaccine with the immune stimulant AS04 compared with the standard 3-dose regimen of Enderix™-B in healthy young adults. *Scandinavian Journal of Infectious Disease*, **34**, 610–614. [1]

Levy, H.L., Milanowski, A., Chakrapani, M., Cleary, M., Lee, P., Trefz, FK., Whitley, C.B., Feillet, F., Feigenbaum, A.S., Bebchuk, J.D., Christ-Schmidt, H. and Dorenbaum, A. (2007) Efficacy of sepropterin dihydrochloride (tetrahydrobiopterin, 6R-BH4) for reduction of phenylalanine concentration in patients with phenylketonuria: a phase III randomised placebo-controlled study. *Lancet*, **370**, 504–510. [11]

Llovet, J.M., Real, M.I., Montaňa, X., Planas, R., Coll, S., Aponte, J., Ayuso, C., Sala, M., Muchart, J., Solà, R., Rodés, J. and Bruix, J. (2002) Arterial embolisation or chemoembolisation versus symptomatic treatment in patients with unresectable hepatocellular carcinoma: a randomised controlled trial. *Lancet*, **359**, 1734–1739. [14]

Lo, E.C.M., Luo, Y., Fan, M.W. and Wei, S.H.Y. (2001) Clinical investigation of two glass-ionomer restoratives used with the atraumatic restorative treatment approach in china: two-years results. *Caries Research*, **35**, 458–463. [1, 5, 10, 12]

Lo, E.C.M., Luo, Y., Tan H.P., Dyson, J.E. and Corbet, E.F. (2006). ART and conventional root restorations in elders after 12 months. *Journal of Dental Research*, **85**, 929–932. [5]

Lobo, D.N., Bostock, K.A., Neal, K.R., Perkins, A.C., Rowlands, B.J. and Allison, S.P. (2002) Effect of salt and water balance on recovery of gastrointestinal function after elective colonic resection: a randomised controlled trial. *Lancet*, **359**, 1812–1818.   [1, 9]

Machin, D., Campbell, M.J., Tan, S.B. and Tan, S.H. (2009) Sample Sizes Tables for Clinical Studies, 3rd edn, Wiley-Blackwell, Oxford.   [1, 3, 9, 10, 12]

Machin, D., Cheung, Y.B. and Parmar, M.K.B. (2006) Survival Analysis: a Practical Approach, 2nd edn, John Wiley & Sons, Ltd, Chichester.   [8]

Machin, D., Day, S. and Green, S. (eds) (2006) Textbook of Clinical Trials, 2nd edn, John Wiley & Sons, Ltd, Chichester.   [1]

Machin, D. and Lee, S.T. (2000) The ethics of randomization trials in the context of cleft palate research. *Plastic and Reconstructive Surgery*, **105**, 1566–1568.   [14]

Machin, D., Stenning, S.P., Parmar, M.K.B., Fayers, P.M., Girling, D.J., Stephens, R.J., Stewart, L.A. and Whaley, J.B. (1997) Thirty years of Medical Research Council randomized trials in solid tumours. *Clinical Oncology*, **9**, 20–28.   [2]

McMurray, J.J.V., Östergren, J., Swedberg, K. Granger, C.B., Held, P., Mivhelson, E.L., Olofsson, B., Yusuf, S., Pfeffer, M.A. (2003) Effects of candesartan in patients with chronic heart failure and reduced left-ventricular systolic function taking angiotensin-converting-enzyme inhibitors: the CHARM-Added trial. *Lancet*, **362**, 767–771.   [14]

Medical Research Council (2002) Cluster Randomised Trials: Methodological and Ethical Considerations, MRC Clinical Trials Series, Medical Research Council, London.   [11]

Medical Research Council Lung Cancer Working Party (1996) Randomized trial of palliative two-fraction versus more intensive 13-fraction radiotherapy for patients with inoperable non-small cell lung cancer and good performance status. *Clinical Oncology*, **8**, 167–175.   [2]

Medical Research Council Whooping-Cough Immunization Committee (1951) The prevention of whooping-cough by vaccination. *British Medical Journal*, **1**, 1463–1471.   [1]

Meggitt, S.J., Gray, J.C. and Reynolds, N.J. (2006) Azathioprine dosed by thiopurine methyltransferase activity for moderate-to-severe atopic eczema: a double-blind, randomised controlled trial. *Lancet*, **367**, 839–846.   [1, 2, 4, 8, 9, 10, 11, 12]

Meyer, G., Warnke, A., Mülhauser, I. and Bender, R. (2003) Effect on hip fractures of increased use of hip protectors in nursing homes: cluster randomised controlled trial. *BMJ*, **326**, 76–78.   [1, 2, 11]

Mitchell, C., Jones, K.P., Shannon, R., Hutton, C., Stevens, S., Machin, D., Imeson, J., Kelsey, A., Vujanic, G.M., Gornall, P., Walker, J., Taylor, R., Sartori, P., Hale, J., Levitt, H.G., Msahael, B., Middleton, H., Grundy, R.G. and Pritchard, J. (2006) Immediate nephrectomy versus preoperative chemotherapy in the management of non-metastatic Wilms' tumour: Results of a randomised trial (UKW3) by the UK Children's Cancer Study Group. *European Journal of Cancer*, **42**, 2554–2562.   [10]

Moher, D., Cook, D.J., Eastwood, S., Olkin, I., Rennie, D., and Stroup, D.F. (1999) Improving the quality of reports of meta-analyses of randomised controlled trials: the QUOROM statement. *Lancet*, **354**, 1896–1900.   [14]

Moher, D., Schultz, K.F. and Altman, D.G., for the CONSORT Group (2001) The CONSORT statement: revised recommendations for improving the quality of reports of parallel-group randomised trials. *Lancet*, **357**, 1191–1194.   [1, 2, 5, 10]

Motzer, R.J., Escudier, B., Oudard, S., Hutson, T.E., Porta, C., Bracardo, S., Grünwald, V., Thompson, J.A., Figlin, R.A., Hollaender, N., Urbanowitz, G., Berg, W.J., Kay, A., Lebwohl, D. and Ravaud, A. (2008) Efficacy of everolimus in advanced renal cell carcinoma: a double-blind, randomised, placebo-controlled phase III trial. *Lancet*, **372**, 449–456.   [10]

Muers, M.F., Stephens, R.J., Fisher, P., Darlison, L., Higgs, C.M.B., Lowry, L., Nicholson, A.G., O'Brien, M. and 8 others (2008) Active symptom control with or without chemotherapy in the treatment of patients with malignant pleural mesothelioma (MS01): a multicentre trial. *Lancet*, **371**, 1685–1694. [13]

National Cancer Institute (2003) Common Terminology Criteria for Adverse Events. (v3.0 CTCAE), National Cancer Institute, Bethesda, www. ctep.cancer.gov/reporting/ctc.html. [3]

National Council for Social Studies (2005) Power analysis and sample size software (PASS): Version 2005, Kaysville, UT. [9]

Newcombe, R.G. and Altman, D.G. (2000) Proportions and their differences. In Statistics with Confidence, 2nd edn (eds D.G. Altman, D. Machin, T.N. Bryant and M.J. Gardner), British Medical Journal Books, London, pp. 45–56. [8]

Nixon, J., McElvenny D., Mason, S., Brown, J. and Bond, S. (1998) A sequential randomised controlled trial comparing a dry visco-elastic polymer gel pad and standard operating table mattresses in the prevention of post-operative pressure sores. *International Journal of Nursing Studies*, **35**, 193–203. [10, 14]

Oliver, P.C., Crawford, M.J., Rao, B., Reece, B. and Tyrer, P. (2007) Modified overt aggression scale (MOAS) for people with intellectual disability and aggressive challenging behaviour: a reliability study. *Journal of Applied Research in Intellectual Disability*, **20**, 368–272. [10]

Palumbo, A., Bringhen, S., Caravita, T., Merla, E., Capparella, V., Callea, V., Cangialosi, C., Grasso, M., Rossini, F., Galli, M., Catalano, L., Zamagni, E., Petrucci, M.T., De Stefano, V., Ceccarelli, M., Ambrosini, M.T., Avonto, I., Falco, P., Ciccone, G., Liberati, A.M., Musto, P. and Boccadoro, M. (2006) Oral melaphalan and prednisone chemotherapy plus thalidomide compared with melphalan and prednisone alone in elderly patients with multiple myeloma: randomised controlled trial. *Lancet*, **367**, 825–831. [4, 9]

Papp, K., Bissonnette, R., Rosoph, L., Wasel, N., Lynde, C.W., Searles, G., Shear, N.H., Huizinga, R.B. and Maksymowych, W.P. (2008) Efficacy of ISA247 in plaque psoriasis: a randomised multicentre, double-blind, placebo-controlled phase III study. *Lancet*, **371**, 1337–1342. [13]

Parmar, M.K.B., Barthel, F.M.-S., Sydes, M., Langley, R., Kaplan, R., Eisenhauer, E., Brady, M., James, N., Bookman, M.A., Swart, A.-M., Qian, W. and Royston, P. (2008) Speeding up the evaluation of new agents in cancer. *Journal of the National Cancer Institute*, **100**, 1204–1214. [4, 14]

PEST (2004) Operating Manual 4.4, MPS Research Unit, University of Reading, Reading. [14]

Peters, T.J., Richards, S.H., Bankhead, C.R., Ades, A.E. and Sterne, J.A.C. (2003) Comparison of methods for analysing cluster randomized trials: an example involving a factorial design. *International Journal of Epidemiology*, **32**, 840–846. [11]

Peto, R., Pike, M.C., Armitage, P., Breslow, N.E., Cox, D.R., Howard, S.V., Mantel, N., McPherson, K., Peto, J. and Smith, P.G. (1976) Design and analysis of randomized clinical trials requiring prolonged observation of each patient (I) Introduction and design. *British Journal of Cancer*, **34**, 585–612. [1]

Peto, R., Pike, M.C., Armitage, P., Breslow, N.E., Cox, D.R., Howard, SV, Mantel, N., McPherson, K., Peto, J. and Smith, P.G. (1977) Design and analysis of randomized clinical trials requiring prolonged observation of each patient (II) Analysis and examples. *British Journal of Cancer*, **35**, 1–39. [1]

Phillips, A. (2006) Flexibility by design, *GCPj*, Informa UK Ltd, July, pp. 13–17, www.GCPj.com [14]

Piaggio, G., Carolli, G., Villar, J., Bakketeig, L., Lumbiganon, P., Bergsjø, P., Al-Mazrou, Y., Ba'aqeel, H., Belizán, J.M., Farnot, U. and Berendes, H. (2001) Methodological considerations on the design and analysis of an equivalence stratified cluster randomization trial. *Statistics in Medicine*, **20**, 401–416. [11, 14]

Piaggio, G., Elbourne, D.R., Altman, D.G., Pocock, S.J. and Evans, S.J.W. (2001) Reporting of noninferiority and equivalence randomized trials: an extension of the CONSORT statement. *Journal of the American Medical Association*, **295**, 1152–1160. [10, 11]

Piaggio, G. and Pinol, A.P. (2001) Use of the equivalence approach in reproductive health clinical trials. *Statistics in Medicine*, **20**, 3571–3577. [11]

Pocock, S.J. (1983) Clinical Trials: a Practical Approach, John Wiley & Sons, Ltd, Chichester. [1, 8]

Pocock, S.J. and Ware, J.E. (2009) Translating statistical findings into plain English. *Lancet*, **373**, 1926–1928. [10]

Pocock, S.J. and White, I. (1999) Trials stopped early: too good to be true? *Lancet*, **353**, 943–944. [7]

Poon, C.Y., Goh, B.T., Kim, M.-J., Rajaseharan, A., Ahmed, S., Thongsprasom, K., Chaimusik, M., Suresh, S., Machin, D., Wong-H.B. and Seldrup, J. (2006) A randomised controlled trial to compare steroid with cyclosporine for the topical treatment of oral lichen planus. *Oral Surgery, Oral Medicince, Oral Pathology, Oral Radiololgy and Endodontology*, **102**, 47–55. [2, 3, 7, 8, 10, 12]

Quaranta, L., Pizzolante, T., Riva, I., Haidich, A.-B., Konstas, G.P. and Stewart, W.C. (2008) Twenty-four-hour intraocular pressure and blood pressure levels with bimatoprost versus latanoprost in patients with normal-tension glaucoma. *British Journal of Ophthalmology*, **92**, 1227–1231. [12]

Redwood, C. and Colton, T. (eds) (2001) Biostatistics in Clinical Trials, John Wiley & Sons, Ltd, Chichester. [1]

Regidor, E., Barrio, G., de la Feunte, L., Domingo, A. and Alonso, J. (1999) Association between educational level and health related quality of life in Spanish adults. *Journal of Epidemiology and Community Health*, **53**, 75–82. [11]

SAS Institute (2004) Getting Started with the SAS Power and Sample Size Application: Version 9.1, SAS Institute, Cary, NC. [9]

Schoenfeld, D. (1982) Partial residuals for the proportional hazards regression model. *Biometrika*, **69**, 239–241. [10]

Scott, N.W., McPherson, G.C., Ramsay, C.R. and Campbell, M.K. (2002) The method of minimization for allocation to clinical trials. *Controlled Clinical Trials*, **23**, 662–674. [5]

Schottenfeld, R.S., Charwarski, M.C. and Mazlan, M. (2008) Maintenance treatment with buprenorphine and naltrexone for heroin dependence in Malaysia: a randomised, double-blind, placebo controlled trial. *Lancet*, **371**, 2192–2200. [13]

Senn, S.J. (2002) Cross-Over Trials in Clinical Research, 2nd edn, John Wiley & Sons, Ltd, Chichester. [12]

Senn, S. (2007) Statistical Issues in Drug Development, 2nd edn, John Wiley & Sons, Ltd, Chichester. [1]

Singapore Lichen Planus Study Group (2004) A randomized controlled trial to compare calcipotriol with betamethasone valerate for the treatment of cutaneous lichen planus. *Journal of Dermatological Treatment*, **15**, 141–145. [10]

Smith, I., Procter, M., Gelber, R.D., Guillaume, S., Feyereislova, A., Dowsett, M., Goldhirsch, A., Untch, M., Mariani, G., Baselga, J., Kaufmann, M., Cameron, D., Bell, R., Bergh, J., Coleman, R., Wardley, A., Harbeck, N., Lopez, RI., Mallmann, P., Gelmon, K., Wilcken, N., Wist, E., Rovira, P.S. and Piccart-Gebhart, M.J. (2007) 2-year follow-up of trastuzumab after adjuvant chemotherapy in HER2-positive breast cancer: a randomised controlled trial. *Lancet*, **369**, 29–36. [1, 5, 10]

Smolen, J.S., Beaulieu, A., Rubbert-Roth, A., Ramos-Remus, C., Rovensky, J., Alecock, E., Woodworth, T., and Alten, R. (2008) Effect of interleukin-6 receptor inhibition with tocilizumab in patients with rheumatoid arthritis (Option study): a double-blind, placebo-controlled, randomised trial. *Lancet*, **371**, 987–997. [10, 13]

Spiegelhalter, D.J., Freedman, L.S. and Parmar, M.K.B. (1994) Bayesian approaches to randomized trials (with discussion). *Journal of the Royal Statistical Society A*, **157**, 357–416. [14]

Sprangers, M.A., Cull, A. and Groenvold, M. (1998) EORTC Quality of Life Study Group: Guidelines for Developing Questionnaire Modules, EORTC, Brussels. [2, 4]

StataCorp (2007) Stata Statistical Software: Release 10, Stata Press, College Station, Texas. [8, 9, 10]

Statistical Solutions (2006) nQuery Advise: Version 6.0, Saugus, MA. [9]

Stevinson, C., Devaraj, V.S., Fountain-Barber, A., Hawkins, S. and Ernst, E. (2003) Homeopathic arnica for prevention of pain and bruising: randomized placebo-controlled trial in hand surgery. *Journal of the Royal Society of Medicine*, **96**, 60–65. [1, 2, 5, 9, 10, 13]

Szefler, S.S., Mitchell, H., Sorkness, C.A., Gergen, P.J., O'Connor, G.T., Morgan, W.J., Kattan, M. and 10 others (2008) Management of asthma based on exhaled nitric oxide in addition to guideline-based treatment for inner-city adolescents and young adults: a randomised controlled trial. *Lancet*, **372**, 1065–1072. [10]

Tan, S.B., Chung, Y.F.A., Tai, B.C., Cheung, Y.B. and Machin, D. (2003) Elicitation of prior distributions for a phase III randomized controlled trial of adjuvant therapy with surgery for hepatocellular carcinoma. *Controlled Clinical Trials*, **24**, 110–121. [14]

Tan, S.B., Dear, K.B.G., Bruzzi, P. and Machin, D. (2003) Strategy for randomised clinical trials in rare cancers. *British Medical Journal*, **327**, 47–49. [14]

Tan, S.B., Wee, J., Wong, H.B. and Machin, D. (2008) Can external and subjective information ever be used to reduce the size of a randomised controlled trial? *Contemporary Clinical Trials*, **29**, 211–219. [14]

Tang, C.-L., Eu, K.-W., Tai, B.-C., Soh, J.G.S., Machin, D. and Seow-Choen, F. (2001) Randomized clinical trial of the effect of open *versus* laparoscopically assisted colectomy on systemic immunity in patients with colorectal cancer. *British Journal of Surgery*, **88**, 801–807. [4]

Tyrer, P., Oliver-Africano, P.C., Ahmed, Z., Bouras, N., Cooray, S., Deb, S., Murphy, D., Hare, M., Meade, M., Reece, B., Kramo, K., Bhaumik, S., Harley, D., Regan, A., Thoma, D., Rao, B., North, B., Eliahoo, J., Karatela, S., Soni, A. and Crawford, M. (2008) Risperidone, haloperidol, and placebo in the treatment of aggressive challenging behaviour in patients with intellectual disability: a randomised controlled trial. *Lancet*, **371**, 57–63. [10, 13]

Ukoumunne, O.C., Gulliford, M.C., Chinn, S., Sterne, J.A.C., Burney, P.G.J. (1999) Methods for evaluating area-wide and organisation-based interventions in health and health care: a systematic review. *Health Technology Assessment*, **3**(5), www.hta.ac.uk/fullmono/mon305.pdf. [11]

van der Meché, F.G.A. and Schmitz, P.I.M. (1992) A randomized trial comparing intravenous immune globulin and plasma exchange in Guillain-Barré syndrome. *New England Journal of Medicine*, **326**, 1123–1129. [10]

Wang, D. and Bakhai, A. (eds) (2006) Clinical Trials. A Practical Guide to Design, Analysis and Reporting, Remedica, London. [1]

Ware, J.E., Snow, K.K., Kosinski, M. and Gandek, B. (1993) SF-36 Health Survey Manual and Interpretation Guide, New England Medical Centre, Boston, MA. [4]

Wee, J.T.S., Tan, E.H., Tai, B.C., Wong, H.-B., Leong, S.S., Tan, T., Chua, E.-T., Yang, E., Lee, K.M., Fong, K.W., Khoo, H.S., Lee, K.S., Loong, S., Sethi, V., Chua, E.J. and Machin, D. (2005) Randomized trial of radiotherapy versus concurrent chemo-radiotherapy followed by adjuvant chemotherapy in patients with AJCC/UICC (1997) stage III and IV nasopharyngeal cancer of the endemic variety. *Journal of Clinical Oncology*, **23**, 6730–6738. [2, 4, 10, 14]

Weng, J., Li, Y., Xu, W., Shi, L., Zhang, Q., Zhu, D., Hu, Y. and Zhou, Z. and others (2008) Effect of intensive insulin therapy on β-cell function and glycaemic control in patients with newly diagnosed type 2 diabetes: a multicentre randomised parallel-group trial. *Lancet*, **371**, 1753–1760. [1, 13]

Whitehead, J. (1997) The Design and Analysis of Sequential Clinical Trials, revised 2nd edn, John Wiley & Sons, Ltd, Chichester. [14]

WHO (2008) WHO International Clinical Trials Registry Platform: Universal Trial Reference Number (UTRN), www.who.int/ictrp/utrn/en/index.html. [6]

Williams, H.C., Burney, P.G., Hay, R.J., *et al.* (1994) The U.K. Working Party's Diagnostic Criteria for Atopic Dermatitis: I. Derivation of a minimum set of discriminators for atopic dermatitis. *British Journal of Dermatology*, **131**, 383–396. [2]

Wright, J.R., Bouma, S., Dayes, I., Simunovic, M.R., Levine, M.N. and Whelan, T.J. (2006) The importance of reporting patient recruitment details in Phase III trials. *Journal of Clinical Oncology*, **24**, 843–845. [2]

Yeow, V.K.-L., Lee, S.-T., Cheng, J.J., Chua, K., Wong, H.-B. and Machin, D. (2007) Randomised clinical trials in plastic surgery: survey of output and quality of reporting (letter). *Journal of Plastic and Reconstructive Surgery*, **60**, 965–966. [1, 2, 7, 13]

Young, T., de Haes, J.C.J.M., Curran, D., Fayers, P.M. and Brandberg, Y. (1999) Guidelines for Assessing Quality of Life in EORTC Trials, EORTC, Brussels. [14]

Zelen, M. (1979) A new design for randomized clinical trials. *New England Journal of Medicine*, **300**, 1242–1245. [14]

Zelen, M. (1992) Randomised consent trials. *Lancet*, **340**, 375. [14]

Zheng, J.-P., Kang, J., Huang, S.-G., Chen, P., Yao, W.-Z., Yang, L., Bai, C.-X., Wang, C.-Z., Wang, C., Chen, B.-Y., Shi, Y., Liu, C.-T., Chen, P., Li, Q., Wang, Z.-S., Huang, Y.-J., Luo, Z.-Y., Chen, F.-P., Yuan, J.-Z., Yuan, B.-T., Qian, H.-P., Zhi, R.-C. and Zhong, N.-S. (2008) Effect of carbocisteine on acute exacerbation of chronic obstructive pulmonary disease (PEACE study): a randomised placebo-controlled study. *Lancet*, **371**, 2013–2018. [10]

Zongo, I., Dorsey, G., Rouamba, N., Tinto, H., Dokomajilar, C., Guiguemde, R.T., Rosenthal, P. and Ouedraogo, J.B. (2007) Artemether-lumefantrine versus amodiaquine plus sulfadoxine-pyrimethamine for uncomplicated falciparum malaria in Burkina Faso: a randomised no-inferiority trial. *Lancet*, **369**, 491–498. [1, 5, 11]

Zwarenstein, M., Treweek, S., Gagniere, J.J., Altman, D.G., Tunis, S., Haynes, B., Oxman, A.D. and Moher, D. (2008) Improving the reporting of pragmatic trials: an extension of the CONSORT statement. *BMJ*, **337**, 1223–1226. [10]

Index

Index compiled by Terry Halliday